Food, Eating and Obesity

Food, Eating and Obesity

The psychobiological basis of appetite and weight control

David J. Mela and Peter J. Rogers

Consumer Sciences Department
Institute of Food Research
Reading, UK

CHAPMAN & HALL

London · Weinheim · New York · Tokyo · Melbourne · Madras

Published by Chapman & Hall, 2–6 Boundary Row, London SE1 8HN

Chapman & Hall, 2–6 Boundary Row, London SE1 8HN, UK

Chapman & Hall GmbH, Pappelallee 3, 69469 Weinheim, Germany

Chapman & Hall USA, 115 Fifth Avenue, New York, NY 10003, USA

Chapman & Hall Japan, ITP-Japan, Kyowa Building, 3F, 2-2-1 Hirakawacho, Chiyoda-ku, Tokyo 102, Japan

Chapman & Hall Australia, 102 Dodds Street, South Melbourne, Victoria 3205, Australia

Chapman & Hall India, R. Seshadri, 32 Second Main Road, CIT East, Madras 600 035, India

First edition 1998

© 1998 Biotechnology & Biological Sciences Research Council

Typeset in 10/12pt Palatino by Columns Design Ltd, Reading, England
Printed in Great Britain by TJ International Ltd, Padstow, Cornwall

ISBN 0 412 71920 7

A catalogue record for this book is available from the British Library

∞ Printed on permanent acid-free text paper, manufactured in accordance with ANSI/NISO Z39.48-1992 and ANSI/NISO Z39.48-1984 (Permanence of Paper).

Contents

Preface

Although the exact prevalence of overweight and obesity are dependent upon the definition used, these conditions are generally accepted to be widespread and increasing problems by health authorities and the public in most western nations. The proportion of the UK and US populations which are overweight or obese, by any measure, has substantially risen over the past decade, and similar increases have been observed in other western nations as well as rapidly modernizing societies (Hodge *et al.*, 1996). The physiological, psychological, and social/environmental factors which may be implicated in the aetiology, maintenance, and treatment of these conditions have been the subject of an extraordinary volume of human and animal research, scientific conferences, and technical and popular literature.

This book focuses specifically on the role of food and eating in overeating and obesity, emphasizing the relationships between people and food which may give rise to positive energy balance, and the potential contributions of specific components, foods, or groups of foods. The intent is to integrate the psychobiological and cognitive psychological aspects of appetite, food preferences, and food selection with physiological and metabolic outcomes of eating behaviours. The ingestion of a particular quality and quantity of food is a voluntary behaviour, and that act, its determinants, features and sequelae are explored here, considering wider academic thought but guided by potential practical implications. There is a very strong emphasis on data from human studies, and relevant animal research is generally cited only where it offers required support or detail, or provides fundamental background information not available in humans. Although we hope that relevant and key papers have been cited, there was no intention to be comprehensive. A basic background familiarity with the biological sciences is assumed.

We would like to make clear that there are several important areas which this book specifically does **not** address. These are largely topics which, in our view, have dominated most other books and conference proceedings on obesity and weight control. Although we explore the nature of hunger and appetite, and the dietary correlates of human obesity, there is no attempt to address in any depth the associated underlying molecular, hormonal, neurophysiological, or cellular events, nor other basic aspects of intermediary metabolism. These are considered only insofar as their outcomes usefully explain how relationships between people and food may influence food intake and weight change. Also, there is no intention to discuss the health implications, pharmacology, or comparative approaches to obesity treatment, although the material here will have implications for behavioural and dietary aspects of the latter.

It is a pleasure to acknowledge all of our colleagues, past and present, who have for many years shaped and challenged our thinking on the issues explored herein. We both feel privileged to have had the opportunity to meet, work with, and learn from so many fine people, and must give particular thanks to our friends and collaborators at the Monell Chemical Senses Center, the Biopsychology group at the University of Leeds, and the Institute of Food Research.

Our hope is that this book will point out the shortcomings of the mind–body dichotomy which still characterizes much of research and thinking in this field, and stimulate students and researchers in the physiological and behavioural sciences to recognize that both disciplines have a critical contribution to make to our understanding of eating behaviour and its outcomes. Indeed, any consideration of overeating and obesity which takes a unidisciplinary approach, or fails to seriously consider the critical interrelationships amongst cognition, learning, and metabolism will always be incomplete.

David J. Mela
Peter J. Rogers

Reading, UK
June 1997

Abbreviations used

BMI	Body Mass Index
BMR	Basal Metabolic Rate
CCK	Cholecystokinin
CCO	Carbohydrate-craving obesity
CHO	Carbohydrate
DEBQ	Dutch Eating Behaviour Questionnaire
FFQ	Food Frequency Questionnaire
FQ	Food Quotient
LH	Lateral hypothalamus
LNAA	Large Neutral Amino Acids
NSP	Non-Starch Polysaccharide
PAL	Physical Activity Level (= TEE/BMR)
PKU	Phenylketonuria
PMS	Premenstrual Syndrome
RMR	Resting Metabolic Rate
RQ	Respiratory Quotient
RRS	Revised Restraint Scale
SAD	Seasonal Affective Disorder
TEE	Total Energy Expenditure
TEF	Thermic Effect of Food
TFEQ	Three-Factor Eating Questionnaire
TRP	Tryptophan
TRP/ΣLNAA	Plasma ratio of Tryptophan to Large Neutral Amino Acids
VMH	Ventromedial nucleus of the hypothalamus

CHAPTER ONE

Control of appetite and energy balance and imbalance

1.1 SOME BACKGROUND AND THE CONCEPT OF HOMEOSTASIS

Obesity develops when, over a sufficiently long period of time, energy intake exceeds energy expenditure. Obesity therefore has to be viewed in terms of the relationships between eating behaviour, and energy use and storage. The origins of modern thinking about this problem are to be found in Claude Bernard's (1878) statement that 'all the vital mechanisms, however varied they may be, have only one object, that of preserving constant the conditions of life in the internal environment', and in Cannon's (1932) subsequent elaboration of the idea and use of the word homeostasis. Derived from two Greek words that mean 'similar to standing still', homeostasis as defined by Cannon is a functional concept in that it specifies outcomes (goals) which are particular steady states (Hogan, 1980). These steady states, or constant conditions, including body temperature and blood volume, and blood oxygen, glucose and calcium concentrations, were held to be maintained by 'coordinated physiological processes'.

In relation to eating behaviour this perspective has generally led to the assumption that appetite is regulated by a homeostatic system that serves to maintain energy balance. Accordingly, attempts to identify the physiological mechanisms underlying energy homeostasis have tended to dominate research in the area, and experimental models of obesity have been studied mainly for their potential to provide insight into these mechanisms. Much of this, though, has been of little direct relevance to human obesity, which, for example, is only very rarely caused by damage to the ventromedial hypothalamus (Section 1.3.1). Some ten years ago Stricker and Verbalis (1987) wrote: 'despite a long history of concern about the causes and consequences of eating, there is little agreement at present regarding how the brain controls food intake or how eating and complementary biological processes form an integrated physiology of caloric homeostasis' (page 3). This is still largely true today; however, as will become clear in later chapters, even if there were major advances in this area, knowledge of human eating behaviour would be far from complete. We are not arguing that the study of physiological mechanisms controlling eating is unimportant, but simply that this should be integrated into a wider context. This context includes taking into account the roles played by learned and cognitive influences guiding behaviour, and ecological constraints and opportunities afforded by the social setting, lifestyle habits, economic circumstances, and culture of the society in which people eat. The resultant systems approach is integrative, providing a framework which acknowledges the interplay of events beneath and outside the skin. A central feature of this systems view is that adjustments in one domain will influence, or be influenced by, the state of components elsewhere in the system. The forces governing appetite control, therefore, are in a constantly dynamic state and encompass biological, psychological and environmental events.

1.2   A NOTE ON TERMINOLOGY

At this point it is probably helpful to clarify the use of certain terms which will appear throughout this book. Terms such as appetite, hunger, satiety and palatability can mean different things to different people. The lack of agreement arises partly because of differing theoretical perspectives, and partly because a term can be used quite legitimately in more than one sense.

Hunger, for example, as used in scientific theory (i.e., in a descriptive or predictive model) is a motivational construct with the status of a mediating or intervening variable (Blundell & Rogers, 1991). In this sense the term refers to an explanatory concept, which is inferred from other directly observable and measurable events. On the other hand, hunger is used in everyday life to describe certain feelings or bodily sensations linked to a desire to obtain and eat food. We use hunger here in both of these ways. Satiety is also a motivational construct, and typically is used to refer to 'a state of inhibition over eating' (Blundell & Rogers, 1991); however, people do not talk about feelings of satiety, though a feeling of fullness is clearly a component of satiety. Sometimes a distinction is made between satiation and satiety, the former being defined as the process leading to the termination of an episode of eating (Blundell, 1979; Blundell & Rogers 1991; Le Magnen, 1992). This is very similar to the distinction between intrameal and intermeal satiety described by Van Itallie and Vanderweele (1981), and accordingly the term 'satiating power of food' (Kissileff, 1984) has two meanings. It can describe the amount of food consumed during the meal (the effect of food on satiation) and the inhibition of further intake after the meal has ended (the effect of food on satiety).

We use palatability and liking to refer to an individual's hedonic or affective response to the taste, flavour, texture, etc. of a food or drink. This, therefore, is a component of the pleasure of eating. The basis of palatability and how it differs from preference is discussed in Chapter 2 (where we also discuss the distinction between taste and flavour).

Appetite is sometimes defined as separate from hunger and satiety. Here, though, we use it as a general descriptive term referring to the disposition to eat. Accordingly, specific appetite (Section 2.2.3) refers to the disposition or desire to eat a specific food. The latter is related to craving, which might be used to indicate a particularly strong desire to eat a specific food. However, we prefer not to give this term a narrow definition because, as discussed in Chapter 9, our interest is in the way in which people use craving to label and explain certain subjective experiences.

Lastly, obesity refers to the excessive accumulation of body fat. Among the simplest (if imperfect) ways to estimate degree of obesity is to use a measure of weight relative to height, such as Body Mass Index (BMI, Table 1.1):

$$BMI = weight~(in~kg)/height~(in~metres)^2$$

BMI is sometimes called Quetelet's Index, after the mathematician who initially used this measure to characterize the relationship between body weight and stature. It is currently the most common proxy measure of fatness used in epidemiological and experimental studies. The advantages and drawbacks (e.g., individuals of the same weight and height can have substantially different proportions of fat to lean tissue) of this measure are well known (Cole, 1991; Garn *et al.*, 1986; Smalley *et al.*, 1990; Garrow & Webster, 1985; Strain & Zumoff, 1992). In turn, the definition of obesity is based primarily on calculations of the relationship between weights-for-height and the likelihood of early death from a variety of chronic diseases. The lowest risk is associated with BMIs in the normal range, with overweight carrying only moderately increased health risks, but severe obesity carrying high risks of, for example, hypertension, coronary heart disease, and diabetes mellitus (WHO, 1990).

Table 1.1 A system for grading human obesity. Adapted from Garrow (1988)

BMI (kg/m²)	Description
<18–20	Underweight
20–24.9	Normal
25–29.9	Overweight
30–40	Obese
> 40	Severely obese

1.3 FEEDBACK CONTROL OF BODY WEIGHT (FAT)

1.3.1 Interaction between brain and body

There was a period when there was a good deal of confidence about the physiological basis of the control of appetite. Results of brain lesion studies on rats showed that destruction of the ventromedial nucleus of the hypothalamus (VMH) resulted in overeating and gross obesity (Hetherington & Ranson, 1942). Conversely, lesions in the area of the lateral hypothalamus (LH) caused animals to refuse to eat and drink, and electrical stimulation of this region was shown to increase eating and drinking (Anand & Brobeck, 1951; Teitelbaum & Epstein, 1962). These observations provided the basis for the proposal that there existed a dual hypothalamic mechanism consisting of interacting 'feeding' (LH) and 'satiety' (VMH) centres which controlled respectively the onset and offset of eating (Stellar, 1954; Brobeck, 1955). In related hypotheses, these brain centres were viewed as critical elements of feedback systems involved in the maintenance of stable body fat sores and glucose homeostasis; the so-called lipostatic and glucostatic theories (Kennedy, 1953; Mayer, 1955).

Subsequent findings forced a reevaluation of these ideas. It soon became clear, for example, that LH lesions cause profound sensory deficits and disrupt many aspects of behaviour. Furthermore, the primary effect of lesions of the VMH actually appears to be on the autonomic nervous system. Specifically, VMH damage results in decreased sympathetic and increased parasympathetic activity, stimulating the secretion of insulin and inhibiting the secretion of glucagon and adrenal catecholamines. Consequently, there is greater storage of ingested energy and also reduced release of nutrients during the postabsorptive phase. Although the animal is storing energy as fat, this is inaccessible for metabolism, therefore it must eat more in order to obtain a continuous supply of metabolizable energy (Friedman & Stricker, 1976). This interpretation of the so-called VMH syndrome was significant in that it represented a shift in emphasis in thinking about the control of appetite from the brain to the gut, liver and adipose tissue. Other evidence suggests that accelerated gastric emptying may also directly encourage the overeating in VMH rats (Duggan & Booth, 1986). The newer focus on peripheral organs has not, however, meant that the central nervous system has been neglected. It is obvious that eating behaviour and the subjective experiences of appetite involve functioning of the central nervous system, and also that metabolic events and stimuli arising from peripheral organs are monitored and integrated by the brain. For modern research on the physiology of appetite control the most important challenge is to understand more about this two-way communication between body and brain (Le Magnen, 1971; Friedman, 1991; Blundell, 1991).

1.3.2 Set-points and settling points

Theorizing about the physiology of appetite (and also thirst) has been closely interwoven with ideas derived from engineering control theory which has provided models of regulatory systems capable of maintaining relatively stable states. Commonly, these homeostatic models of motivation have incorporated a set-point and negative feedback. The system is assumed to contain a representation of the ideal level or reference value of the variable it regulates. This ideal level is the set-point. The actual level is compared continuously with this set-point and the difference is measured, producing an error signal. If the actual level is below the set-point motivation arises and, conditions permitting, food (or water) ingestion occurs. This eventually restores the deficit, thereby switching off the motivation (Toates, 1986). Accordingly, behaviour is controlled by cycles of depletion and repletion. A textbook analogy for such a system is the regulation of room temperature by a thermostatically controlled heater (Carlson, 1994).

Set-point models can account for the maintenance of energy balance and the observation that in adulthood there is rather little long-term variation in body weight. Associated with this is the idea of the defence of body weight, or more realistically the defence of the level of body fat, and crucially, the notion that the origins of obesity lie in the pathological functioning of the set-point control system. For example, obese people might have a high body weight set-point, which could explain why most weight loss diets fail (e.g., Keesey, 1978), and perhaps even why many obese people claim to be continuously hungry (Nisbett, 1972). Nisbett suggested that because of a desire to be slim obese people normally tend to restrict their food intake, thus driving their weight to below set-point and in turn causing an elevation of hunger (Section 8.3.1).

There is other evidence, however, which is clearly inconsistent with the existence, in a strict sense, of a set-point for body weight or body fat. In particular, there are some simple dietary manipulations which can markedly affect energy intake and body weight. These studies have been carried out on animals, mainly rats, but the results appear to be highly relevant to human eating behaviour and obesity. When switched from a standard laboratory diet to a high fat diet or to a 'cafeteria diet' (consisting of a variety of foods such as bread, chocolate, cheese and breakfast cereals) rats overeat and become grossly obese. Although the degree of obesity differs according to the strain of rat (e.g., Schemmel *et al.*, 1970), implicating a significant genetic component in the control of energy balance in relation to particular environmental circumstances (Chapter 4), this dietary-induced obesity can reach impressive proportions (Figure 1.1).

Although dietary-induced obesity contradicts a body fat set-point model, the results shown in Figure 1.1 are consistent with a negative feed-

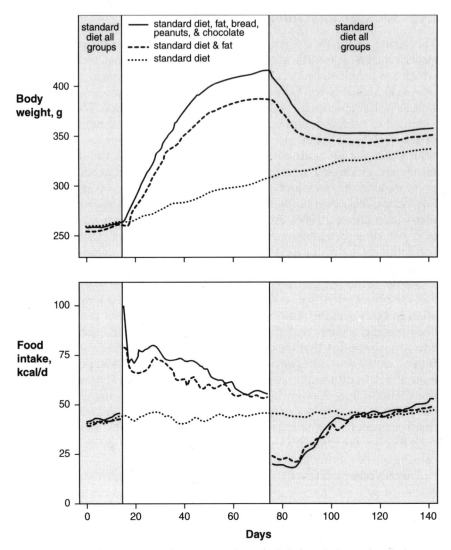

Figure 1.1 Body weights and energy intakes of adult female Lister-hooded rats before, during and after being fed a cafeteria or high-fat diet, and in a control group fed a standard laboratory diet throughout (n = 7 per group). Increased body fat content accounted for 75% of the excess weight gained during cafeteria feeding. Adapted from Rogers (1983).

back effect of body fat on appetite. As body weight (fatness) increased there was a decline in food intake, until a point was reached at which a new stable weight was maintained. This suggests a reduction in appetite with fattening which, physiologically, could be due to the increase in fat mobilization (lipolysis) or a related signal such as leptin that changes in proportion with the accumulation of body fat (Booth & Mather, 1978;

Friedman, 1991; Sorensen *et al.*, 1996). Computer models suggest that only a small background influence feeding back to suppress food intake is sufficient to provide a marked long-term stabilizing effect on body weight and fat (Booth & Mather, 1978).

Of course, the phenomenon of dietary-induced obesity raises the question as to what factors related to the diet are responsible for the very substantial differences in energy intake and body weight. This is what a large part of this book is about. One answer is that eating is increased because of the greater palatability of cafeteria diets and diets high in fat (e.g., Sclafani, 1980; Louis-Sylvestre *et al.*, 1984; Rogers & Blundell, 1984). Food variety, as available in cafeteria diets, also appears to play a significant role in stimulating food intake, perhaps at least partly by increasing the likelihood that individual food preferences are catered for (Blundell & Rogers, 1991). In terms of control theory models these influences can be represented as external factors having a positive input into the system, thereby tending to stimulate eating. Together with an inhibitory effect proportional to body fat content, this can account for the cycle of fattening and weight loss that occurs when rats are given a cafeteria diet which is then subsequently withdrawn. That is, the initial overeating stimulated by the more palatable diet is in due course limited by the increase in weight. On return to the less palatable diet the accumulated weight causes undereating, until the ensuing weight loss and weakening negative feedback signal allows intake to recover sufficiently for weight to re-stabilize. [Actually, Figure 1.1 shows that the diet-induced increase in weight was not completely reversed following the rats' return to the standard diet, suggesting that the cycle of weight gain was accompanied by persisting physiological or behavioural changes (Rolls *et al.*, 1980; Rogers, 1985; Ramirez, 1990)].

As we discuss later (Chapters 2, 5 and 6), the statement that food palatability is a cause of obesity is not a very revealing suggestion, unless there is an understanding of the basis of palatability. For example, if palatability is measured by the amount eaten, then an explanation of overeating based on the effects of palatability is entirely circular. For the present purposes, however, we use palatability as part of a model only to illustrate how feedback control can account very well for observations on food intake (appetite) in relation to body weight. Such a model is represented in Figure 1.2. Sometimes the term 'settling point' is used to describe the behaviour of this model (Wirtshafter & Davis, 1977; Pinel, 1993), the idea being that weight appears to be regulated around a point at which the various factors that influence its level achieve equilibrium. This contrasts with the notion of a fixed reference or 'desired' level that is usually implied in discussions of set-point models (although some models might be said to contain a set-point which is influenced by, for example, diet palatability; see discussion by Reddingius, 1980).

Unlike rats, human beings also exert a degree of deliberate control

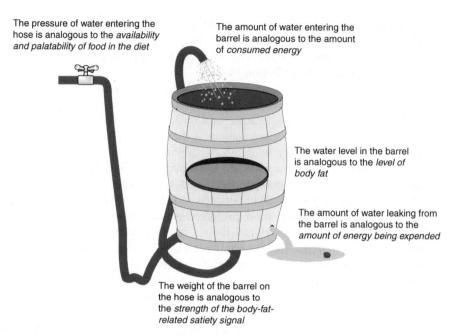

The pressure of water entering the hose is analogous to the *availability and palatability of food in the diet*

The amount of water entering the barrel is analogous to the amount of *consumed energy*

The water level in the barrel is analogous to the *level of body fat*

The amount of water leaking from the barrel is analogous to the *amount of energy being expended*

The weight of the barrel on the hose is analogous to the *strength of the body-fat-related satiety signal*

Figure 1.2 Leaky barrel model illustrating eating and body weight control. Adapted from Pinel (1993), with permission, copyright Allyn and Bacon.

over their eating, most typically in order to lose weight or prevent weight gain. An individual's preferred weight, shape, waist size etc. derived from cultural norms can be viewed as a 'cognitive set point' (Booth, 1978). Deviations from this set-point are detected when the individual notices a change in fit of their clothes, an increase in measured weight, or a perception of chubbiness when looking in a mirror, causing her or him to try to eat less in an attempt to eventually restore weight to the desired level. Actually, although cognitively restrained eating and dieting are common, they are not always successful and can even prove counterproductive (Chapter 8). In contrast, other individuals such as weight-lifters and body-builders deliberately try and increase their weight and body size by eating more or by altering their food choices.

Finally, it should be noted that appetite in growing people and animals can be influenced markedly by requirements for protein. This influence is less important in adults, except under fairly extreme conditions where, for example, protein intake is very low or protein is consumed in excess (reviewed by Millward, 1995; see also Section 9.3).

1.3.3 Passive feedback

Even without negative feedback inhibition of appetite, changes in body weight (fat) tend to be self-limiting. This is because of changes in body mass, including fat content, are accompanied by increases or decreases in energy expenditure due to changes in both resting metabolic rate and the energy cost of moving the body (Jéquier & Schutz, 1983). Thus a sustained increase in energy intake without any change in physical activity would lead to a self-limiting weight gain; the initial rate of weight gain progressively diminishing until a new asymptote is reached (Van Itallie & Kissileff, 1990; Section 3.3.1). Note from Figure 1.1, that after the initial period of rapid fattening, a greater energy intake was required to maintain the higher asymptotic weight levels of the cafeteria-fed and high-fat fed rats.

An analogous effect is present in the leaky-barrel model. Imagine that the hose is removed from beneath the barrel. If there is now an increase in the rate of water flowing into the barrel this will cause the water level to rise; however, due to the resulting increase in water pressure, the rate of outflow will also increase. Eventually, the amount of water in the barrel will attain a new equilibrium level (provided that the rate of inflow is not too high, in which case the barrel will overflow). This is an example of passive feedback. Although the system cannot be represented diagrammatically without using a feedback loop, it is not an 'intentional' part of the system, at least not in the sense that a thermostatically activated room heating system is a feedback controller purposely designed to work in that way (Toates, 1975; Reddingius, 1980).

1.4   AN ECOLOGICAL AND EVOLUTIONARY PERSPECTIVE ON ENERGY BALANCE

The evidence and models discussed above show that there are several types of mechanisms which can contribute to homeostasis. Stability of body fat and body weight in adulthood is achieved in part through a negative feedback effect on food intake; however the stable level is not fixed, it moves up or down according to shifts in the balance of a variety of exogenous and endogenous influences. Significantly, in the case of body fat, stability can occur within a very wide range of levels. This is because of the enormous storage capacity of adipose tissue, and the fact that the feedback inhibition of appetite is rather weak (and fat gain is associated with only relatively small increases in energy expenditure). In this section we argue that these characteristics evolved to buffer longer-term uncertainties in food supply.

1.4.1   Predisposition to obesity as an adaptation to conditions of feast and famine

Information from the study of human dietary prehistory shows that over the past tens of thousands of years our ancestors have subsisted on a wide variety of diets (Garn & Leonard, 1989). Therefore, it is not possible to be precise about how the nutritional composition of the 'natural' human diet, that is, the diet to which modern human beings are genetically adapted, compares with the contemporary western diet. Some degree of selection may have taken place relatively recently, with the development of agricultural practices and the domestication of animals, but the extent of this is unclear. It is fairly certain, though, that we are descendants of omnivores and that throughout much of our past cyclic food shortages and also famine were (and tragically in some Third World countries still are) commonplace (Brown & Konner, 1987; Garn & Leonard, 1989). These factors have, in turn, helped to shape human biology in a number of ways.

For example, three priorities for the omnivore are, first to select a diet which satisfies nutritional requirements, second to avoid ingesting harmful substances, and third to exploit resources efficiently (Rogers & Blundell, 1991). Rozin (1977) has discussed the first two of these in terms of the 'omnivore's paradox': balancing the need to seek sustenance from among a large number of potential food sources, few if any of which are capable of providing all the nutrients needed in sufficient amounts, with the need to take care to avoid ingesting environmental toxins. Accordingly, learning appears to play a major role in guiding appropriate food choice (Section 2.3.3).

As we have already suggested, the problem for our ancestors of obtaining enough to eat (i.e., the first priority in the list above) appears to be one of substantial variation in food availability both on a day-to-day and seasonal basis. This is based on fossil and archaeological evidence, which together with anthropological studies also points to the tendency to gorge when the opportunity arose. In particular, this is characteristic of the hunter–gatherer lifestyle where the subsistence component of the diet is of low to moderate energy density, supplemented relatively infrequently with highly prized energy-dense foods, including depot fat, organ meats, fatty insects and honey. The capacity to store such excess intake efficiently into body fat which can then be mobilized during periods of food shortage (Chapter 3) would clearly provide a key survival advantage. Subsequently, these adaptations are likely to have been maintained or even selected for more strongly in the early agriculturalists (Garn & Leonard, 1989; O'Dea, 1992). Note that there exists a variety of animal adaptations for overcoming short and longer-term variations in food supply, including food hoarding (storage), migration and hibernation (e.g., Collier, 1985).

Adipose tissue (body fat) has an impressive ability to store large amounts of energy efficiently – it can expand to an enormous size, and compared with other body tissues it is highly energy-dense (Table 3.2). Estimates show that the 'average' modern human being has a body fat content of about 15 kg (20 to 25% of total body weight). The energy content of fat is 9 kcal/g (37 kJ/g), so this store amounts to 135,000 kcal (555 MJ) which at a typical daily energy expenditure is sufficient for 55 days of life (Frayn, 1996). This average person has a BMI of 24 kg/m^2. Recalculating these figures for an obese person of the same height, with a BMI of 34 kg/m^2, and assuming that 75% of their extra weight is fat (Forbes, 1987a), gives a body fat content of 37 kg having an energy value of 333,000 kcal (1369 MJ), or sufficient for 137 days of life! Actually these may be underestimates, since they do not take into account the body's protein content, which increases with obesity, and can provide a significant source of energy during starvation. Also, there will be a considerable decline in obligate energy expenditure with prolonged starvation. It should be pointed out that body composition in adulthood, as well as being influenced by diet and food intake, varies substantially according to, for example, age, sex and level of physical training (Forbes, 1987).

Further evidence that energy storage is the primary function of adipose tissue comes from comparative anatomical studies (Pond, 1992). For example, polar bears feed almost exclusively on seals, and rapidly become obese in the winter and spring when conditions favour predation. In summer, however, food availability is poor and they remain active for several months without feeding. It is possible the increase in body fat also serves as an adaptation contributing thermal insulation, but comparisons of polar bears with temperate-zone and tropical carnivores show a similar partitioning of adipose tissue between superficial and intra-abdominal depots. In other words, there is little to suggest that the distribution of adipose tissue in this winter-active species is specially adapted to the cold climate.

Nonetheless, the metabolic properties of adipose tissue vary substantially according to its site (Pond, 1992). The superficial depots, which describe adipose tissue that accumulates between the superficial muscles and the skin, and the intra-abdominal depots can expand very considerably and are relatively metabolically inert compared with the usually smaller intermuscular depots. Therefore, although an oversimplification, it is tempting to suggest that the former provide a longer-term storage function, while the intermuscular depots contribute more to routine, day-to-day glucose and energy homeostasis, acting as a local energy source for adjacent muscles.

1.4.2   Now we have a 'continuous feast'

The arguments above lead to the conclusion that human beings and other mammals have evolved a predisposition to become obese under appropriate environmental conditions. However, the behavioural, metabolic and anatomical traits which favour overeating and the storage of surplus energy in the form of body fat in times of plenty conflict with relatively very recent human socio-cultural and economic developments. In modern industrialized societies food availability rarely or never limits intake, and the prevalence of obesity is high and constitutes a major public health concern. The changes in food intake patterns from human prehistory to the present have been characterized as a progression from feast and famine for the hunter–gatherer, to subsistence and famine for the early agriculturalists, and finally to continuous feast for people from modern 'western' societies (O'Dea, 1992). Coupled with this are changes in the energy density and nutrient composition of the diet and in levels of energy expenditure, which further encourage the development of obesity.

Contrary to these tendencies, though, the cultural preference in economically and technologically advanced societies is for a thin body shape, and especially for women, who have a proportionally higher body fat content than men. On the other hand, in societies where it is easy to remain lean, cultural standards of beauty favour plumpness. What underlies this paradox, of wanting to be thin in a fat society and fat in a thin society, is the greater investment of economic resources and individual effort that is required to achieve the desired standard in the different contexts (Brown & Konner, 1987). In its context each standard involves a display of wealth or achievement, even if this achievement relates only to the successful self-control of eating (Section 8.3). In turn, however, attempts to attain a biologically unrealistic thin body shape are implicated in the aetiology of the eating disorders anorexia nervosa and bulimia nervosa (e.g., Polivy & Herman, 1985; Hill, 1993; Section 8.5.2), which like obesity are also associated with significant morbidity and mortality.

1.5 SUMMARY

The study of eating behaviour has tended to be dominated by the notion that appetite is controlled by a homeostatic system that serves to maintain energy balance. Evidence, for example from studies on dietary-induced obesity in rats, contradicts the existence of a body weight or body fat set-point, but nevertheless suggests there is a negative feedback influence of body fat on appetite which tends to stabilize body weight. However, because the storage capacity of adipose tissue is very large and the feedback inhibition on appetite is rather weak, stability of body weight can occur within a very wide range of values. These characteristics probably evolved to buffer uncertainties in food supply. In most natural habitats food supplies are unpredictable or may vary seasonally. The storage of energy in the form of body fat in times of plenty can reduce the impact of food shortages, but where food availability rarely or never limits intake this adaptation will encourage the development of obesity.

More generally, the need for precise control of nutrient intakes is avoided by sophisticated metabolic regulatory mechanisms. Excesses are dealt with by metabolic transformation, storage and excretion (Frayn, 1996). Consequently, at the level of behaviour, the nutritional priorities for omnivorous species are to select a diet that meets certain minimal nutritional requirements, and in doing so avoid ingesting harmful substances. An appropriate way to view the goal of this whole system, therefore, is in relation to the anticipation of needs and the long-term sufficiency of nutrient supplies, rather than in terms of the maintenance of energy balance. Within this framework the next chapter discusses physiological and learned influences that control eating from one meal to the next.

Hunger, palatability and satiation: physiological and learned influences on eating

2.1 APPETITE AND PLEASURE

The Creator who made man such that he must eat to live, incites him to eat by means of appetite and rewards him by pleasure.

Brillat-Savarin, 1755–1826

This chapter is about what arouses and satisfies appetite, and what determines the pleasure of eating. These questions are addressed primarily with human experiences of eating in mind; however, we also draw heavily on the insights provided by studies of the physiological and learned bases of animal eating behaviour.

Eating occurs in bouts called meals, and food intake can vary according to the number and/or size of meals eaten. 'Snacks' can contribute substantially to nutrient intake and are probably best considered as small meals, since the distinction between meals and snacks appears to be based mainly on social convention rather than any substantial differences in the processes controlling eating (Section 7.2.1). The meal, therefore, can be considered as the basic unit for the analysis of eating behaviour. In turn, meals may be divided into three phases: namely, the initiation, maintenance, and termination of eating. Here we examine the processes underlying the control of these phases of the meal, and consider how the integration of meal-to-meal influences on eating and food choice influence the longer-term stability of nutrient intake.

2.2 MEAL INITIATION

2.2.1 Depletion or absence of satiety as a stimulus for hunger

As discussed earlier (Section 1.3.2), the biological basis of appetite control has for a long time been considered in terms of homeostasis and homeostatic behaviour. According to this perspective the bodily energy deficit that accumulates as time passes since the last meal causes eating motivation to increase, leading the individual to obtain and consume food, which in turn removes the energy deficit. This focuses on the individual's internal state as the primary motivating factor for eating – a 'hunger drive' which increases as a result of food deprivation and is reduced by food intake. It is clear, though, that this simple depletion–repletion model of motivation does not adequately account for eating behaviour (even of laboratory rats which were the source of many of the data collected to test these ideas). At the very least it is also necessary to consider the motivational effects of the presence of food and the quality or palatability of that food and the effort required to obtain it, which additionally influence the decision to eat and how much is eaten (Toates, 1986). The way in which these external influences (incentives) and internal influences combine to affect eating are considered in detail below (Sections 2.3.5 and 2.4), while the remainder of this section examines evidence concerning the role of depletion as a stimulus for hunger and the initiation of eating.

An early observation reported from studies on the free-feeding patterns of laboratory rats was that meal size is relatively strongly correlated with the length of the postmeal interval ('postprandial pattern'), but poorly correlated with the premeal interval ('preprandial pattern') (Le Magnen & Tallon, 1966). Arguably, this finding is consistent with depletion-driven eating in that it suggests that eating is initiated in response to the depletion of the food energy consumed in the previous meal (but see Stricker, 1984 for a different interpretation). In other words, if the preceding meal is large then, all else (e.g., energy expenditure) being equal, depletion of reserves will take longer and the onset of the next meal will be relatively delayed.

Accordingly, the physiological stimulus for hunger can be expected to be related primarily to short-term depletion. Indeed, a fairly simple model based on estimates of stomach capacity and emptying rates can account quite well for meal patterns in the freely fed rat. Specifically, postprandial correlations can be explained if it is assumed that eating is initiated when the stomach empties to below a certain threshold (Snowdon, 1970; de Castro, 1981). However, rather than stomach emptiness itself, the critical variable is more likely to be, for example, changes in glucose metabolism associated with the rate of energy flow from the gut (Booth, 1978; Le Magnen, 1992; Section 2.3.4). This in turn will be related to the rate at which food empties from the stomach to the intestines, which is influenced by, among other factors, the energy content of the stomach (Hunt & Stubbs, 1975).

Actually, another way to describe this relationship between metabolism and eating behaviour is to say that the initiation of eating occurs when the inhibitory effects of repletion dissipate. According to this reasoning hunger equates to the absence of satiety. Although there is no real distinction here, it does give a somewhat different perspective on the control of appetite (*cf.* Stricker, 1984). One of the advantages of avoiding the term 'depletion of reserves' is that, as suggested above, the predominant influence on satiety in the postmeal interval is the amount and composition of the food consumed in the previous meal. It is unlikely that the energy economy of the whole body can have much impact in the short term, because for adult rats and human beings depletion from one meal to the next is typically very small compared with total bodily energy reserves (Sections 1.4.1 and 3.3). The level of these reserves (body fat content) does exert an influence on appetite, but the action of this relatively weak negative feedback effect will only be apparent over the longer term (Section 1.3.2). Figure 2.1 proposes how these influences combine to determine hunger/satiety at different times after eating.

Finally, the suggestion made here that increased adiposity tends to influence postmeal hunger/satiety rather than processes controlling eating within meals (satiation) is supported by observations on the meal patterns of dietary obese rats. It was found that the decline in energy intake during the development of obesity in cafeteria rats (see Figure 1.1) was due entirely to a decrease in meal frequency, which closely paralleled the increase in body weight (Rogers & Blundell, 1984). This suggests the view that the low meal frequency which is sometimes found to be a feature of human obesity is a consequence of the obesity, and not one of its causes as claimed by some authors (e.g., Fábry & Tepperman, 1970; see Chapter 7).

2.2.2   Effects of constraints on eating

Thus far in this review of factors controlling the initiation of eating we have considered evidence coming largely from studies on freely feeding subjects. In this situation there is unhindered access to food throughout the day and night, which clearly is often not the case in natural environments where opportunities to eat are constrained by food availability and competing priorities. Such constraints can have a dramatic impact on feeding patterns. For example, when the cost (i.e., amount of work to be done) to gain access to a meal is increased, the frequency of meals is reduced and their size increases in compensation (Collier, 1985). This provides a simple example of optimal foraging; that is, at least within certain limits, behaviour adapts to maximize the ratio of the benefit to cost of exploiting food resources.

Another consequence of reducing access to food is to alter the relationships between intermeal interval and meal size. De Castro (1988) found that giving rats access to food at 5 fixed times each day caused them to decrease their meal frequency to an average of 3.2 meals per day compared with around 10 meals per day when given continuous access. Daily food intake stabilized to only a slightly lower level on the restricted

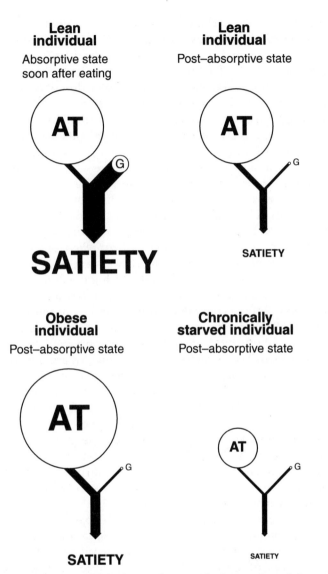

Figure 2.1 A highly simplified scheme showing the integration of the influences of the energy contents of the gut and adipose tissue on satiety. Together, the signals generated by the presence of food in the gut and the energy supplied from this food are relatively strong but dissipate rapidly (Section 2.3.4), while the body fat-related signal is weak but acts chronically (Section 1.3.2). Note that the strength of the output signal, depicted by the thickness of the arrow, is relatively little affected by obesity or starvation. Not shown is how these influences interact with energy expenditure, which for example is higher in obese individuals, necessitating a higher energy intake to maintain the obese state (Section 3.3.1). Underlying this higher intake might be an accelerated supply of food energy from the previous meal, resulting in a faster decay of the net satiety signal in the postmeal interval (see also Section 1.3.2). AT = adipose tissue, G = gut.

access regimen; however, these rats now showed a preprandial pattern of intake (meal size significantly correlated with premeal interval) in contrast to the postprandial pattern during free feeding (see also Levitsky, 1974). Does this shift in feeding pattern contradict the scheme shown in Figure 2.1? Probably not, because the results described by de Castro (1988) can be modelled by introducing a fairly minor change in feeding strategy. Specifically, it is assumed that under conditions where opportunities to eat are relatively infrequent, the subject eats simply until the gut is full. As a result meal size is determined by the amount of food in the gut at the beginning of the meal, and there is a positive correlation between meal size and the length of the preceding interval, because a longer wait before eating would leave less food in the gut thus allowing greater intake in that meal (de Castro, 1988).

This conclusion is further supported by the finding that rats show only small short-term increases in food intake when subjected to more extended periods of food deprivation (Le Magnen, 1992). For instance, an analysis of the pattern of feeding of rats during the first 24 hours following 18 hours of food deprivation revealed a mere 10% or 6 kcal (26 kJ) increase in food intake compared with the intake of non-deprived controls (Rogers, 1983). Furthermore, most of the increase was accounted for by a larger intake during the first 4 hours (comprising 2 to 3 meals) after food was returned. This increase, even allowing for a reduction in energy expenditure during deprivation, indicates a sluggish compensatory response in relation to the amount of food missed [an estimated 38 kcal (160 kJ); these data are for rats fed a standard laboratory diet, but parallel results were obtained for rats maintained on a more energy-dense, cafeteria diet – *cf.* Figure 1.1]. In terms of total body energy stores, however, the energy deficit resulting from the food deprivation was trivial. Therefore even when eating behaviour is placed under fairly severe constraints the short-term control of food intake still appears to be dominated by the effects of food consumed in the previous meal.

Analyses of the meal patterns of human subjects (North Americans) showed a stronger preprandial than postprandial pattern, at least when the correlations were calculated without the overnight fast included in the intermeal intervals (de Castro & Kreitzman, 1985). Furthermore, significant correlations were found between estimated premeal stomach content and premeal hunger ratings, and in turn these variables predicted meal size. The evidence from the studies on rats suggests that the pattern of infrequent eating (3 to 4 meals per day on average) adopted by these human subjects can help explain the preprandial correlations, with food intake being influenced by the level of premeal hunger determined by factors related to gut content (de Castro, 1988; 1996). If the overnight fast is taken into account, however, it might be concluded that the pattern is more mixed. Typically, the largest meal of the day is eaten in the evening (de Castro, 1996) and this anticipates the longest intermeal interval.

2.2.3 Effects of external cues associated with eating

There is evidence, therefore, that despite the complexity of the eating environments that exist in affluent, modern societies, human eating patterns to some extent exhibit the same orderly relationships found for the meal patterns of rats living in simple and unchanging laboratory environments. This is consistent with the action of persistent physiological influences on eating (de Castro, 1996; Section 2.4). Nevertheless, it is also clear that for any individual eating opportunity there are many other factors which will influence the decision of whether or not to eat (and what and how much to eat). On its own, the idea that hunger is generated by internal physiological signals related to energy or nutrient depletion fails to account for many aspects of eating. For example, appetite can be stimulated by the offer of an unexpected treat, a person's desire to eat may fade in the afternoon even though they were too busy to eat lunch, and many people regularly do not eat breakfast despite the fact that this meal follows the longest fast of the day. These and other observations show that external (environmental) stimuli, including the sight and smell of food and learned contextual cues such as location and time of day, play a major role in motivating eating.

The earliest systematic investigations of the role of learning in the control of appetite were carried out by Pavlov (1927). These showed that arbitrary external cues, such as the sound of a bell or buzzer, paired with the presentation of food to a food-deprived dog eventually gained the capacity to elicit eating-related responses (salivation) in the absence of food. Since that time the importance of Pavlovian or classical conditioning in guiding behaviour has been widely recognized and, as discussed below, this is one of the basic processes through which food preferences and aversions are acquired. Nonetheless, the full extent to which conditioning influences eating motivation has only recently begun to be appreciated.

An example relevant to the initiation of eating is revealed by the results of studies carried out on rats by Weingarten (1983; 1984a). The rats were fed a liquid diet on a preprogrammed schedule of 6 irregularly spaced meals per day giving a total daily intake of 70% of their *ad libitum* intake. During this training phase each meal was signalled with a buzzer and light (the conditioned stimuli, CS+) presented for 4 minutes before and 30 seconds after the meal was made available. In the test phase the CS+ was presented again, but the rats were no longer food restricted since in addition to these signalled meals a bottle of the same liquid food was available *ad libitum*. The rats, nonetheless, responded 'robustly and rapidly' to the CS+ by taking a substantial meal, and this behaviour was maintained throughout many subsequent days of testing. In contrast, they did not respond to another stimulus (a steady tone, the CS−) which had been present exactly midway in each intermeal interval. These results show that external stimuli previously associated with food consumption can reliably motivate eating in the absence of immediate nutritional deprivation. Responding was reduced only if the animal had eaten very recently prior to a presentation of the CS+. Note that although Pavlov was interested primarily in salivary and gastric secretory responses, he also observed that presentation of the CS+ caused behavioural effects. For example, the dogs would strain in their harnesses attempting to approach the source of the CS+.

The extent to which this learning depends on the fairly severe level of food restriction imposed during initial exposure to the association between the CS+ and food delivery was not tested in these experiments. Parallel studies on human subjects (children aged between 3 and 5 years), however, showed some evidence for the control of meal initiation by learned cues without there being any restriction on food access during either conditioning or testing phases (Birch *et al.*, 1989). This is significant because potentially it widens the relevance of the effects of learned cues to include most eating situations.

Another basic question arising from Weingarten's (1983; 1984a) observations concerns the specificity of the effects of external stimuli conditioned to eating. One possibility is that exposure to these stimuli triggers certain physiological responses in preparation for eating, including salivation, insulin release and gastric acid secretion (the so-called cephalic phase of digestion), the consequences of which feed back to the brain where they are interpreted as an internal signal for hunger. Against this, though, is the finding that pharmacological blockade of cephalic-phase responses with atropine does not disrupt the initiation of eating in response to learned cues (Weingarten, 1984b). Alternatively, rather than a general state of hunger, the presentation of stimuli which have become associated with consumption of a food may elicit a desire to eat that specific food (Weingarten, 1985).

This last suggestion has not been adequately tested, but it does coincide with the observation that appetite tends to be food and context specific. For instance, it is typical to have a desire to eat cornflakes or toast, but not prawn cocktail, for breakfast. Why is this? The latter is inappropriate for this time of day, at least in British gastronomic culture; however, the idea of learned specific appetites suggests that if this convention was ignored, a habit of eating (and wanting to eat) prawn cocktail at breakfast could be relatively easily established. Similarly, choosing to eat breakfast cereal at other times of day could be expected to increase the frequency of appetite for this particular food. Another example which provides an analogy for this question is to consider visiting the cinema where in the past you have usually eaten popcorn. What is the effect of exposure to this eating-related setting? Does it trigger a general feeling of hunger, or a specific desire to eat popcorn?

An extension of these ideas is that specific appetites might also become conditioned to salient internal stimuli, for example, accompanying particular emotional states. In fact, more probably this would involve associations formed between eating and a configuration of both internal and external stimuli evoking the emotional response (*cf.* Robbins & Fray, 1980; Wardle, 1990; Booth, 1994). Such a mechanism might underlie mood- and stress-induced eating, and in turn help explain effects of mood on eating at an individual level, since these relationships would be shaped according to a person's own particular learning history (Chapter 8). Also if specific appetites are based on learned associations then presumably they can be unlearned (i.e., 'extinguished'), for instance, through unreinforced exposure to the context in which the appetite or craving is experienced. This technique, which is called cue exposure, has shown some success in the treatment of binge eating in bulimia nervosa (Jansen *et al.*, 1992).

2.2.4 'Hunger' during prolonged food restriction

Following on directly from the discussion above, there is also evidence that the extinction or weakening of learned appetites can occur during voluntary dieting, particularly when eating is severely restricted. Thus, contrary to what is predicted by a simple energy depletion–repletion model of appetite control, rated hunger and desire to eat is often found to be hardly increased at all or even diminished during extended periods of dieting and weight loss (Coronas *et al.*, 1982; Rosen *et al.*, 1982; 1985; Wadden *et al.*, 1985; 1987; Lappalainen *et al.*, 1990; de Graaf *et al.*, 1993a; see also Harvey *et al.*, 1993). In part the results might be explained by the high protein content of the energy-restricted diets used in most of these studies, since protein has a greater satiating efficiency than either carbohydrate or fat (Section 5.1). In some instances protein intake was actually higher than before dieting. Nevertheless, the planned energy deficits were substantial [≥ 1,000 kcal (4.2 MJ)], and typically hunger ratings were higher during the first compared with subsequent weeks of dieting.

Especially remarkable are the results obtained by Lappalainen *et al.* (1990). They studied a small group of obese individuals treated on an outpatient basis and advised to consume a 200 kcal/d (0.8 MJ/d) liquid only diet. This 'fast' was maintained for 19 days, the subjects having reduced their intake in steps during the preceding 3 days. Although weight loss was substantial (mean = 7.9 kg), the reported frequency of hunger and food craving, and 'reactivity to food stimuli' decreased very significantly during the fast. This contrasted with much smaller changes on these measures among subjects who lost an average of 2.0 kg while consuming a 'regular' 1,600 kcal (6.7 MJ) diet over the same period. The technique used to assess reactivity to food stimuli is particularly relevant as it involved subjects rating their hunger before and after being shown slide pictures of food items. These findings, therefore, appear to be consistent with the view that the reduction in appetite that may occur during food restriction is due to the extinction of associations between eating-related cues and food intake. According to this explanation, appetite decreases more rapidly with fasting than partial food restriction because during fasting there is a higher frequency of unreinforced exposure to stimuli previously paired with eating (Lappalainen *et al.*, 1990).

These conclusions have practical implications for the treatment of obesity. For example, appropriate modification of eating behaviour, including confining eating to very restricted times and places, could be expected to achieve improved appetite control without the need for severe fasting, which is associated with high a rate of loss of lean body mass, marked reduction in basal metabolic rate, and other undesirable effects. The results are also relevant to the problem of anorexia nervosa. Anorexics apparently do not experience overwhelming levels of 'hunger', even though they reduce their food intake often to the point of extreme emaciation (both of these issues are examined in more detail in Chapter 8).

It should be noted finally, however, that under certain circumstances moderate to severe food restriction is associated with greater hunger and increased preoccupation with food. In Keys' *et al.* (1950) well-known study on the effects of chronic semi-starvation marked and sustained increases in complaints of hunger were evident during underfeeding (although it was further reported that 'some subjects suffered relatively little distress from hunger', page 829). This is also illustrated vividly by the following passage by Primo Levi describing the starvation he experienced during his incarceration in Auschwitz during 1944–5.

> We were not normal because we were hungry. Our hunger at that time had nothing in common with the well-known (and not completely disagreeable) sensation of someone who has missed a meal and is certain that the next meal will not be missed: it was a need, a lack, a yearning that had accompanied us now for a year, had struck deep, permanent roots in us, lived in our cells, and conditioned our behaviour. To eat, to get something to eat, was our prime stimulus, behind which, at a great distance, followed other problems of survival, and even still farther away the memories of home and the very fear of death.

From *The Periodic Table* by Primo Levi (1986, page 140)

Taken together these observations demonstrate that food restriction does not invariably provoke increased feelings of hunger. The individual response will be determined by cognitive as well as physiological and learned influences, and will differ according to, for example, whether the restriction is enforced, is rigidly self-imposed, is a casual attempt at dieting, or is part of a therapeutic programme to reduce overweight.

2.3   THE MAINTENANCE AND TERMINATION OF EATING

Once the meal begins, eating is controlled moment to moment predominantly by the orosensory and postingestive effects of the food consumed.
Typically, the overall contribution of the effects in the mouth is stimulatory, while the net effect of the entry of food into the stomach and
intestines is inhibitory (Smith, *et al.*, 1990; Rogers, 1993). Figure 2.2 shows
these positive and negative feedback influences combining to produce a
cumulative intake curve similar to that observed in studies of the
microstructure of human eating (Spiegel & Jordan, 1978; Westerterp-
Plantenga *et al.*, 1990). Of course similar output curves can be obtained
with stimulatory and inhibitory influences varying in a number of different ways; so, for instance, there may be some decline in the strength of
positive feedback during the meal (indicated by the dashed lines in
Figure 2.2, see Section 2.3.5).

The positive feedback arising from orosensory contact with food probably plays an essential role in keeping behaviour 'locked in' to eating.
Simulations show that without positive feedback there is a tendency for
behaviour to oscillate or dither between activities (Houston & Sumida,
1985; McFarland, 1971). This stimulation of eating by eating would
appear to be consistent with subjective experience – '*l'appétit vient en
mangeant*' or 'appetite comes with eating' (see also Yeomans, 1996). In
addition, there are behavioural data which support the existence of such
an effect. A good example comes from Wiepkema's (1971a; 1971b)
detailed analysis of feeding in the mouse, which led him to propose a
model very similar to that shown in Figure 2.2. At the beginning of a
spontaneous meal a large increase in the length of successive feeding
bouts was observed, while the length of non-feeding intervals was
unchanged during this part of the meal. Furthermore, the strength of the
positive feedback effect was found to depend on the quality of the sensory stimuli (i.e., palatability). When bitter, less preferred food – the standard food adulterated with sucrose octoacetate – was offered, the early
increase in feeding-bout length was much reduced. Therefore, consumption of highly palatable foods can be expected to have a powerful positive
feedback effect thereby strongly stimulating eating and increasing meal
size.

The operation of negative feedback during normal eating is demonstrated by the results of studies on sham feeding. Rats fitted with a
chronic gastric fistula eat (drink) vastly increased amounts when the liquid food is allowed to drain out of the open fistula, compared with when
the fistula is closed (Smith *et al.*, 1974). In other words, satiety does not
occur if ingested food fails to distend the stomach or enter the small intestine – thus excluding taste, other oral stimuli, pharyngeal and
oesophageal movements, and the contact of food with the gastric mucosa
as potent stimuli for satiation. Although the sham-fed rat does eventually

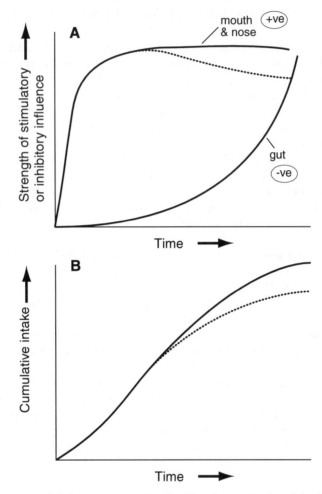

Figure 2.2   Model illustrating positive (+ve) and negative (−ve) feedbacks oper-
ating on eating during a meal. (A) Stimulatory and inhibitory effects of orosensory and gut-mediated signals. (B) Resulting cumulative amount of food eaten
during the meal. Adapted from Rogers (1993), with permission, copyright John
Wiley and Sons Ltd.

stop eating, this is likely to be due to fatigue or the effects of the digestion
and absorption of a portion of the ingested nutrients (Sclafani &
Nissenbaum, 1985). Other evidence shows that the postingestive and
postabsorptive effects of food ingestion which influence meal size and
the maintenance of satiety in the post-meal interval include filling of the
gastrointestinal tract, release of regulatory hormones such as cholecystokinin and the detection of nutrients absorbed into the systemic circulation (e.g., Forbes, 1988).

    In order, therefore, to predict food choice and intake during the meal it is necessary to understand the basis of palatability and the processes underlying satiation and satiety. These issues are discussed in the following three sections.

2.3.1 Palatability: the hedonic response to food

A dictionary definition of palatable is 'agreeable to the taste' (*Collins English Dictionary*, 1986), and this is the sense in which we use it here. However, because the term has been applied inconsistently and sometimes more broadly in the scientific literature, the first part of this discussion will take a closer look at what palatability is and is not.

To begin with, palatability is not merely an aspect of the stimulus properties of food such as its taste, aroma, texture and temperature – on their own these are simply categories of orosensory stimuli. And at the other extreme, palatability is not the final common pathway determining food intake, ingestive movements or food preference. Instead, as suggested above, palatability refers to the individual's hedonic or affective response to orosensory stimuli (e.g., Young, 1959; Rogers, 1990), and can therefore be identified with food liking and pleasantness.

The following example illustrates the difference between palatability and food preference. Consider a person choosing between margarine and butter; she may eat more margarine because of price or perceived health benefits, but she may like the 'taste' of margarine less than that of butter. As measured by the amount consumed she would show a preference for margarine, although on a hedonic measure butter would score higher. That is, although preference will generally be strongly affected by palatability, it is also subject to other separate influences.

Having said this, much of the evidence concerning the determinants of palatability has actually been obtained from studies measuring food preference. This is because many of these studies have been carried out using animals as subjects. It has been claimed that an animal's affective response to a food stimulus (and therefore palatability) can be inferred from observing fine details of its behaviour (e.g., Grill & Berridge, 1985). Nevertheless, it is considerably more straightforward to assess food preference, for instance, by measuring the relative intake of two foods offered simultaneously. An advantage of studying human subjects is that they can be asked to state on standardized rating scales how pleasant a food tastes or how much they like it. The ratings can be then used to indicate palatability. However, since reporting on hedonic experience relies on the individual's conscious introspection and an agreement as to what constitutes this experience, liking and pleasantness ratings should be treated with caution. In other words, such ratings do not directly measure either palatability or affective experience. This is a problem to which we will return to below (Section 2.3.5) in a discussion of the relationship between palatability and satiation.

2.3.2 Palatability: innate influences

Perceptions of the sensory characteristics of foods and drinks are derived from combinations of sensations mediated via gustation, olfaction, and chemesthesis ('trigeminal' system or 'common chemical sense') (Table 2.1). These sensory modalities are largely distinct in anatomy and physiology, and activation of the oral and olfactory reception systems provides diverse and widespread input to the brain (Smith et al., 1990). It should be noted that use of the word 'innate' to characterize sensory responses present at birth and/or universal in humans may be confusing. 'Innate' responses are not necessarily genetically endowed, and might in many cases be best explained as a function of *in utero* or very early neonatal experiences (Sclafani, 1995; Mela & Catt, 1996).

Table 2.1 Neuroanatomical processes mediating sensory responses to oronasal stimuli

Process	Sensations mediated
Gustation	Taste: sweet, sour, salty, bitter (umami?, others)
Olfaction	Odour (aroma, smell): unlimited number
Chemesthesis	Touch, Temperature, Nociception/Irritation, Proprioception

The qualitative attributes of taste stimuli are commonly grouped into 4 or 5 'basic' dimensions, although there continues to be debate over the foundations for such distinctions (Delwiche, 1996). Despite the lingering controversy, this classification scheme has guided (and arguably simplified) much of taste research, which typically makes use of compounds which are believed to be representative of these distinct categories.

There have been a large number of studies examining various aspects of responsiveness to basic chemosensory stimuli (simple tastes and odours) by newborn infants. These indicate that humans are born with positive hedonic responses to at least one sensory quality, sweetness, and probably a dislike for bitter and sour tastes (Beauchamp et al., 1991b). Human newborns show marked facial reactions indicating acceptance and a positive hedonic response to sweet stimuli, while bitter stimuli evoke rejection coupled with negative expressions (Steiner, 1987; see also Tatzer et al., 1985). Similar reactions can be elicited in rats (Grill & Berridge, 1985; Section 2.3.3). The adaptive value of these congenital biases have been interpreted in terms of, for example, avoiding ingestion of toxic substances such as bitter tasting alkaloids in certain plants, and the facilitating effect of sweetness on the infant's early acceptance of its mother's milk (Beauchamp, 1994; Blass, 1991; Booth 1991). Studies on human newborns have also shown an acceptance response to monosodium glutamate, which appears to be distinct from the reaction to sweet tastes (Steiner, 1987). The taste of monosodium glutamate and the 5'-ribonuleotides is characterized as 'umami' or savoury, and it has been suggested that this serves as a signal for protein-rich foods (Ikeda, 1909; Deutsch *et al.*, 1989). In contrast, responses to salt appear to be undeveloped at birth, although by about 4–6 months of age human infants strongly prefer saline solutions compared with water. This developmental change is thought to be due to maturation of the sensory responsiveness to salt rather than to learning (Beauchamp *et al.*, 1986).

It is logical to presume that the normal neonatal hedonic responses to these basic taste qualities are truly unlearned: the types of stimuli which give rise to these taste sensations are shared by many common biological compounds, there are relatively specific receptor elements and/or transduction mechanisms for each of these taste qualities, and related animal species show hedonic responses broadly similar to those of human beings. That clearly does not, however, exclude the possibility that these innate responses might be modified by later experience.

The powerful action of sweet taste is further demonstrated in studies by Blass and his colleagues (Blass, 1991; Blass & Hoffmeyer, 1991; Smith *et al.*, 1990). In one experiment 2–3-day-old human infants were given 2 ml of 12% sucrose solution to drink immediately prior to blood collection made using a heel lance. Compared with the same volume of water, the sucrose substantially reduced the initial amount and duration of crying in response to the painful blood collection procedure. Sweet taste rather than a direct nutritional effect was implicated, since the response was very rapid and the small volume of sucrose was presumably nutritionally insignificant. These observations have been confirmed and extended in subsequent work (Barr *et al.*, 1994; Miller *et al.*, 1994a). The latter of these experiments used the cold presser test (in which one arm is immersed in cold water) and found analgesic effects of oral sucrose in 8–11-year-old children. Similar studies in the rat have indicated that this antinociceptive and/or calming property of sucrose, and possibly other food materials including fats, is mediated by the activation of central opioid mechanisms (Blass *et al.*, 1987; Blass, 1991).

In contrast to the apparently limited gustatory repertoire, the number of unique odours or aromas human beings can discern appears to be essentially unlimited, and although there have been many attempts to organize these sensations into a limited set of categories (like the 'basic' tastes), no single odour classification scheme has ever received general endorsement. Humans invariably describe odours in terms of familiar, specific sources (e.g., 'popcorn', 'rose', 'vomit'). Specific anosmias, the inability to smell particular compounds, have been described for a number of odours (Rogers & Mela, 1992). These may be genetically based, but also involved there appear to be interactions of genetics, experience, and developmental effects (Beauchamp & Wysocki, 1990). There is little evidence to support the existence of universal unlearned odour preferences. Recent studies have suggested a possible inborn attraction of newborns for the odour of lactating breasts, but these have not discounted the possibility that this reflects an outcome of learning which occurred *in utero* (Porter *et al.*, 1991; Varendi *et al.*, 1996; Mela & Catt, 1996). In addition, it is apparent that human infants can express and retain conditioned responses to specific odours within days of birth (Sullivan *et al.*, 1991; Davis & Porter, 1991), and readily respond to food flavours transmitted through breast milk (Menella, 1995).

It is by their volatile odours, sensed retro-nasally (generated from food present in the mouth and passing through nasal passages during exhalation) that most individual foods are perceived and recognized as unique. For example, many fruits taste sweet, but only one has the aroma of strawberry. Accordingly, the perception of the 'flavour' of a food or drink depends on the integration of inputs from all of the systems summarized in Table 2.1. Because foods are felt on the tongue and in other parts of the mouth and there is no tactile experience associated with the olfactory receptor region, sensations of food-related aromas are generally referred to the mouth, with the consequence that the terms 'taste', 'smell' and 'flavour' are often confused or used interchangeably in colloquial speech (Rozin, 1982). However, the diversity and specificity of volatile odours (as opposed to tastes) has critical implications for the acquisition of food preferences through learned associations.

Tactile, thermal and nociceptive (pain) sensations on the surfaces of the lips, mouth and nasal cavity, together with proprioceptive information (muscle/joint position), are mediated by nerve fibres which are distinct from gustatory and olfactory receptor cells, and mediate oronasal chemesthesis (Green, 1996). Activation of these fibres is primarily responsible for experiences such as the chemical 'burn' from chili and alcohol, the 'cooling' of menthol and wintergreen, and the irritation from ammonia and other vapours. Reflex response to stimulants of this system include sneezing, salivation, sweating, watering of the eyes, flushing and momentary interruption of breathing.

There appear to be a number of substantial, genetically based individual differences in human olfactory and also gustatory sensitivity. The most well studied example of the latter is the differential response of 'tasters' and 'non-tasters' to bitter thioureas such as phenylthiourea and propylthiouracil. Many studies have attempted to relate taste reactions to these compounds to food preferences and intake, with rather mixed success. However, recent studies have refined the distinction of taster status, with additional identification of a group of 'supertasters', who may be particularly sensitive to a range of other bitter and non-bitter compounds (Bartoshuk, 1979; Bartoshuk *et al.*, 1996).

2.3.3   Palatability: learned influences

The effects of experience on food preference are demonstrated dramatically by the well known finding that animals learn to avoid a food when consumption of that food is associated with gastrointestinal discomfort (Garcia *et al.*, 1974; and see Forbes & Rogers, 1994). This has been investigated experimentally using, for example, exposure to X-rays and injections of lithium chloride, known to induce nauseous feelings in most vertebrates. For instance, when paired with red food (the conditioned stimulus or CS) injection of lithium chloride (the unconditioned stimulus or UCS) induces avoidance of that colour by chickens, which like many other birds rely heavily on vision to locate and select among food sources (Martin *et al.*, 1977). Rats, in contrast, learn aversions more readily when these manipulations are paired with flavour cues.

The occurrence of food aversions in human beings has been examined in retrospective questionnaire surveys (e.g., Garb & Stunkard, 1974; Logue *et al.*, 1981; Mattes, 1991), and in relation to acute and chronic illness and cancer chemotherapy (Bernstein, 1994). The findings suggest that human beings can acquire food aversions through the same Pavlovian conditioning processes as other species, with the result that aversions are sometimes acquired despite the person's awareness that the food did not cause the illness. The typical features of food aversion learning, that is, rapid (one-trial) learning, learning despite long delays (up to several hours) between food ingestion and the onset of symptoms of illness, and persistence of the learning (up to 50 years!) are very clearly evident in these studies. Learned aversions are also more likely to be formed if the food is novel and has a strong (salient) taste or odour. Nevertheless, even though typically a large percentage (up to 65%) of people report at least one acquired food aversion, this phenomenon can only account for a tiny proportion of the variance in human food preferences.

In the same way that animals can learn to associate the sensory properties of a food with malaise caused by that food they can learn to prefer foods which are metabolically satisfying. Sclafani and his colleagues (e.g., Elizalde & Sclafani, 1988; 1990b) have shown, for example, strong long-lasting conditioned preferences in rats for flavours paired with intragastric infusions of Polycose®, a partially hydrolysed corn starch. The success of these studies derives from a number of clever procedural features which, among other things, reduced the possibility of aversive consequences arising from the infusions. Other findings show that rats can also acquire preferences based on the postingestive, nutritive properties of fats (Sclafani, 1990) and proteins (Baker *et al.*, 1987). Studies investigating the nature of the visceral stimuli (produced by the nutrients) underlying flavour preference conditioning have revealed that the reinforcing effect of Polycose® infusions is eliminated if carbohydrate absorption is inhibited (Elizalde & Sclafani, 1988). Therefore a postabsorptive site appears to be involved, which is consistent with evidence suggesting that fuel oxidation in the liver can provide the unconditioned stimulus for such nutritional or calorie-based learning (Tordoff & Friedman, 1986; Tordoff *et al.*, 1990). Tordoff and Friedman (1986) paired jugular infusions of glucose into rats with one flavour of food and infusions of saline with another flavour and found no subsequent preference for either flavour. However, in animals infused with glucose into the hepatic portal vein (which depresses intake much more than glucose infusion into the jugular vein), there was subsequent preference for the flavour which had been paired with glucose infusion. Other evidence suggests that preabsorptive, probably intestinal, effects are also involved in nutrient conditioning (Sclafani, 1995). Furthermore, rats can discriminate between the postingestive consequences of protein and carbohydrate, and modify their preferences accordingly (e.g., Pérez *et al.*, 1994). Altogether, though, rather little is known at present about the nature or source of the signals generated by food that reinforce conditioned food preferences.

Increases in flavour preference controlled by the postingestive effects of nutrient manipulations have also been found in a smaller number of studies on human subjects. Examples include results showing conditioned preferences in children and adults for flavours associated with high carbohydrate content (Booth *et al.*, 1982; Birch *et al.*, 1990) and high fat content (Johnson *et al.*, 1991; Kern *et al.*, 1993). These acquired preferences appear to persist over time. It is claimed that they also tend to be state-dependent, such that preferences are more readily acquired if initial exposure (i.e., conditioning) occurs during a state of hunger, and are subsequently expressed more strongly when the individual is hungry compared with when they have recently eaten.

It also appears that the medicinal effect of a food containing a needed nutrient can condition a positive preference for that food (Garcia *et al.*, 1974). An example of this is provided by the finding that chicks showed a significant preference for food of the colour which was paired with ascorbic acid supplementation when the requirement for ascorbic acid was increased by heat stress (Kutlu & Forbes, 1993). Otherwise, when kept in thermoneutral temperatures, at which they can synthesize sufficient ascorbic acid, they preferred the colour of unsupplemented food.

Other consequences that follow the ingestion of a food or drink are due to the effects of pharmacologically active compounds. Here the most significant substances are caffeine, alcohol and perhaps carbohydrate (Rogers, 1995; Section 9.3.). It is fairly certain that human beings are not born with, for example, preferences for coffee or tea, at least partly because these drinks contain bitter constituents (including caffeine) and bitterness is disliked at birth. Instead it appears that preferences for coffee, tea, beer, wine etc. are reinforced by their psychoactive constituents. This has been tested directly in studies in which caffeine ingestion was paired with the consumption of novel-flavoured fruit juices. Caffeine was given either in the drink or in a capsule swallowed with the drink. A drink of a different flavour was given without caffeine or with a placebo capsule containing a non-pharmacologically active substance such as cornflour. The design of these studies is, therefore, similar in principle to methods used in the work on flavour preferences conditioned by nutrient manipulations, and the straightforward prediction is that if caffeine has beneficial effects on for example mood, then pairing the drink with the consumption of caffeine should promote increased preference for that drink (actually based on subjects' ratings of pleasantness of the 'taste' of the drinks). The results showed that caffeine can act both as a negative reinforcer, by removing or alleviating the negative effects of overnight caffeine withdrawal (Rogers *et al.*, 1995b), as well as a positive reinforcer (Richardson *et al.*, 1996). Results of an earlier study found similar effects in rats (Vitiello & Woods, 1977).

An implication of these findings is that caffeine will have a positive influence on the consumption of caffeine-containing drinks only after a pattern of fairly frequent, perhaps daily, intake of these drinks has already been established. Initially, therefore, other factors must operate to promote the habit (Cines & Rozin, 1982; Zellner, 1991). Thirst may motivate consumption on some occasions, but in general most people consume tea and coffee, together with other beverages, well in excess of what is needed to maintain adequate fluid balance. Alternatively, preferences for coffee and tea could be acquired through association with the nutritional benefit derived from added milk, cream and/or sugar, or through a flavour–flavour conditioning process whereby preference for a neutral or even disliked flavour is modified as a result of being paired with a liked flavour or sweet taste (Zellner *et al.*, 1983; Baeyens *et al.*, 1990). If nothing else, the use of sweeteners, milk and cream may provide an immediate way of improving the sensory appeal of the beverage for the novice coffee or tea drinker.

Yet a further possibility is that contextual influences on mood play a role in reinforcing preferences for certain foods and beverages. Coffee, tea and indeed many drinks are typically consumed in social contexts and during, for example, breaks from work or other activities. Pairing the positive shifts in mood occurring in such situations with consumption of a drink could result in a conditioned increase in preference for that drink (Zellner, 1991; Rogers & Richardson, 1993).

Preferences and aversions reinforced by the after-effects of eating and drinking as described above appear to be characterized by changes in palatability or liking (i.e., alterations in the individual's affective response to the food's flavour, see Section 2.3.1). Thus Booth has said that 'conditioned aversion is a nasty taste, not merely or at all the refusal to take something because it is perceived as dangerous' (Booth, 1979, page 566). Similarly, Sclafani (1995) proposes that pairing a flavour (CS+) with intragastric nutrient infusion produces 'changes in the rat's evaluation of the flavour' (page 422). This is suggested by several results, including the observation that rats continue to prefer the previously reinforced flavour (CS+) to the CS− flavour (previously paired with intragastric infusion of water) for many weeks after all intragastric infusions have been discontinued. Note that intragastric water infusion does not make the rats averse to the CS− flavour (Elizalde & Sclafani, 1990b). The best direct evidence, however, that altered palatability underlies conditioned aversions and preferences comes from studies of the taste-elicited, fixed-action patterns displayed by rats (Grill & Berridge, 1985). In these experiments solutions are infused into the animal's mouth through a fixed intraoral catheter, and its behaviour is recorded on video tape for subsequent detailed analysis. Aversive reactions, for example, to innately disliked bitter tastants, include gaping movements, chin rubs, head shakes and paw wipes, varying in intensity and frequency. Aversions established by flavour–illness pairings result in a shift away from acceptance reactions towards this aversive pattern even for the innately liked taste of sucrose (e.g., Spector *et al.*, 1988; Ossenkopp & Eckel, 1995), which has been interpreted as showing not that this taste is now perceived as bitter, but simply as unpleasant (Berridge, 1996). Furthermore, it is also argued that the assignment of positive or negative values to conditioned stimuli is a basic feature of all Pavlovian conditioning (Martin & Levey, 1994).

The evidence reviewed in this and the previous section shows that palatability is partly preprogrammed and also strongly altered by learning. Accordingly, it plays a critical role in motivating the choice and consumption of foods in relation to their biological utility. Because palatability is modified by associations with the metabolic and other after-effects of ingestion, it also follows that influences of palatability and nutrient content on food intake cannot be readily separated (Rogers, 1990). Nevertheless, it is fairly certain that, for example, the high energy density of fat encourages 'overeating' to a large extent independently of its effects on palatability (Chapter 5), while sweetness can promote liking and consumption irrespective of the nutritive value of the food or drink with which it is associated (e.g., Sclafani *et al.*, 1996).

2.3.4   Satiation and satiety

During the meal, effects of accumulation of food in the gastrointestinal tract are the major source of the negative feedback signals which underlie feelings of fullness. Although it may seem obvious that stomach distension contributes to satiation, this factor by itself is probably relatively unimportant unless the food is of very low energy density (Forbes, 1988). Inflating a balloon in the stomach produces an uncomfortable sensation of gastric pressure, rather than the usually pleasant feelings of fullness and satisfaction experienced during and after eating. More normal feel-

ings of fullness are experienced, however, if fat is infused into th
num at the same time the stomach is distended by the balloon
Read, 1992). In obese persons, food consumption is considerably reduce
by the presence of a gastric balloon, and this can assist weight loss, but
this appears to be due more to·the discomfort it causes than to the
enhancement of normal satiation and satiety (Read *et al.*, 1994).

Further studies have shown that infusion of fat into the small intestine
before and during a meal induces premature feelings of fullness and a
reduction in food intake. In contrast there were no effects on satiation
when the same lipid emulsion was infused into a peripheral vein (Welch
et al., 1985; see also Greenberg *et al.*, 1989). Such evidence suggests that
fat and indeed other nutrients (Forbes, 1988; Read *et al.*, 1994; but see
Friedman *et al.*, 1996) act on pre-absorptive gastrointestinal receptors
(Mei, 1985) to inhibit eating. At least one of the mechanisms through
which this occurs involves the hormone cholecystokinin (CCK) (Smith &
Gibbs, 1992). This peptide is produced from endocrine cells scattered
throughout the duodenal and jejunal mucosa (Johnson, 1991) and its
release is potently stimulated by the presence of fat, peptides and amino
acids (e.g., Liddle *et al.*, 1985). In human beings, slow intravenous infusion of low doses of CCK reduced appetite and food intake (Stacher *et
al.*, 1979; 1982; Kissileff *et al.*, 1981), while the CCK-A antagonist MK-329
(i.e., an antagonist for the form of CCK found largely outside the brain;
A = alimentary) has been reported to increase ratings of 'hunger'
(Wolkowitz *et al.*,1990). CCK has multiple physiological effects, including modulation of gastric emptying and gall bladder, ileal and colonic
motility. Evidence from studies on animals suggests that the satiating
effects of CCK are mediated by the abdominal vagal nerves, activated
both indirectly by CCK-induced gastric distension and by direct stimulation of vagal nerves by CCK (McHugh & Moran, 1992). There are, in
addition, various other gastrointestinal hormones, for example,
glucagon-like peptide-1 (Ranganath *et al.*, 1996) and gastrin-releasing
peptide (Kirkham *et al.*, 1995), which can be considered as good candidates for satiety agents.

Also during the meal, and even in anticipation of eating (Section 2.2.3),
there is a sharp rise in the level of circulating insulin, which serves to stabilize blood glucose concentration both as eating continues and in the
early postmeal interval. Destruction of the insulin-secreting beta cells of
the pancreas results in chronically increased eating (Stricker, 1982).
Conversely, insulin injection causes the early termination of eating. This
occurs even in sham feeding rats·(Section 2.3), and the result cannot be
explained simply by aversive effects of the treatment, because when the
insulin administration was paired with the consumption of a distinctive
flavour the rats subsequently preferred that flavour (Oetting &
Vanderweele, 1985). Glucagon levels in the blood also increase during
eating, and there is good evidence that this hormone can influence

satiation and satiety, probably through its glycogenolytic action in the liver and activation of a vagal pathway to the brain (Forbes, 1988).

Indeed, many results are consistent with a major role for the liver as a source of signals controlling appetite (reviewed by e.g., Anil & Forbes, 1987; Forbes, 1988; Friedman, 1991). The liver is well placed to monitor the flow of nutrients from the digestive tract, and its function in smoothing out this erratic supply to maintain more stable blood levels must mean that it is able to detect concentrations or the rate of uptake of metabolites such as glucose and amino acids. Furthermore, there are intimate two-way neural connections between the liver and brain. The critical evidence includes the finding that glucose infusion into the hepatic portal vein depresses food intake to a much greater extent than infusion into the jugular vein, and the demonstration that this effect is blocked by vagotomy.

Results from sham feeding experiments show that learning also contributes to the control of meal size. A large increase in meal size is not seen on the first occasion that rats are sham fed. Instead there is a suppression of eating during initial sham feeds due to learned satiety (Weingarten & Kulikovsky, 1989). During normal feeding the visual and orosensory properties of the food become associated with the postingestive effects experienced, and this provides anticipatory control of meal size. On the first sham feed, meal size is modulated according to the 'expected' postingestive effects, but with continued sham feeding this learning extinguishes and meal size increases. The learned control of meal size by flavour cues has also been demonstrated in studies on human adults and children (Booth *et al.*, 1982; Birch & Deysher, 1985). Potentially, the learned anticipatory control of meal size is a refinement which could help overcome the problem posed by the delay between the moment of eating and the major postingestive and postabsorptive effects of food (Booth, 1977). It is not clear, though, whether this mechanism can operate effectively where meals are composed of many tastes and flavours. Additionally there is the problem that there is not always a consistent relationship between the orosensory characteristics and the energy content of foods or drinks. For instance, a food sweetened with an intense sweetener such as aspartame can have a much lower energy content than the same food sweetened with sugar. On the other hand, product labels supply information on nutrient composition and energy content, and potentially therefore this unpredictability might be offset by the cognitive control of intake (Chapter 8). Finally, another example of how decisions made in advance of eating can affect meal size is when a particular amount is loaded onto the plate. A clean plate is a strong cue for satiety, but then the amount eaten may have been determined by someone else in the family, a friend or perhaps the restaurant chef!

It should be recognized that the various effects of eating described above have different but overlapping time courses. Food intake can therefore be seen as triggering a cascade of events, some of which will exert an inhibitory influence primarily during eating, thereby bringing the meal to an end, while others will be more important in maintaining satiety in the postmeal interval (e.g., Le Magnen & Devos, 1984; Stricker & Verbalis, 1987; Blundell & Rogers, 1991). For example, at the time lunch is started most of the food eaten at breakfast will have emptied from the stomach. Satiety during this intermeal interval is maintained by the effects of food in the intestines and then increasingly by the continued action of absorbed nutrients. Finally, perhaps when the flow of nutrients from the intestines reaches a certain minimum, events such as a transient decline in blood glucose level may signal the end of satiety (Campfield *et al.*, 1996). Usually, however, the timing of the next meal will not be determined simply by internal signals, because the opportunity to eat is often constrained or stimulated by external factors (Sections 2.2.2 and 2.2.3). Under these circumstances the amount eaten in the previous meal will influence satiation in the current meal. This is shown, for example, by studies in which human subjects are fed a 'preload' followed after a fixed interval by an *ad libitum* 'test meal'. Covert manipulations of the energy content of the preload have been found to affect test meal intake, sometimes even to the extent that there is complete caloric compensation (e.g., Rogers & Blundell, 1989b; Section 5.1.1).

Ultimately, information concerning the food filling the gut during eating and remaining there after the meal has ended, together with information from learned cues and about liver metabolism and the status of body fat reserves (Section 1.3.2) is integrated by the brain. That is, signals for satiation and satiety originate from the periphery (though see e.g., Woods *et al.*, 1986) – the brain itself being well protected against the 'ebb and flow' of calories from these different sources (Stricker & Verbalis, 1987). The neurotransmitters and hormones involved and the complexity of this integration, which occurs at different levels in the brain, including the medulla and pons, the hypothalamus and the limbic forebrain, is enormous and has only relatively recently begun to be appreciated (e.g., Blundell, 1991; Rowland *et al.*, 1996). A strong stimulus underlying currently increasing efforts to understand these systems is the possibility of developing new pharmacological interventions for appetite and weight control.

As for dietary influences on eating and obesity, a critical question is what characteristics of food influence satiation and satiety, and in particular what determines satiating efficiency (i.e., degree of inhibition of eating per calorie consumed). These characteristics include macronutrient composition, energy density, physical properties such as osmolarity, viscosity and particle size, and palatability (e.g., Kissileff & Van Itallie, 1982; Holt *et al.*, 1995; Prentice, 1995b), and their effects on short-term and longer-term energy intake are examined in detail in Chapter 5.

2.3.5　Hunger, palatability and satiation

It is often argued that hunger (lack of satiety) and satiation influence palatability, so that food 'tastes' better when the eater is hungry than when he or she is full. Therefore as well as providing information about the nutritive value, safety, etc. of the food (Sections 2.3.2 and 2.3.3), palatability might contribute to the control of eating by reflecting the individual's state of repletion. The evidence on this subject suggests, however, that hunger and satiation act largely independently from palatability (Rogers, 1990).

To begin with, in studies on animals it has been observed that altering palatability, for example, by adulterating the food with a bitter tastant, led to a change in the length of uninterrupted eating bouts, whereas food deprivation affected mainly the duration of non-eating intervals within the meal (Wiepkema, 1968; 1971a; Rogers, 1983). Experiments on human volunteers have shown that opioid antagonist drugs such as naloxone and nalmafene reduce the intake and pleasantness ratings of preferred foods and/or sweet and high fat foods. At the same time, however, these compounds have minimal effects on self-reported hunger, and perception of the intensity of orosensory stimuli is also unchanged (e.g., Yeomans *et al.*, 1990; Yeomans & Wright, 1991; Drewnowski *et al.*, 1992a; Drewnowski, 1992). Similarly, in studies of rats sham feeding sucrose, naloxone did not alter the latency to approach food and initiate eating, but appeared to reduce the rate of intake in a manner that corresponded to the effect of lowering the concentration of sucrose (Kirkham & Cooper, 1988). In contrast, the serotonergic drug fenfluramine reduced pre-meal hunger ratings and food intake, although it was found not to affect the pleasantness of a sweet taste (Blundell & Hill, 1988). Results from animal lesion studies together with further pharmacological evidence supporting this distinction between the effects of hunger and palatability are discussed in detail by Berridge (1996), who uses the terms 'wanting' and 'liking' to refer to these separable components of motivation.

Most relevant to the present discussion, though, are findings showing that during a meal rated hunger decreases and fullness increases, while ratings of the pleasantness of foods remain relatively unchanged (e.g., Hill & Blundell, 1990). Normal eating, in other words, is not accompanied by decreased palatability. Nevertheless, some evidence it has been argued contradicts this. For example, infusion of sucrose into a rat's mouth through an intraoral catheter (Section 2.3.3) initially elicits characteristic acceptance reactions. These decline in number as the amount ingested increases, and the decline is more rapid in animals that have been recently fed. This has been interpreted as indicating a shift in the palatability of sucrose (Grill & Berridge, 1985). However, what is being measured may be merely a lack of interest in ingestion: as the infusion continues eventually the rat allows the fluid to drip passively from its mouth, or even actively expels it (Berridge, 1995). It does not necessarily follow that the sucrose tastes less pleasant. Instead it is just as likely that fullness of the gut is responsible for inhibiting ingestion in this situation. When allowed to freely feed, the satiated rat would simply no longer take food into its mouth (see below).

Similarly, there is ambiguity in the studies on human subjects which have been claimed to demonstrate decreases in the pleasantness of sweet tastes following caloric loading (known as 'alliesthesia', Cabanac, 1971; 1992), or changes in pleasantness specifically of foods recently eaten ('sensory-specific satiety', Rolls *et al.*, 1981; 1984; Hetherington *et al.*, 1989). One of the problems here is that the answers subjects give to questions about appetite, hunger, fullness and food pleasantness tend to be highly correlated. While this may be explained by an underlying connection between these feelings (Booth, 1987), there is also the possibility that the rating scales used are not generally measuring what they are intended to because subjects are rather indiscriminate in expressing changes in their desire to eat. In particular, if questions are asked only or mainly about food pleasantness (e.g., Cabanac, 1971; Rolls *et al.*, 1981; 1984; Hetherington *et al.*, 1989), then a decrease in appetite – whatever its cause – will tend to be rated as a decrease in food pleasantness. Furthermore, the discussion above and earlier in this chapter (Section 2.3.1) suggests that it is necessary to distinguish between the pleasantness of the flavour of food in the mouth (influenced by palatability) and the pleasantness of eating or ingesting that food, which presumably is influenced both by palatability, and hunger and satiation (fullness of the stomach, etc.). This is the difference between how good the food 'tastes' and how good it is to eat (*cf.* Mook, 1987).

When subjects were asked both these questions while they ate a meal of cheese sandwiches to satiety, their ratings of the pleasantness of eating the sandwiches decreased markedly, whereas the pleasantness of the 'taste' of the sandwiches was unaltered two-thirds through the meal and thereafter showed only a relatively small decrease (Rogers & Blundell, 1990). A very similar result was obtained in a replication of this experiment using chocolate as the test food. From Figure 2.3 it can be seen that many subjects rated the pleasantness of the 'taste' of chocolate as highly at the end of the meal as at its beginning. Other subjects' ratings showed fairly large changes in both eating and taste pleasantness, but this could not be explained by differences in the amount of chocolate eaten, their initial liking for chocolate or their feelings of fullness. We suggest, therefore, that this was because these latter individuals failed to report accurately on these subtle but nonetheless real differences in experience between the pleasantness of the taste of the food and their desire to eat it.

Finally, Mook and Votaw (1992) simply asked individuals to give the reasons why they usually stop eating at the end of a meal. Feelings of

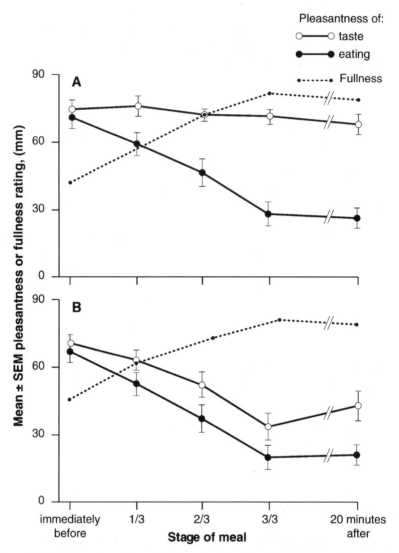

Figure 2.3 Changes in ratings of fullness and ratings of the 'pleasantness of the taste' and the 'pleasantness of eating' milk chocolate. The chocolate was consumed to satiety by 6 men and 18 women, aged between 18 and 40 years, none of whom were highly restrained eaters (Chapter 8). The pleasantness ratings were made on 100 mm line scales labelled 'extremely unpleasant' (left hand end = 0) and 'extremely pleasant' (right hand end = 100). The fullness scale was labelled 'not at all' and 'extremely'. (A) results for subjects showing less than the median change in the pleasantness of taste at the end of the meal. (B) subjects showing greater than the median change in the pleasantness of taste at the end of the meal. There was no significant difference in the amount of chocolate eaten by these two groups of subjects: means (± standard errors) were 553 ± 55 kcal (2.31 ± 0.23 MJ) and 521 ± 57 kcal (2.18 ± 0.24 MJ), respectively. Unpublished data from J.S. David and P.J. Rogers.

fullness and reasons such as 'the food is all gone' and 'I've had all I'm allowed' were chosen much more often than reasons indicating a change in palatability such as 'the food tastes less good'. In other words, people do not generally perceive changes in food liking to be striking features of meals.

Taken together these various findings support the view that palatability changes little if at all during eating, which is consistent with a minimal reduction in positive feedback from eating as depicted in Figure 2.2. That is, orosensory contact with liked food is always stimulatory, and contributes little to the development of satiation and satiety. Even after a large meal food remains palatable, but feelings of fullness prevent further eating – if there is no 'room' left the cheese or the extra piece of chocolate cake will not be eaten however delicious it tastes.

2.4   INTEGRATION OF INFLUENCES ON EATING BEHAVIOUR

The discussion in this chapter has focused on the basic psychobiological processes controlling appetite and food preference. These processes are common to all human beings, but they operate in interaction with social, cultural and economic influences which shape the individual's experiences with food through constraints on food selection and eating behaviour. Thus cultural forces are the major determinants of cuisine and food attitudes (Rozin, 1996). Additionally, an individual's eating is affected by many psychological (e.g., mood), social and environmental factors, resulting in for example daily, weekly and seasonal variations in food intake (Schlundt *et al.*, 1990; de Castro, 1996). In particular there is strong social facilitation of eating. Recent studies have found that individual intake is much greater in meals eaten with company than in meals eaten alone, and furthermore that intake increases as the number of other people increases (de Castro & Brewer, 1992; Redd & de Castro, 1992; Clendenen *et al.*, 1994).

How then, amidst the complexity of these external influences, is eating regulated to achieve longer-term energy balance and stability of body weight, and what does this reveal about the causes of obesity? Physiological stabilizing factors include an inhibitory effect on appetite of body fat and recent energy intake (Figure 2.1), and a 'passive' feedback effect due to the greater energy cost associated with increased body mass (Sections 1.3.3 and 3.3.1). There are also limitations placed by the physical capacity of the digestive system to accommodate and process food. Nevertheless, the physiological system does not exert precise control over energy intake in relation to expenditure. Indeed, the ability in times of plenty to 'overeat' and store the excess energy as body fat is an adaptive trait, but one which predisposes the susceptible individual to harm in environments where energy-dense food is always in surplus (Sections

1.4.1 and 1.4.2). Within this context, conscious dietary restraint and micro-environmental influences (i.e., short-term influences acting on the individual) have a major impact on eating, so that food intake may vary very substantially across the day, from day to day and even in the longer term. Crucially, however, when viewed over sufficiently long periods of time their net effect will be constant (de Castro, 1996). This is because exposure to these external influences is regulated by the individual's lifestyle. It follows, therefore, that significant changes in adult body weight will tend to be associated with changes in lifestyle, such as occur when leaving home for college, after marriage or retirement, or when changing jobs (*cf.* Rodin & Slochower, 1976; Section 8.2).

Although the physiological system controlling appetite is fairly permissive in its response to undereating and overeating, it possesses a variety of features which, together with learned habits and the tendency for the individual's external environment to remain constant, typically ensure long-term stability in energy balance.

2.5 SUMMARY

Eating occurs in bouts or meals, and food intake can vary according to the number and/or size of meals eaten. Meal initiation is identified with appetitive states such as hunger and food cravings which direct behaviour towards eating and perhaps particular foods. Internal cues related to, for example, the dynamics of blood glucose can provide a reliable stimulus for the initiation of eating; however, the role of energy depletion in meal initiation should not be overemphasized. In fact, the energy reserves of the whole body are depleted very little between one meal and the next, and a greater influence on hunger is the amount and composition of the food most recently eaten. Additionally, eating is motivated by external stimuli previously associated with food consumption, such as the sight and smell of food and contextual cues.

During the meal, eating is controlled by the orosensory and postingestive effects of the food consumed. The latter are mainly inhibitory and arise from, for example, filling of the gastrointestinal tract, the release of regulatory hormones such as cholecystokinin, and the detection of nutrients absorbed into the systemic circulation. Orosensory contact with food stimulates eating in proportion to its palatability. Palatability is essentially equivalent to liking and pleasantness, and refers to an individual's hedonic or affective response to orosensory stimuli (i.e., the taste, smell, texture, etc. of the food or drink). There are innate biases in reactions towards certain tastes, such as a liking for sweet tastes and a dislike of bitter tastes, but palatability is also modified strongly by learning, so that aversions are acquired for foods causing sickness and preferences are increased for foods producing certain nutritional and other beneficial after-effects. On the other hand, palatability does not appear to be much affected by immediate satiation – food remains palatable even at the end of a large meal.

These basic processes underlie individual 'nutritional wisdom'. Within the social and cultural context, they adapt preferences according to the 'benefit' or otherwise of consuming particular foods, and influence food intake and eating patterns, usually ensuring long-term balance between energy intake and expenditure.

CHAPTER THREE

Energy intake and expenditure: basic concepts and issues

This chapter is intended to provide a relatively brief and basic introduction to some of the concepts and terms relating to energy metabolism, as background material for later chapters. We also explore several broad, general issues relating to energy intake and expenditure in obesity.

3.1 DIETARY ENERGY SOURCES

Food provides a source of energy (measured in [kilo]calories, kcal, or [kilo]Joules, kJ, or [Mega]Joules, MJ, equal to 1000 kJ) for life and activity, available from the oxidation of macronutrients: fats (primarily triglycerides), carbohydrates (sugars and starches), proteins, and alcohol (ethanol). For most purposes and most diets, across a wide range of cultures and climates, energy in human diets is predominantly (80 to 90%) derived from a mixture of carbohydrate and fat, with a relatively lower and less variable protein intake, and perhaps modest (or occasionally immodest) ingestion of alcohol. Thus, most of the discussion on energy intake and metabolism here and elsewhere tends to focus on fat and carbohydrate.

For each macronutrient, the metabolizable energy value (**physiological fuel value**) basically reflects its potential for chemical oxidation, minus normal losses in faeces (digestibility) and urine. The values given in Table 3.1 are approximations generally applicable to mixed human diets, though not necessarily accurate for more specific purified foods or macronutrients (Livesey, 1991). Technically, the actual values are dependent upon the exact chemical composition of the macronutrients (for example, not all fats are identical) and are also influenced by other constituents of the food matrix (e.g., through influences on bioavailability). The value for alcohol in particular could be somewhat lower than stated, depending upon the the route of oxidation and other metabolic effects (Prentice, 1995a; Rumpler *et al.*, 1996; Lands & Zakhari, 1991; Lieber, 1991). Taking all macronutrients together, the overall concentration of energy within foods and diets is often expressed in terms of calculated **energy density**, e.g., as kcal (or kJ) per 100 grams.

Table 3.1 Approximate human physiological fuel values of macronutrients in mixed diets

Nutrient	kcal/gm	kJ/gm
Fat	9	37
Carbohydrate	4	16
Protein	4	16
Alcohol	7	29

In addition to these major macronutrients, there are dietary constituents present in smaller quantities which may have intermediate fuel values. These include certain oligo- and polysaccharides and sugar alcohols, which are increasingly appearing in foods as ingredients for replacement of sucrose or fat, along with resistant starches (i.e., starch in a physical or chemical form not accessible to normal digestive processes) and non-starch polysaccharides (**NSP**, dietary **fibre**) (Champ, 1996). Some of these may undergo variable degrees of bacterial fermentation in the large colon, yielding a range of metabolizable by-products. The physiological fuel values of these and other specific materials may be difficult to determine with precision (Livesey, 1991; Van Es, 1991). This is generally not a major concern in determining the energy value of total diets, but can become more important for specific food items. In addition, much of the resistant starch and NSP is excreted intact, but might still have a significant impact on energy balance through effects on hunger and satiation (Section 5.1.3). Energy values for all of these, as well as the major macronutrients, can also differ considerably between animal species due to differences in digestion and metabolism.

3.2 ENERGY EXPENDITURE

3.2.1 Components of energy expenditure

Changes in energy balance reflect intake minus expenditure (oxidation). This basic rule of energy metabolism means that storage of energy in the body (primarily as fat) will depend on the difference in food energy consumed and the energy expended via the routes described below. In a period of energy stability, where there is no net storage (positive energy balance) or loss (negative energy balance), the oxidation of ingested and stored macronutrients is equivalent to the intake of metabolizable energy. **Total Energy Expenditure** (TEE) is generally viewed as comprising 3 components:

Basal or Resting Metabolic Rate (BMR or RMR) – This is the energy expenditure required for basic resting physiological functioning, including maintenance of structural and neural components and body temperature. (BMR and RMR differ technically, but for practical purposes the terms are interchangeable, and the former will be used here.) BMR typically accounts for about 60 to 75% of TEE for sedentary to moderately active individuals. Within a large population, between-person variance in BMR is almost fully explained by body mass, particularly lean body mass, age, and sex, and can be determined by actual measurement or estimated from age and sex-specific equations (e.g., Department of Health, 1991). Larger individuals invariably have higher absolute BMR expenditure (kcal/day) (Prentice *et al.*, 1996a), though not necessarily greater metabolic rates when corrected for metabolically active (lean) tissue mass (e.g., kcal/kg fat free mass). BMR does, however, decline significantly shortly after the onset of a significant negative energy balance, disproportionately to and preceding any meaningful weight loss, which may be blunted by this physiological response (see Jebb, 1995; Leibel *et al.*, 1995). The possible relationships between BMR and obesity are discussed further in Section 3.3.1 below.

Thermic Effect of Food (TEF) – This is a transient rise in energy expenditure above BMR which occurs following food consumption. Over time, this averages to about 10% of energy intake (and therefore about 10% of TEE under conditions of energy balance), but differs somewhat at extremes of macronutrient composition and metabolic state. In general, TEF is correlated with the energy content of mixed meals, but it is somewhat variable, even for within-person repeat measures under controlled conditions (Ravussin *et al.*, 1986; Ravussin & Swinburn, 1993). TEF is generally the term in current use, but in some literature this same component of energy expenditure is also called 'Specific Dynamic Effect' or 'Specific Dynamic Action', or (confusingly, since the term also has other meanings) 'Diet-Induced Thermogenesis'.

Physical activity – This is proportionally the most variable portion of energy expenditure, and includes the only significant voluntary component. Physical activity typically represents about 15 to 30% of TEE, but can rise to extreme values with prolonged labour or endurance exercise. To the extent that an activity requires movement of body mass, the energy cost of performing a similar activity can be moderately to substantially higher for heavier vs lighter individuals (Prentice *et al.*, 1996b). Notably, unplanned or unintentional and 'involuntary' movements, such as restlessness and fidgeting, can make a significant contribution to physical activity energy expenditure (Ravussin *et al.*, 1986).

In addition to the established components of TEE above, there has been a long history of investigation of the putative existence and mechanisms of dissipation of excess energy intake through energy-wasting thermogenic (heat-producing) processes (see Bray, 1995 for a historical perspective). These would work to defend the body against weight gain, and the effect has been termed 'Adaptive', 'Facultative' or 'Diet-Induced' Thermogenesis, or 'Luxuskonsumption'. If it were to exist, it would appear as a rise in BMR occurring with overfeeding. Although there is evidence in support of such phenomena in certain animal species, both current research and inspection of older data lead to the conclusion that this is not significant in human energy metabolism, and that all of the changes in body composition occurring in response to overfeeding human subjects – lean or obese – can be accounted for by measurement of energy intake and its expenditure in BMR, TEF and physical activity (Schoeller, 1996; Bray, 1995).

3.2.2 Quantifying energy expenditure and macronutrient utilization

TEE and its individual components can be estimated by a variety of methods, either directly (actual heat production, now rarely used) or indirectly (by measurement of the chemical substrates and products of metabolism) (Bray, 1997; Blaxter, 1971; Ravussin & Swinburn, 1993; Heymsfield *et al.*, 1995; Whitehead & Prentice, 1991). Methodological advances in the past decade, especially the use of doubly-labelled water, have made it possible to fairly precisely assess the energy expenditure of free-living individuals engaging in normal activities, over extended periods. This has led to a range of experiments not previously possible, and has also generated doubts about the interpretation of certain types of data collected earlier and by less sophisticated techniques.

The **Physical Activity Level** (PAL) is a useful measure used to express relative TEE over an extended period of time, in multiples of BMR (and therefore largely corrected for age, sex and weight) (James *et al.*, 1988).

PAL = TEE/BMR

The minimum PAL compatible with sustaining energy balance, under totally inactive 'survival' conditions, has been estimated as approximately 1.27. This means that an individual with a BMR of 1500 kcal/day (6.3 MJ/day) would have an absolute minimum TEE of about 1.27×1500 = 1905 kcal/day (8.0 MJ/day), and sustained intakes below this level will generate a continuous negative energy balance until a new equilibrium is achieved (through weight loss or other reduction in BMR). Typical PAL values for maintenance of energy balance amongst sedentary, moderately and highly active individuals have been respectively estimated at about 1.55, 1.7, and 1.8 to 2.1 (with values all slightly lower for females and higher for males) (World Health Organization, 1985).

These concepts and numerical values have had application not only in developing criteria for assessing adequacy of nutriture and feeding programs internationally, but also for evaluating the individual diets and the validity of self-reported dietary intake data (Goldberg *et al.*, 1991; Black *et al.*, 1991; Section 3.3). For example, sedentary individuals not losing weight but reporting sustained energy intakes below certain PAL cut-offs (e.g., PAL < 1.4) are unlikely to be reporting their true, habitual intake level.

3.3 ENERGY INTAKE AND EXPENDITURE IN OBESITY

Up until the early 1990s, one of the more disquieting problems in nutritional studies of obesity was the frequent failure to identify any apparent differences between the (self-reported) energy intakes of the obese and their lean counterparts (e.g., Bandini *et al.*, 1990; Kulesza, 1982; Lissner *et al.*, 1989; Manocha & Gupta, 1985; Baecke *et al.*, 1983; Miller, 1991; Rolland-Cachera *et al.*, 1986). Indeed, many studies found the opposite, *viz.*, lower energy intakes were related to fatness, at least for some groups of subjects (e.g., Baecke *et al.*, 1983; Braitman *et al.*, 1985; Miller *et al.*, 1990; Eck *et al.*, 1992a; Bandini *et al.*, 1990; Kromhout, 1983; Rolland-Cachera *et al.*, 1990; Slattery *et al.*, 1992). Although the likelihood of systematic under-reporting of energy intakes of obese subjects was well known (e.g., Baecke *et al.*, 1983), the results from dietary intake studies nevertheless led many investigators to conclude that 'obesity is not associated with overeating' (Miller, 1991, p. 280), and contributed to what may now be seen as largely misguided efforts to identify marked 'defects' in energy expenditure amongst obese individuals (Prentice *et al.*, 1989; Prentice & Jebb, 1995). In fact, it appears the energy economies of lean and obese individuals are qualitatively fairly similar, and that TEE rises with body weight, but there is considerable evidence that self-reported dietary and activity patterns do not provide an accurate record of habitual behaviours.

3.3.1 Energy expenditure, body weight and obesity

As detailed above, it is accepted as fact that absolute basal metabolic expenditure (kcal or kJ/day) tends to rise with increasing body weight. This has been shown consistently in a large number of studies, and is particularly well documented in a meta-analysis by Prentice *et al.* (1996a) (Figure 3.1). The relationship between BMR and lean body mass is generally linear; however, because adipose tissue is less metabolically active than most body tissues, and the ratio of fat:lean tissue is increased in obesity, the slope of the relationship between BMR and total weight tends to become flatter (but, importantly, still rises) with greater fatness (Ravussin & Bogardus, 1989).

Although a number of investigations found evidence of reduced TEF in the obese, these reports are balanced by many others indicating no substantial difference in this component (see Table 1 of Ravussin & Swinburn, 1993), and low TEF has not been found to predict later weight gain. Although the matter is still debated, the current consensus view is that any defects in TEF might result from (rather than cause) obesity, and that variation in TEF is unlikely to be a meaningful contributor to observed variance in body weights (Prentice, 1996; Astrup, 1996; Ravussin & Swinburn, 1993; D'Allessio *et al.*, 1988; Prentice *et al.*, 1989). If

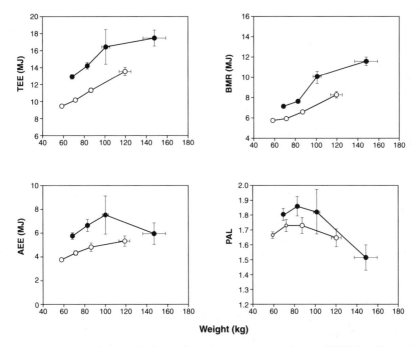

Figure 3.1   Mean (± standard error) total energy expenditure (TEE), basal metabolic rate (BMR), activity energy expenditure (AEE), and physical activity level (PAL) in relation to body weight among 319 free-living males (●) and females (○). From Prentice *et al.* (1996a) with permission.

differences exist, they are small, and may be expressed only under certain conditions.

Figure 3.1 illustrates relationships of body weight with physical activity and basal metabolic energy expenditures, and these relationships are clearly described in several studies (Welle *et al.*, 1992; Prentice *et al.*, 1996a, Schultz & Schoeller, 1994). Activity levels appear to be similar across a wide range of body weights (as indicated by the constant PAL values), and therefore absolute physical activity energy expenditure tends to rise modestly with increasing body weight, due to increased metabolic costs associated with greater body size (Blair and Buskirk, 1987; Prentice *et al.*, 1996b). Although significantly reduced activity levels (in terms of time and movement) seem to characterize extreme obesity, total energy expended on activity is not dramatically reduced in this group.

Despite this body of evidence, there remains debate over whether a relatively lower BMR and/or TEF expenditure contributes to a predisposition for weight gain or in some groups or individuals, including weight regain in post-obese subjects (Astrup, 1996; Ravussin, 1995; Foster *et al.*, 1997; Saltzman & Roberts, 1995; Dietz, 1996; Section 4.2.2). There can be quantitatively significant individual differences in BMR, and Taratino &

Ravussin (1995) have estimated the variance in RMR within a large, heterogenous population at 168 kcal/day (700 kJ/day), after controlling for age, sex and lean body mass. They suggest that this residual variance may be related to differences in relative organ sizes, and muscle fibre metabolism and structure. Any or all of these factors may contribute to the significant genetic component of BMR (Section 4.4.2). However, it is not certain whether such variation ultimately translates into practically meaningful explanations for variance in obesity. There is clearly not a direct relationship between BMR and obesity: many normal weight individuals have lower BMRs than others who are or become obese (e.g., Ravussin *et al.*, 1985; Amatruda *et al.*, 1993; Sipiläinen *et al.*, 1997). Furthermore, although Ravussin *et al.* (1985) are widely cited for observing that low BMR was a predictor of subsequent weight gain amongst Pima Indians genetically predisposed for obesity, the senior author (Ravussin, quoted in Astrup, 1996, p. 172) has noted that this still explains very little of the degree and variance of obesity actually observed, and states: 'Metabolic efficiency alone cannot explain obesity.' Also, the children of Pima Indians do not apparently exhibit any evidence of unusually low BMR (Fontvieille *et al.*, 1993).

Previously obese individuals who have lost weight are known to be at high risk of subsequent weight regain and re-establishment of obesity. Many recent studies have found no evidence for a reduced BMR or other alterations in energy metabolism among long-term post-obese subjects (e.g., de Peuter *et al.*, 1992; Amatruda *et al.*, 1993; Weinsier *et al.*, 1995) and, indeed, energy expenditure does not seem to be a strong predictor of weight regain in that group (Amatruda *et al.*, 1993). However, in a review of these studies, Astrup (1996) shows that a slightly reduced BMR relative to controls is always observed, and suggests that most studies reported no significant effects largely because they lacked statistical power. Some discrepancies between studies might also be attributable to an extended duration of the known reduction in BMR occurring during undereating in slimming programmes (Jebb, 1995; Leibel *et al.*, 1995).

More intriguing results have been derived from recent studies of restrained eaters, who may be (or at least perceive themselves to be) at risk of difficulties with weight control (Chapter 8). Tuschl *et al.* (1990) reported that 14-day TEE (determined by doubly-labelled water) of female restrained eaters averaged a remarkable 620 kcal/day (2.6 MJ/day) lower than unrestrained women of the same age and weight. Differences of this magnitude must be largely attributed to physical activity (not measured), because it so greatly exceeds normal variance in BMR or TEF (Taratino & Ravussin, 1995; Ravussin & Swinburn, 1993), and weight and body composition did not change over the period of study. In a follow-up study, Platte *et al.* (1996) reported a 150 kcal/day (630 kJ/day) lower RMR among female restrained eaters, compared with matched controls. Subject selection criteria and further experimentation ruled out acute or chronic dieting history as a cause of the discrepancy, and none of the subjects had previously been obese. They also reported slightly but not significantly higher TEF in the restrained eaters, while Westerterp-Plantenga *et al.* (1992) found that restraint was negatively correlated with TEF. It therefore seems plausible that restrained eaters may be at greater risk of low energy expenditure, although Lawson *et al.* (1995) carried out a much more extensive characterization of the eating behaviour of subjects, and found no effects of restraint or disinhibition (measured by the Three Factor Eating Questionnaire, Chapter 8) on TEF or RMR corrected for lean body mass.

On the basis of diet records alone, de Castro (1995) and Laessle *et al.* (1989b) concluded it was likely that restrained eaters had lower energy requirements. While the metabolic studies cited above offer some mixed support for this possibility (though not necessarily low BMR or TEF), self-reported intakes are notoriously suspect (Section 3.3.2). Studies specifically focused on groups of self-reported 'small eaters' and 'large eaters' have suggested possible metabolic differences which might predispose 'small eaters' toward their perceived tendency for weight gain (Clarke *et al.*, 1995), but these groups generally have not been found to exhibit meaningful differences in parameters of energy expenditure (McNeill *et al.*, 1989; Clark *et al.*, 1993; 1994; Tremblay *et al.*, 1991b; Lichtman *et al.*,1992).

Overall, low absolute BMR seems unlikely to be a major contributor to aetiology or widespread maintenance of obesity in the general population (Prentice, 1996; Amatruda *et al.*, 1993); indeed, while low BMR expenditure might generate modest weight differences (assuming it has no influence on food intake), the changes in BMR which accompany changes in body weight ultimately should act to passively reconcile intake and expenditure, and stabilize body weight (an example of this is described in Section 3.5). Taking all components together, recent studies using accurate methodology to measure energy expenditure of free-living individuals show quite clearly and consistently that TEE generally rises with body size (Figure 3.1) (Welle *et al.*, 1992; Prentice *et al.*, 1996a; Schultz & Schoeller, 1994).

Although there is significant individual variation, there is no evidence that obesity in otherwise healthy individuals is associated with gross impairments of energy expenditure, a 'thrifty' metabolism, greater metabolic efficiency, or any other other physiological defect which would cause absolute energy expenditure to be substantially reduced relative to lean individuals of the same height. In order to maintain the obese state at this high TEE, therefore, energy intake must also be elevated.

3.3.2 Energy intake and obesity

The preceding sections show that, within groups and individuals (over a reasonable period of time), energy intake should quite closely match energy expenditure; substantial deviations will produce significant weight loss or gain. Thus, the actual energy expenditure of free-living subjects, which can be measured quite accurately, provides a proxy measure of habitual energy intakes, which cannot be readily measured.

Experimental feeding studies indicate that weight gain and loss is largely predicated by established metabolic and thermogenic principles, and the parameters associated with these are broadly similar in lean and obese subjects (e.g., Ravussin *et al.*, 1985; Diaz *et al.*, 1992; Klein & Goran, 1993; Forbes, 1990; McNeill *et al.*, 1989; Prentice *et al.*, 1989; Roberts *et al.*, 1990; Tremblay *et al.*, 1991b; 1992a; 1992b). Although it is common to hear anecdotal reports of individuals who claim to eat massive amounts without gaining weight, and their counterparts who gain weight 'just by looking at food', there is little objective support for such such marked individual variation in energy metabolism. Data from studies on groups of 'small eaters' and 'large eaters' provide detailed support for the view that self-described 'small eaters' primarily suffer from substantial misimpressions and inaccurate reporting of their habitual energy intakes and expenditures (McNeill *et al.*, 1989; Clark *et al.*, 1993; 1994; 1995; Tremblay *et al.*, 1991b; Fricker *et al.*, 1992; Lichtman *et al.*, 1992).

Accessing the intakes of free-living individuals in their usual environment inevitably relies upon some form of self-report methodology, and mis-reporting of dietary intakes has long been a concern in studies using such self-report data. In addition to errors intrinsic to dietary analyses (such as variation between foods and the accuracy of nutrient databases), the major sources of error may stem from the specific behaviours of subjects. First, subjects may simply forget to record certain items, or make unintentional errors in item descriptions or portion size estimates. Second, the process of recording may prompt subjects to alter their usual dietary habits, either to facilitate the recording process, or to consciously or unconsciously project a different (e.g., 'healthier') eating pattern to the investigators. Lastly, subjects may intentionally misrepresent their actual intake, by deliberately not recording certain items, or recording items not actually eaten. PAL values can be used as a rough indicator of the degree of mismatch between reported intakes and estimated or actual energy requirements (Goldberg *et al.*, 1991). This gives some indication as to whether the records provide a plausible estimate of usual energy intake, but cannot identify whether the reported intake is actually correct .

Studies of reported energy intakes vs. measured expenditure have verified the actual extent of under-reporting of energy intakes, which is now clearly documented in a very large number of publications (e.g., Livingstone *et al.*, 1990; Schoeller, 1995; Black *et al.*, 1991; Lichtman *et al.*, 1992; Heymsfield *et al.*, 1995; Bandini *et al.*, 1990; Lissner *et al.*, 1989). The reporting of implausibly low total energy intakes has been suggested to be particularly notable amongst overweight and obese subjects

(Heymsfield *et al.*, 1995; Lissner *et al.*, 1989; Sawaya *et al.*, 1996; Johnson *et al.*, 1994; Heitmann & Lissner, 1995). However, it is clearly also very common amongst normal weight individuals (Livingstone *et al.*, 1990; Schoeller, 1995; de Vries *et al.*, 1994), and has even been observed in records from highly motivated and experienced study participants (Martin *et al.*, 1996; Lichtman *et al.*, 1992). It appears that dietary restraint (Chapter 8) and other measurable subject characteristics might be more sensitive than body weight status as predictors of likelihood and degree of low reported energy intakes (Mela & Aaron, in press; Ortega *et al.*, 1996; unpublished data from Gatenby *et al.*, 1994). This may relate best to more specific measures of eating behaviour and restraint (Section 8.5.1); nevertheless, despite the results of metabolic studies (Section 3.3.1) and the reassurances given by investigators (e.g., de Castro, 1995), self-reports of low energy intakes from restrained eaters should continue to be interpreted very cautiously. Estimates based on published dietary intake data from restrained eaters (De Castro, 1995; Laessle *et al.*, 1989b) suggest untenably low group PAL values.

It must be accepted that self-reported diet records provide an inaccurate measure of habitual energy intakes. The question then arises as to whether changes from habitual diet are generally occurring across the entire diet, or are more directed towards particular eating occassions, foods, or macronutrients. Evidence relating to this issue is sparse, in part because (unlike total energy intake), there are no readily available objective measures of actual intakes of macronutrients other than protein. Based on their analyses of the Dietary and Nutritional Survey of British Adults (Gregory *et al.*, 1990), Pryer *et al.* (1994) indicated that low reported energy intakes were not randomly distributed across all food groups, and tended to be directed towards items with a poor 'health image'. Our own (unpublished) analyses of that data set confirmed an extremely high prevalence of low reported intakes, and suggested that sugars intakes were particularly reduced among apparent under-reporters. While Lissner & Lindroos (1994) concluded that under-reporting did not appear to be macronutrient specific in lean or obese subjects, Heitmann & Lissner (1995) found evidence that protein intakes were being relatively over-reported (actually, less under-reported), and suggested that under-reporting was particularly directed at energy-dense (fatty and high carbohydrate) foods, and perhaps snack-type food items ~~undereating~~ (cf. Section 9.4.2). A similar conclusion (under-reporting of fats, sugars, ~~during~~ and snacks) was reached by Fricker *et al.* (1992) in a study of obese 'small ~~study~~ eaters'. In a consumer survey, we found that many people not only overtly indicated that they would change their eating behaviour during a diet recording period, but also stated that they would specifically eat fewer 'fatty foods' (most specifically cakes, pastries and confectionery) and more fruits and vegetables (Mela & Aaron, in press).

Although it is difficult to distinguish whether discrepancies in intake vs. expenditure are due to honest and fully recorded but atypical intakes during the reporting period, or to incomplete or fraudulent records, our research and experience suggest the former is more common (Mela & Aaron, in press). That is, subjects tend to (knowingly) change their eating behaviour and provide investigators with honest records of that behaviour; records which then are not representative of habitual or usual intakes. Thus, the phenomenon might be better characterized as 'under-eating', rather than 'under-reporting'.

These problems with self-reported dietary information will be raised again in conjunction with discussions of epidemiological relationships presented in Chapters 6 and 7.

3.4   MACRONUTRIENT UTILIZATION

3.4.1   Quantifying macronutrient utilization

The energy available in ingested macronutrients can be released by oxidation or, with limitations (see below and Table 3.2), stored. The metabolism of different macronutrients requires different amounts of oxygen consumption relative to carbon dioxide production, and these can be measured during different activities and diets. By appropriate procedures, and with some caveats, the **Respiratory Quotient** (RQ) can provide a measure of the mix of macronutrient fuels being metabolized over a given time and conditions. The RQ is defined as:

$$RQ = \frac{\text{Volume of } CO_2 \text{ produced}}{\text{Volume of } O_2 \text{ produced}}$$

For oxidation of pure carbohydrate, RQ will be close to a value of 1.0; for oxidation of pure long-chain triglycerides, the RQ will be close to a value of 0.7. (The average RQ for mixed proteins is about 0.83.) The formation of fat from carbohydrate (de novo lipogenesis), if it occurs, would theoretically generate an RQ exceeding 1.0, although disposal of carbohydrate through this pathway appears to be quantitatively negligible in humans under most physiological and dietary conditions (Section 5.3). Within the range of 'normal' diets, the 24-hour non-protein RQ is generally in the range of 0.78 to 0.88, with higher values indicative of greater relative utilization of carbohydrate vs fat.

Given the macronutrient composition of a food or diet, its **Food Quotient** (FQ) can be calculated, based on the requirement for oxygen and generation of carbon dioxide which would be involved in oxidation of its constituent parts. Because of the relative inconvertibility of macronutrients under most conditions (Jéquier, 1992), it becomes appropriate to think of overall energy balance as reflecting the balancing of intake and utilization of each macronutrient.

There is a clear difference in the necessity and capacity for oxidizing or storing specific macronutrients, and this becomes apparent from the information summarized in Table 3.2. There is no storage capacity for alcohol, and it is toxic; hence it must be (and is) completely oxidized within a fairly short period following ingestion. There is a large pool of structural and functional protein in the body, but body protein content is relatively constant (except under conditions of growth). Thus, utilization of protein is closely controlled, and will generally match intake over a period of days. Although a high proportion of energy is derived from carbohydrate, storage capacity (as glycogen) is quite limited, so that carbohydrate oxidation is also closely constrained, and must ultimately rise with higher carbohydrate intakes. Disposal of carbohydrate through lipogenesis, as noted, appears to be negligible for humans under most conditions, although it does occur with very high carbohydrate intakes in excess of energy requirements (Acheson *et al.*, 1982; 1988; Hellerstein, 1996; Section 5.3).

Because there is limited storage capacity for alcohol, protein and carbohydrate, oxidation of each of these must reflect their intake over a period of time. Fat storage capacity, however, is extremely large; hence there is no physiological need to match fat oxidation to fat intake and, indeed, it is not observed (Flatt *et al.*, 1985; reviewed by Jéquier, 1992). As shown by Abbott *et al.* (1988), this means that dietary fat is largely stored and later utilized to make up differences between energy expenditure and the energy generated from other macronutrient sources. A corollary of this is that high intakes of other macronutrients will suppress mobilization and oxidation of fat. A range of experiments have confirmed and extended these findings (Bennett *et al.*, 1992; Thomas *et al.*, 1992; Tremblay *et al.*, 1989; 1991a).

Regardless of diet composition, RQ fluctuates over the course of a day, particularly in response to food consumption (when RQ rises). However, given that macronutrients are not readily interconverted, then over a longer period of time (e.g., several days) in which energy balance is achieved, the average intake and oxidation of each separate macronutrient will also be individually balanced. This principle means that the average RQ of an individual in energy balance over that period must equal the FQ of their diet; i.e., RQ/FQ = 1, and differences between intake and expenditure will reflect fat storage or oxidation. For mixed diets, RQ/FQ < 1 implies that endogenous lipid is being oxidized (i.e., the fuel mix being used by the body is higher in fat than the food consumed). An RQ/FQ > 1 indicates that more fat is being consumed than oxidized, and implies a positive fat balance, or net fat storage. Chronically sustained, this is the dietary and metabolic route to obesity.

Table 3.2. Characteristics of macronutrient storage and balance in adult humans (modified from Ravussin & Swinburn, 1993)

		Macronutrient		
Characteristics	*Alcohol*	*Protein*	*Carbohydrate*	*Fat*
Stores				
Storage form	none	Protein	Glycogen	Fat
Approximate energy density of storage form (kcal/gm)	–	1	1	9
Storage capacity	–	Small	Tiny	Large
Daily variability in size	–	Small	Large	Tiny
Potential for expansion	–	Small	Tiny	Immense
Degree of regulation	–	High	High	Low
Balance				
Typical daily intake as % of body stores	–	1–1.5%	25–75%	<1%
Oxidation stimulated by intake	Yes	Yes	Yes	No
Potential for long-term imbalance	No	No*	No	Yes

*Net gain of body protein can occur as a result of pharmacological effects, exercise and weight gain.

3.4.2   Macronutrient utilization and obesity

Current views of energy metabolism imply that under a broad range of dietary conditions, energy balance is only achieved when the fuel mix oxidized matches the fuel mix consumed. Recent work has investigated the possibility that defects in macronutrient utilization, generating a consistent mismatch between RQ and FQ, may contribute to the development and maintenance of obesity, and susceptibility to particular diets and sedentary lifestyle. Specifically, this view holds that a predisposition to obesity is associated with an elevated RQ, such that there is a comparatively enhanced tendency to oxidize dietary carbohydrate relative to fat. The reduced capacity for raising fat oxidation, commensurate with moderate or high fat intakes, would therefore tend to promote relatively greater fat storage on such diets. Fat balance would ultimately be re-established by increased fat oxidation secondary to the expansion of body fat stores. The background and supporting evidence for this has been reviewed by several of the major research groups involved (Flatt, 1995; Astrup, 1993; Schutz *et al.*, 1989; Schutz, 1995; Astrup *et al.*, 1996). This will be referred to here as the 'nutrient utilization' model of obesity.

Interest in this concept was stimulated by the observation that higher RQs were predictive of 3-year weight gain in Pima Indians, independent of energy expenditure (Zurlo *et al.*, 1990). Similarly, measures of (high) RQ, but not BMR, predicted 10-year weight gain in a relatively heterogeneous group of white men (Seidell *et al.*, 1992), although this result could be an artifact of differing diets. Groups of subjects who might be considered 'at risk' for obesity have also been found to show evidence of elevated RQs under certain dietary conditions. Raben *et al.* (1993) reviewed studies showing that, compared with never-obese controls, formerly obese subjects do not exhibit differences in RQ on relatively high carbohydrate test meals. However, Lean & James (1988) had reported that RQ was markedly elevated among post-obese subjects following fasting or a high-fat diet. This effect of diet was specifically addressed by Astrup *et al.* (1994a), who found that raised RQ amongst their post-obese subjects was only apparent on a diet of 50% (as opposed to 20 or 30%) energy from fat. A similar pattern of response to diet manipulation was also observed in non-obese restrained eaters compared with unrestrained controls (Verboeket-van de Venne *et al.*, 1994). Raben *et al.* (1994a) also found that post-obese subjects exhibited markedly elevated carbohydrate and diminished fat oxidation in response to a single high-fat meal, and the observation of relatively reduced fat oxidation in post-obese subjects has now been confirmed in other studies (Larson *et al.*, 1995; Buemann *et al.*, 1994).

Insufficient fat oxidation relative to intakes causes a positive fat balance, and fat storage. Flatt (1987a; 1987b) proposed that the expansion of fat stores would prompt increased fat oxidation, leading to re-establishment of fat (and energy) balance at a higher body weight. A critical aspect of this hypothesis was confirmed by Schutz *et al.* (1992) and Astrup *et al.*, (1994b), who provided evidence of positive quantitative relationships between body fat mass and fat oxidation. Thus, lipolysis (release of fatty acids from body fat stores, and their utilization as a metabolic fuel) tends to increase with the expansion of fat stores and related changes in metabolism which characterize obesity. In contrast to non-obese (pre-obese?) individuals at risk of weight gain, obese individuals could therefore tend to have high levels of fat oxidation relative to lean controls, although they may still exhibit a relatively sluggish response to changes in diet composition (Thomas *et al.*, 1992). Thus, it is proposed that obesity is an adaptive response to a high fat diet, with the necessary equilibration of fat intake and oxidation being achieved through expansion of fat stores (Astrup *et al.*, 1994b; Schutz, 1995) (or perhaps through increased physical activity [Flatt, 1987; Tremblay & Alméras, 1995]). An interesting prediction of this is that obesity-prone individuals would be much more likely to express their propensity for weight gain on a high-fat diet (Astrup *et al.*, 1994). There is supportive epidemiological evidence (Heitmann *et al.*, 1995; Section 4.2.4), but little prospective experimental data addressing this point.

The 'nutrient utilization' model and proposed mechanisms must of course still operate within the 'rules' of overall energy metabolism, and therefore these events could only result in chronic weight gain if they were linked to or resulted in an overall positive energy balance. This has not been demonstrated empirically. Flatt (1987a; 1987b; 1995) proposed that factors related to carbohydrate stores might provide potent controlling signals for hunger and food intake. This would suggest that the mix of nutrients consumed could exert an important influence on appetite control due to their post-prandial utilization. In particular, high carbohydrate diets would generate more potent signals for controlling (suppressing) intake. Although many features of this proposal seemed to hold high explanatory power, its predictions have not been supported when directly tested in human studies (Stubbs *et al.*, 1993; Shetty *et al.*, 1994).

Friedman (1995; Friedman & Stricker, 1976; also Russek, 1981) has described a model of appetite control integrating nutrient partitioning, oxidation and intake, which might provide a connection between nutrient utilization and subsequent eating behaviour. An essential feature of this model is that partitioning of ingested energy into storage fat (e.g., because of relatively reduced fat oxidation) diverts it from participating in the sequence of metabolic events which would lead to suppression of eating (cf. Figure 2.1). It is proposed that hepatic fuel oxidation could generate the signal which controls appetite, such that high hepatic fuel oxidation (e.g., after eating, or greater lipolysis from expanded fat stores) would suppress intake, while utilization of nutrients elsewhere in the body (e.g., by thermogenesis or exercise) would stimulate intake. The control of energy intake could be mediated through a common pathway, which does not distinguish between dietary or endogenous fuels, or their chemical nature. Many features of the 'nutrient utilization' hypothesis are consistent with this view of appetite control. The model does not clearly assign a special role to any macronutrient, since it relates to overall storage and oxidation, but the tendency for passive overconsumption of energy-dense foods could be readily accommodated within it.

A greater liking and selection for fat in association with the predisposition to obesity (Chapter 6) seems to be a potentially important feature of the model for obesity outlined by Astrup *et al.* (1996). That is not a necessary feature, however, if the 'normal' dietary environment contains sufficiently high fat content to exceed the oxidative capacities of susceptible individuals. Nevertheless, an appealing but completely speculative scenario might consider a common underlying psychobiological mechanism, generating both a heightened sensory responsiveness to high-fat, energy-dense foods, as well as predisposing individuals to gain weight on such a diet, perhaps mediated by variations in nutrient partitioning and utilization (Mela, 1996b; Astrup, 1996). It may be possible to test this experimentally by seeking links between characteristics of metabolism (e.g., measures of fat oxidation) and the existence or acquisition of preferences.

The 'nutrient utilization' hypothesis, as described here, has generated considerable research interest, and seems to bring together observations from biochemical, metabolic, genetic, and nutritional epidemiological studies. However, there are many features which have not yet been fully tested or resolved, and potential pitfalls relating to proof of cause and effect (e.g., Prentice *et al.*, 1994). Furthermore, from the evidence presented in Chapter 5 and elsewhere in this volume, it is not obvious that a specific 'biogenetic' [as opposed to 'biobehavioural' (Schlundt *et al.*, 1990)] explanation is required to understand the high prevalence of overeating and obesity under prevailing environmental conditions of modern western societies.

3.5   ENERGY BALANCE AND BODY WEIGHT: PRACTICAL APPLICATIONS

In general, the loss or gain of 1 kg of adipose tissue (fat plus associated lean tissue) represents a positive or negative energy balance of roughly 7000 kcal (30 MJ; approximately the amount adults in western societies consume in a 2 to 4 day period). Although one often sees calculations suggesting that a tiny intake 'error' consisting, for example, of an excess of only 20 kcal/day (84 kJ/day) generates the considerable weight gain of 10 kg per decade [20 kcal/d $\times$ 365 d/y $\times$ 10 y = 73000 kcal (305 MJ), equivalent to about 10 kg of adipose tissue gain], such calculations generally make the error of assuming no concurrent change in energy expenditure.

However, as noted above, when all else is kept constant, BMR and TEE tend to rise or fall with increasing and decreasing weight, respectively, such that a fixed change in energy intake does not result in a constant gain or loss of body weight. Instead, energy balance is ultimately re-established at a higher or lower weight.

Figure 3.2 illustrates this type of relationship for a 75 kg, 40-year-old man consuming an average of 200 kcal/day (840 kJ/day) less than the level of intake required for maintaining energy balance at his initial weight, given a consistent PAL of 1.6. Based solely on weight-related changes in TEE, he loses about 6 kg in a year rather than the calculated 10 kg [200 kcal/d × 365 d = 73000 kcal (305 MJ)], and the rate of weight loss slows as energy requirements approach the new level of intake. For this same man, a 20 kcal/day (84 kJ/day) rise in intake above maintenance intake at 75 kg would be offset by the rise in TEE associated with a body weight gain of about 1.0 kg. Any further or continuous weight gain (assuming no change in PAL) would require continuously greater energy intakes, always exceeding the rising requirements for weight maintenance at greater and greater body weights.

Positive or negative energy balance implies predictable weight loss or gain in the long term, but this may differ in the shorter term, between individuals, and as a result of their starting characteristics and the type of diet and lifestyle changes used to alter energy balance (Forbes, 1987b; 1990; Jebb, 1995). Apart from any individual metabolic 'adaptations' to changes in energy balance, the composition of tissue gained or lost will

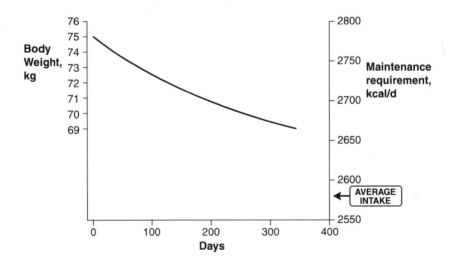

Figure 3.2 Example of predicted changes in body weight and maintenance energy requirements over 1 year, for a 40 year old man with initial 75 kg body weight, having a constant energy intake of 200 kcal (840 kJ) below initial requirements, and total energy expenditure at 1.6 × BMR.

affect the relationship between body energy stores and actual body weight. Protein and carbohydrate stores are highly hydrated, and therefore markedly lower in energy density than body fat (Table 3.2). This discrepancy between units of weight and their energy equivalents also has some important implications.

In the short term, significant weight change (1 to 3 kg) can occur with relatively little change in overall energy balance, primarily due to the loss or gain of water in highly hydrated storage tissues. Compared with other storage forms, losing or gaining 1 kg of fat will require a substantially greater energy deficit or excess. Forbes (1990) makes the point that individuals may vary in the relative deposition of excess energy into fat vs. lean tissue when in positive energy balance, leading to an outcome of different rates of actual weight gain despite similar energy balance. Those gaining or losing relatively more non-fat tissue will show a greater weight change for a similar change in energy balance. Given that the proportion of fat gained or lost rises with a higher proportion of body fat, Forbes (1990) concludes that obese individuals should therefore actually gain body weight less easily than thin people. The corollary, however, is that it should also take longer for the obese individuals to lose weight at the same caloric deficit.

3.6 SUMMARY

With some caveats, current knowledge of energy metabolism is generally consistent with the view that 'the propensity to become obese or maintain the obese state is not related to low energy expenditure' (Amatruda *et al.*, 1993, page 1241). This apparently bold statement has considerable support as a generality, but may mask significant individual differences in metabolism, and meaningful interactions with diet and lifestyle.

Fundamental principles of energy metabolism establish a series of rules which guide and set limits to the possible effects of variations in food consumption or physiological mechanisms which might influence weight gain and loss. Most central to this is the fact that the energy derived from macronutrients in food (protein, fat, carbohydrate, and alcohol) must be expended (by oxidation) or stored, and long-term weight change only occurs when the intake of energy consistently differs from its expenditure.

There is a clear hierarchy in the necessity and capacity for oxidizing or storing specific macronutrients. In particular, there is no storage of alcohol, and little capacity for additional net protein or carbohydrate storage. There also appears to be little disposal of protein and carbohydrate through conversion to body fat under a wide range of dietary conditions. This relative inconvertibility of alcohol, protein, and carbohydrate means that, averaged over a period of time, the oxidation of each will closely match intake. In contrast, the capacity for storage of fat is extremely large, and fat oxidation is not tethered to fat intake. Since intake and expenditure of other macronutrients must always be balanced, net fat oxidation or storage reflects an energy imbalance (the difference between energy intake and expenditure). High intakes of other macronutrients will suppress fat oxidation. Long-term changes in energy balance and weight gain or loss thus largely represent fat balance; i.e., weight change occurs when fat oxidation does not match fat intake.

The utilization of energy (Total Energy Expenditure, TEE) occurs through 3 routes: basal metabolism, Thermic Effect of Food (TEF), and physical activity. There is no clear support for the existence of any other substantial energy dissipating processes in human beings, which might actively protect against weight gain. For sedentary and moderately active individuals, the main component of TEE is basal metabolism, which is largely determined by (lean) body mass. Basal Metabolic Rate (BMR) and (assuming similar activity patterns) TEE therefore tend to be higher in larger individuals, and this is borne out by a large quantity of data indicating no meaningful defects in the routes of energy expenditure amongst overweight and obese individuals. Based upon comparison with data on energy expenditure, analyses of self-reported dietary intakes show a high prevalence of implausibly low energy intakes, and this is more apparent for obese than for lean subjects. Such dietary records cannot reflect true, habitual energy intake, but it is not clear whether or how relative macronutrient intakes might also be biased.

Recent hypotheses have been developed which implicate 'defects' in macronutrient utilization in the aetiology of obesity. These suggest that a basic feature of susceptibility to obesity might be a reduced capacity to oxidize fat relative to carbohydrate. According to this view, low fat oxidation, in conjunction with high fat intakes, would tend to promote fat storage. The resulting rise in fat storage would eventually cause increased fat oxidation, so that fat and energy balance could be re-established (at an elevated body weight). This is an attractive hypothesis, and there is a growing body of circumstantial evidence to support it. However, a number of details have not been tested or fully resolved, and it is not clear how this is linked to or causes a positive overall energy balance (excessive intake).

Experimental feeding studies indicate that all of the changes in body composition occurring in response to over- or underfeeding human subjects – lean or obese – can be accounted for by measurement of energy intake and expenditure through established routes. The rise and fall of energy expenditure with increasing and decreasing body weight means that a fixed change in energy intake does not result in a constant weight gain or loss. Instead, changes in BMR tend to passively offset differences between intake and expenditure, and energy balance is ultimately re-established at higher or lower body weights. For this reason, continuous weight gain would require continuous increases in energy intakes, always exceeding the rising requirements for weight maintenance at greater and greater body weights.

Energy storage exists in relatively limited amounts in lean body mass forms (protein and glycogen), and in relatively unlimited amounts as fat. Long-term weight loss or gain (as fat) is relatively predictable from knowledge of long-term energy intake and expenditure. However, there may be discrepancies in the shorter term, and a number of causes for differences between individuals. In the short term, significant weight fluctuations (1 to 3 kg) can occur with relatively little change in overall energy balance, primarily due to the loss or gain of water in non-fat storage forms, which are highly hydrated. Initial body composition may also influence responses, by affecting the relative deposition of energy into (and from) fat vs. lean tissue, leading to an outcome of different rates of actual body weight gain despite quantitatively similar actual energy (im)balances.

Obesity is at least maintained, and probably caused, by excessive eating and fat deposition in the face of normal or elevated energy expenditure.

CHAPTER FOUR

Genetics of obesity and energy balance

4.1 OBESITY: NATURE OR NURTURE?

It has long been recognized that overweight and obesity tends to run in families, although estimates of the differential contributions of genetic and of various environmental influences to adult fatness have varied widely, depending upon the population used and the methodology applied. The observed familial trends in weight status have both genetic and non-genetic components, and the genetic component is itself quite complex and not fully resolved. A direct or interactive role of environment cannot be questioned: obesity is a disease which is ultimately dependent upon voluntary behaviours (eating, physical activity), and is only widely prevalent in mechanized societies where energy-dense foods are readily and continuously available. However, this fact does not diminish the potential importance of inborn predispositions toward behavioural or metabolic characteristics which would make certain individuals much more likely to become overweight or obese under permissive environmental conditions.

It is now widely accepted that genetic heritage explains far more of variance in measures of adult fatness than specific features of childhood and family environment. This statement may be surprising to anyone not familiar with this area, or based on anecdotal observation of family eating behaviours, but the research support for this view is strong and consistent. This was in large part stimulated by the work of Stunkard and colleagues (Stunkard et al., 1986a; 1986b; Sørensen et al., 1989; Stunkard et al., 1990), who used data sets which allowed for greatly improved capacity to distinguish genetic factors and family environment. In a landmark paper, Stunkard et al. (1986b) examined a very large and complete database on biological and adopted children and their parents, and concluded that 'genetic influences have an important role in determining human fatness in adults, whereas the family environment alone has no apparent effect'. Although that work was commonly misinterpreted as suggesting that obesity was entirely genetically determined (i.e., pre-destined), with little or no environmental influence, a direct or interactive role of environment is clearly acknowledged in that report. But the influences of environment must operate either at a very individual or at a broad population level, rather than specifically within families. Shared family environment therefore may have little direct relationship with measures of adult relative weight status, except insofar as it reflects a more general environmental condition (e.g., social class). Lifestyle behaviours such as smoking and certain dietary habits may also be imparted from parents to children, but together this within-family variance explains a relatively low proportion of variance in adult weight status. It should be noted here though, that regardless of cause, there is also significant (if imperfect) individual tracking of relative BMI and overweight between childhood and adult status (see Guo *et al.*, 1994; Valdez *et al.*, 1996).

The view that shared family environment has relatively low or negligible influence on adult measures of fatness and obesity has strong and wide support from a variety of other studies (Stunkard *et al.*, 1990; Sallis *et al.*, 1995; Fabsitz *et al.*, 1992; Grilo & Pogue-Geile, 1991; de Castro, 1993a; 1993b; Herskind *et al.*, 1996). Grilo and Pogue-Geile (1991), in a comprehensive survey of environmental influences, concluded that shared family environment is relatively unimportant in contrast to effects of unshared environment. In summarizing their findings, they state that 'experiences shared among family members do not play an important role in determining individual differences in weight, fatness, and obesity', and 'it is remarkable that individuals within families who apparently share similar diets resemble each other so little in weight'. The documented support for their conclusion is clear and extensive. Vogler *et al.* (1995) also reported no evidence for effects of shared family environment on adult BMI, and stated that 'all familial resemblance in adults can be attributed to genetic influences'. From a behavioural perspective, the observation of a weak role of family environment in weight status is not necessarily anomalous. Grilo & Pogue-Geile (1991) and Stunkard *et al.* (1986b) cite parallels with the apparent lack of effect of shared childhood environment on other personality and behavioural characteristics (Scarr *et al.*, 1981; Plomin & Daniels, 1987).

It is important to reiterate that these views do not negate an important influence of environmental factors, but simply indicate that within-family, shared (early) home environment seems to account for little of variance in (later) adult weight status. Environmental conditions unique to individuals and particularly those influences present at a wider population level beyond families, are clearly a significant factor in adult weight status, and are considered in subsequent chapters.

Recent large studies of twins appear to produce relatively consistent estimates that genotype can explain about 60–70% of variance in BMI (Price & Gottesman, 1991; Allison *et al.*, 1996; Table 5 of Herskind *et al.*, 1996) and also adipose tissue distribution (Carey *et al.*, 1996). However, studies of twins generate higher estimates of genetic transmission than do studies of nuclear families. Based on their studies, Bouchard and colleagues (1993; Bouchard & Pérusse, 1993) have assigned considerably lower estimates for the heritability of BMI, and propose that much of the variance in measures of overall adiposity (e.g., BMI or % body fat) is not accounted for by either genetic or specific cultural transmission, but is nontransmissible. This is ascribed to the fact that different body tissues or regulatory and metabolic processes (energy intake, energy expenditure, response to overfeeding) may all have different patterns of transmission, independently contributing to varying origins for a range of possible obese phenotypes, which may in turn have differing susceptibilities to environmental conditions. According to this analysis, although the overall heritability of obesity in a population may be modest, the risk of obesity (e.g., proneness to overeating or fat deposition) may be more influenced by genetic factors, and obesity in a given individual may be strongly rooted in their genetic makeup (Bouchard, 1991b). Clearly, however, a genetic predisposition is not absolutely necessary for the development of obesity, since lean individuals will gain weight predictably and can become obese if intentionally overfed (Sims *et al.*, 1973; Diaz *et al.*, 1992; Roberts *et al.*, 1990; Klein & Goran, 1993; Bouchard *et al.*, 1988; 1990).

One point of agreement is that even a high estimate of genetic influences does not mean that certain individuals are predestined to be obese, but that it is **susceptibility** to becoming obese that may be genetically transmitted, and this may hinge on particular environmental conditions for expression. This is immediately apparent from the recent within-population changes in the prevalence of obesity (which cannot be attributed to changes in the gene pool), the broader geopolitical distribution of obesity in humans, and studies of socioeconomic status and obesity within specific cultures (Sobal and Stunkard, 1989; Dowse *et al.*, 1996). The food supply and lifestyle of most western nations would appear to provide an environment in which a predisposition for obesity can be readily expressed. Indeed, when close to half of a nation's population are overweight or obese, and the proportion is still increasing (as in the UK and USA at this writing), it suggests that one or more environmental factors have been changing in a way which allows for the threshold for expression of a widespread predisposition for excessive fatness to be increasingly exceeded. The environmental factors associated with food and eating are explored elsewhere in this book.

4.2 INHERITED ASPECTS OF ENERGY BALANCE

In the context of this book, perhaps the most pressing question relates to **what is inherited?** Polymorphisms (variations) in a number of genetic loci have been associated or linked with predisposition to obesity in humans (see Roberts & Greenberg, 1996; Pérusse *et al.*, 1997), although many of these may only be markers, and not specifically involved in the etiology of the condition. Current research is oriented toward identifying the actual contribution of specific genes, the size of the populations affected, and the environmental conditions in which they are expressed. Even for known human genetic abnormalities which include obesity as part of the clinical features, the extent to which these particular gene loci are linked to obesity in otherwise normal individuals remains to be established (Reed *et al.*, 1995). The additive effects of a large number of loci appear to be involved in the genetic transmission in most forms of human overweight, although there is indirect evidence for contributions of major single-gene defects (Pérusse & Bouchard, 1996).

A genetic contribution to obesity implies that variations in energy or nutrient intakes or expenditure, or perhaps macronutrient partitioning or utilization, have genetic origins. Given the apparent mix of additive (interactive) and non-additive (dominant and recessive) genetic effects linked to various biochemical, behavioural, and anthropometric characteristics, it is likely that individuals will vary in their predisposition to a broad range of potential contributors to high or low BMI. Nevertheless, the identification and prevalence of specific 'defects' is important insofar as it may guide selection of specific prevention or treatment strategies. As throughout this book, the discussion below emphasizes human behavioural and physiological observations, but not their ultimate biochemical or neurophysiological basis.

4.2.1 Genetics and energy intake

There are major problems in establishing a genetic basis for variability in energy intakes determined from diet records, including the high random measurement error, and a high prevalence of overall and possibly non-random mis-reporting by human subjects (see Section 3.3.2). Even where the validity of intake data is established, interpretation of results must consider other fundamental determinants of energy and total macronutrient intakes, particularly tendencies toward particular body weight and physical activity levels, which may have greater or lesser independent genetic determinants.

In their study of nuclear families, Pérusse *et al.* (1988c) found no evidence for independent genetic effects on absolute or adjusted (for body weight or energy intake) intakes of total energy or macronutrients. They reported a significant cultural (non-genetic parent to child) inheritance, but a considerably greater nontransmissible variance component. The conclusion of this work was that strong family resemblances in nutrient intakes were apparent, and largely due to environmental conditions shared by families. However, the study was carried out over a short period amongst family members living together, conditions which may

have favoured the expression of shared influences over individual preferences.

Studies of twins have had some mixed results, but generally found
evidence for significant genetic contribution to variance in nutrient
intakes (Fabsitz *et al.*, 1978; Wade *et al.*, 1981; de Castro, 1993a; 1993b). De
Castro (1993a; 1993b) reported strong, significant heritability for energy
intakes, with no evidence of any effect of shared common (family) environment. That research concluded that there was considerable genetic
component to variance in total daily energy intake and average meal size,
independent of body weight, which was not significantly correlated with
energy intakes. The latter result is somewhat problematic because, as
detailed in Section 3.3, body weight is normally positively correlated
with TEE, and therefore should also be reflected in the approximate level
of habitual energy intake (Prentice *et al.*, 1996a). Such apparently inconsistent results raise basic questions about the validity and interpretation
of self-reported nutrient intake data and their analysis in relation to body
weight. However, mis-reporting or other errors in the dietary data should
not have contributed to the substantial genetic effects observed (de
Castro, 1993b). In that work, apparent genetic influences on intakes of
specific macronutrients appeared to be a secondary outcome of the effects
on total energy intake.

4.2.2   Genetics and energy expenditure

Although variance in BMR across a population is almost fully explained
by body mass (particularly lean body mass), age, and sex, the remaining
variance could represent a quantitatively meaningful amount of energy
expenditure, which appears to have a significant genetic component
(Fontaine *et al.*, 1985; Bogardus *et al.*, 1986; Bouchard *et al.*, 1989;
Sipiläinen et al., 1997). Similarly, TEF following a fixed caloric load has
been shown to have a significant heritability (Bouchard *et al.*, 1989).
However, these findings do not directly implicate these routes as a basis
for genetic variance in fatness. For example, Sipiläinen *et al.* (1997)
describe a genetic polymorphism which is associated with reduced BMR,
but not with measures of fatness. Despite a very large literature which
has considered whether obesity is at least partly attributable to low or
impaired BMR or TEF (Ravussin & Swinburn, 1993), a causal role has not
been established, and it is apparent that both BMR and total energy
expenditure rise with body weight (see Sections 3.3.1 and 3.5).

Longitudinal studies of infants and young children have been undertaken to clarify cause–effect relationships of energy intake and expenditure characteristics and subsequent weight gain. Roberts *et al.* (1988)
reported that infants who became overweight by the age of 1 year had
manifested low TEE but normal energy intake and metabolic rate at 3
months of age. Although non-genetic explanations are considered, these

data were interpreted as supportive of a genetically based, early-onset of low physical activity, linked both to maternal characteristics and actual weight gain. However, larger subsequent studies found no links between TEE at 12 weeks of age and fatness at 2 to 3 years of age (Davies *et al.*, 1991; Wells *et al.*, 1996), and have also found no relationship between parental BMI and energy expenditure of infants or children (Davies *et al.*, 1995; Goran *et al.*, 1995). Similarly, there is no clear evidence of unusually low absolute or adjusted BMR amongst pre-adolescent children of Pima Indians, a relatively genetically homogeneous group extraordinarily highly prone to obesity (Fontvieille *et al.*, 1993).

The results of the studies above, and others showing reduced physical activity levels of overweight infants and children, are perhaps more consistent with a view that fatter infants are (or become) less active infants, rather than the reverse. There is other evidence from children and adults, and also epidemiological analyses, which support low physical activity as a precursor to excessive weight gain (see Roberts, 1995; Dietz, 1996), and indications that spontaneous physical activity levels (but not necessarily exercise participation) may be influenced by genotype. Analyses of survey and experimental data have suggested significant familial correlations in activity levels, and provided mixed support for a genetic component (Bouchard *et al.*, 1993; Pérusse *et al.*, 1988a; 1988b; 1989; Moore *et al.*, 1991).

The links to weight status may be further complicated by diet–activity interactions: Lissner and Heitmann (1997) have reported evidence that a high fat diet was associated with 6-year weight gains in women, but the effect was most pronounced in sedentary subjects. Prentice & Jebb (1995) have documented how the prevalence of obesity has risen dramatically in Britain over a period when *per capita* energy intakes declined and macronutrient composition of the diet remained roughly stable, facts which can only be reconciled by implicating reduced physical activity as a causal factor. However, the role of inactivity as a fundamental cause of obesity, and its interactions with diet and genetics, remain unsettled.

4.2.3 Genetics and fat deposition

In studies in which identical twins were overfed fixed energy loads for extended periods, Bouchard and colleagues (1988; 1990) found a wide range of individual body weight and fat mass gains, but a high degree of similarity for these measures, and fat distribution, within twin pairs. Studies by other groups prior to this time had also revealed considerable individual variation in responses to overfeeding, and the twin data shows strong support for a genetic component to this apparently differing sensitivity to weight gain. The physiological basis for this variation to fixed loads is, however, not immediately apparent.

Substantial differences in dissipation of excess energy intake through rises in energy-wasting thermogenic processes does not seem likely (Schoeller, 1996; Bray, 1995; Section 3.2.1). In general, there also is no strong support for significant defects in thermogenesis as a major cause of most human obesity (see Prentice 'et al., 1989; Schoeller, 1996 and Section 3.3.1). It is conceivable that (unmeasured) differences in spontaneous physical activity could explain a significant part of the differences in overfeeding responses (Diaz et al., 1992). Rises in physical activity energy expenditure have been reported to be a significant adaptive response to overfeeding, even where subjects have ostensibly limited access to opportunities for unregulated exercise (Ravussin, 1985; Klein & Goran, 1993; Liebel et al., 1995).

Bouchard and colleagues (1990; Bouchard, 1991b) suggest that the genetic differences observed in their overfeeding studies could be attributable to individual variation in relative partitioning of excess macronutrients into lean vs fat tissue. A tendency toward the latter would then be a basis for susceptibility to becoming overweight. Unfortunately, this intuitively appealing explanation becomes less convincing with closer scrutiny. In overfeeding studies, leaner individuals have a greater tendency to add excess body mass as lean relative to fat tissue, whereas fatter individuals show a greater relative tendency to gain body fat (Forbes, 1990; Section 3.5). Thus, the type of tissue gained during experimental overfeeding may primarily be a result, rather than a cause, of body composition which itself has a strong genetic component. There is clearly limited capacity to energy storage as lean tissue, so incoming nutrients must either be diverted elsewhere (into fat) or oxidized. Lean individuals also do not have greater mass or turnover of lean tissue relative to the obese; indeed, total lean tissue mass is invariably also greater in the obese (Forbes, 1987a). Because of the lower energy content (kcal/g) and higher metabolic activity of lean vs fat tissue, leaner individuals should tend to gain more weight than obese subjects, and show a greater rise in absolute BMR when overfed by a fixed amount. Thus, without complete information regarding the initial body composition and TEE of subjects in overfeeding studies, it is difficult to determine the degree to which individual responses in fat deposition are actually secondary to other, more fundamental genetic influences.

4.2.4   Genetics and macronutrient utilization

The notion that certain individuals are genetically predisposed to overweight and obesity due to differential macronutrient utilization (rather than a primary defect in thermogenesis or partitioning into lean tissue) is extremely attractive. This hypothesis has now been the focus of considerable investigation in cross-sectional studies and experimental trials (detailed in Section 3.4.2), and could potentially resolve many separate pieces of research on metabolism, genetics, and food intake.

Zurlo and Ravussin (1992; Zurlo *et al.*, 1990) proposed that a relatively low ratio of fat to carbohydrate oxidation is a predictor of weight gain which might contribute to familial aggregation of obesity. At present, there is modest evidence for a signficant genetic influence on RQ from studies of twins and nuclear families, although it is fully possible that some of this relationship is secondary to genetic influences on food selection and macronutrient intake (Astrup *et al.*, 1996). However, Heitmann *et al.* (1995) have reported that consumption of a high fat diet was associated with a striking rise in BMI of adult females over a 6-year period only amongst overweight subjects with a family history of obesity (at least 1 obese parent). There was also some evidence for this amongst normal weight women with a strong family history (2 obese parents). These and other data (Section 3.4.2) suggest that RQ might be a primary rather than secondary factor in the etiology of obesity amongst susceptible individuals. Confirmation of this in other groups, and data relating specifically to the possible mode and strength of heritability of the relative utilization of fat and carbohydrate, will undoubtedly be a subject of future research.

4.2.5 Recent advances and the molecular genetics of obesity

In recent years, tremendous advances have been made in the molecular biology of the gross obesities associated with single gene defects in specific animal models, raising hopes for applications in understanding and treating the human condition. This work will only be touched upon, here and in other chapters, for two reasons. First, the speed of advances is proceeding at such a pace that any detailed discussion today will be rapidly outdated. Second, and more importantly, while this represents valuable basic science, the implications of this work for the understanding, prevention and treatment of the common forms of human obesity remain unclear. In the animal models, many of the single-gene defects are associated with physiological symptoms not necessarily associated with human obesity, as well as body composition changes which are markedly different from the human condition (Forbes, 1987a). As of this writing, there is also limited evidence for a link between the physiological basis for obesity in these animal models and any similar defects in human obesity syndromes. Nevertheless, the possibility that a limited number of major genes may contribute to a high proportion of the heritability of human obesity spurred the search for these, and the genes established as defective in animal models have provided an obvious focus for the search. Identification of genetically based molecular mediators predisposing certain individuals to obesity could arguably lead to opportunities for early detection and more targeted interventions.

Although a galaxy of hormones, neurotransmitters and peptides have been implicated in feeding behaviour and weight regulation (see Blundell, 1991; Rowland *et al.*, 1996), recent work has particularly focused on a signal-receptor system implicated in obese rodent models. Zhang *et al.* (1994) reported the identification and sequencing of the obese (*ob*) gene associated with development of gross obesity in a strain of mice ('*ob/ob*') homozygous for a defect in this gene. The product of the *ob* gene from normal mice and humans is a secreted protein, leptin, with a sequence largely conserved between species. A series of subsequent studies showed that administration of mouse or human leptin prompts decreases in food intake in *ob/ob* mice and, apparently, a stimulation of thermogenesis and activity, leading to substantial loss of body weight (Pelleymounter *et al.*, 1995; Halaas *et al.*, 1995; Campfield *et al.*, 1995). Similar treatment of mice made obese by means of a high-fat diet was found to generate significant reductions in food intake and body weight. Leptin adminstration to lean mice also appears to produce reduced food intake and significant changes in body composition. Other genetically obese animal models have a normally functioning *ob* gene and leptin sequence, but defects in the encoding of the hypothalamic leptin receptor, which also shares a common structure between mice and humans (Tartaglia *et al.*, 1995). Together with a range of other studies, this body of work has provided strong support for the current view that leptin functions as a peripheral signal from adipose tissue, and acts centrally to modulate feeding behaviour and energy balance.

The original work with leptin in *ob/ob* mice prompted speculation that at least some forms of human obesity might also be due to analogous deficiencies in the quantity or function of leptin. However, subsequent work has generally not found specific abnormalities of leptin structure associated with obesity, and serum leptin levels are strongly positively correlated with fatness in humans (Considine *et al.*, 1995; 1996a; Lonnquist *et al.*, 1995; Hamilton *et al.*, 1995; Rönnemaa *et al.*, 1997). Nevertheless, extreme obesity in a subset of human subjects may be associated with variants of *ob* or nearby genes (Duggirala *et al.*, 1995; Reed *et al.*, 1996; Clement *et al.*, 1996), although this is not a consistent finding (Norman *et al.*, 1995; Niki *et al.*, 1996; Bray *et al.*, 1996; Maffei *et al.*, 1996; Carlsson *et al.*, 1997) and there is no evidence to date that these variants are generating a specific functional defect. One report poses the possibility that variants of the human *ob* gene might have an independent, perhaps primary influence on the psychiatric and behavioural correlates of obesity, in addition to any effects on appetite regulation (Comings *et al.*, 1996). Current work has also focused on possible alternatives, e.g., that certain human obesities are attributable to defective leptin receptor or post-receptor mechanisms, or to diminished leptin transport into the brain. There is preliminary support for the latter (Caro *et al.*, 1996), but analyses of hypothalamic tissue from lean and obese humans has revealed no evidence of any specific defects in the leptin receptor (Considine *et al.*, 1996b).

The 'leptin system' clearly appears to function in body weight and energy balance regulation, but this is also true of many other hormones and neurotransmitters, where pharmacological treatments or genetic variants in production or reception can be shown to have a marked impact on weight status. Variation in relevant genes for several of these has been linked to predisposition for obesity in humans (Roberts & Greenberg, 1996). Current evidence is consistent with a view that high leptin levels, perhaps like high insulin levels, may largely occur as a secondary response to weight gain, rather than reflecting a special role in individual genetic susceptibility toward obesity. Indeed, leptin levels appear to be largely normalized, in parallel with insulin levels, by weight loss in obese humans (Havel *et al.*, 1996; Geldszus *et al.*, 1996), although those investigators suggest that weight loss-induced reductions in leptin levels may contribute toward the tendency for weight regain. While there will continue to be a great volume of research activity in this area, current research has not found strong evidence that inheritance of a predisposition for obesity in humans is commonly an outcome of variance in leptin function or sensitivity. The search continues, although the orientation of this body of work is clearly more focused toward pharmacological treatment than toward prevention though public health programmes.

4.3 SUMMARY

Obesity tends to run in families, and a wide range of studies support the existence of strong genetic component to its development. However, it is clear that it is not obesity *per se* that is inherited, but a **susceptibility** toward becoming obese, and this will depend upon particular conditions for its possible expression. There is relatively good agreement in the literature that, quite contrary to popular assumptions, the influence of the shared family environment is relatively unimportant in contrast to genetic transmission and other, unshared, environmental influences. A sedentary lifestyle and an abundant supply of food, particularly food high in fat or energy density (Chapter 5), appear to be important, perhaps necessary, though not always sufficient conditions.

There are many candidates for the functional outcome of genes associated with the development of chronic positive energy balance leading to excess fat deposition. Studies have quantified significant, specific genetic contributions to a multitude of physiological and behavioural responses, any and all of which might contribute to the expression of overeating and obesity under appropriate circumstances. These include selection and utilization (oxidation and/or deposition) of ingested fuels, overall energy intake, thermogenesis, and voluntary activity levels. Given the apparent contribution of many genes, this broad range of potential influences is not necessarily surprising, and their relative importance in the aetiology of obesity (and therefore potentially also its prevention) seems likely to differ between individuals. Recent research into the molecular biology of obesity may help to characterize those differences between individuals.

In terms of interaction with diet availability and composition, certain potentially genetically mediated factors are of particular interest. A genetic predisposition toward certain selection of a particular macronutrient mix, perhaps mediated through responsiveness to characteristic sensory and food preferences, would be consistent with other relevant experimental and epidemiological data (Chapters 5 and 6). The hypothesis that a propensity for obesity may derive from relatively reduced rates of fat oxidation is consistent with other evidence suggesting that dietary fat may be particularly implicated in excessive weight gain. However, it is also reasonable to consider that more generalized inherited psychological traits may confer a heightened responsiveness to particular types of food or other environmental stimuli.

Stunkard *et al.* (1986b) make an analogy between obesity and phenylketonuria (PKU), a disease with clear genetic determinants, but which can be prevented by relatively simple manipulation of diet in

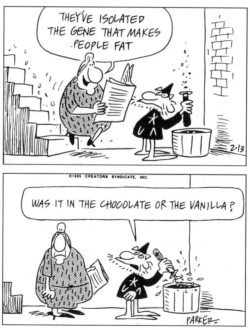

Figure 4.1 The integration of the molecular genetics of obesity with behavioural research on food composition and palatability. By permission of Johnny Hart and Creators Syndicate, Inc.

infancy and childhood. Unlike PKU, however, obesity may occur, and must therefore be prevented or controlled, throughout the lifespan. Furthermore, PKU does not have a broad range of etiologies and susceptibilities, and is therefore amenable to genetic testing and a specific intensive therapeutic regimen. It seems that obesity can have many determinants, and that many of these may in turn involve one or more genetic factors. With the prevalence of obesity rising rapidly, and half of the population overweight in some nations, changes in the permissive environmental conditions becomes much more efficacious and appropriate than the search for and treatment of individual defects. This then leads to the question of what environmental influences are relevant, and their possible roles in promoting and maintaining the overweight condition.

CHAPTER FIVE

Food composition, food intake and energy balance

Explanations for differential effects of food composition on energy balance may be seen as largely falling into 3 classes (Warwick & Schiffman, 1992): effects on hunger and satiation, food acceptance, and metabolism. These largely fall along the following respective lines of reasoning: 1) differences in the satiety value of macronutrients and effects of bulk volume tend to promote or suppress energy intakes; 2) high and low energy density (high and low fat) diets differ in acceptability or 'palatability', and therefore different amounts are eaten; and 3) differences in post-prandial metabolism attributable to changes in food composition alter the efficiency or degree of energy expenditure or fat deposition.

5.1 MACRONUTRIENTS, ENERGY DENSITY AND ENERGY INTAKE

5.1.1 Short- and medium-term laboratory studies

Information on the relationships of dietary composition and energy intake come from a wide range of sources. In particular, there are a large number of studies assessing the influences of variations in specific macronutrients and other dietary constitutents on appetite and energy intake, mostly under short-term (1 to 2 days) or medium-term (3 days up to 2–3 weeks) controlled conditions, generally based in the laboratory and/or using covert manipulations of preloads or foods.

Studies of short-term regulation of food intake have typically focused on two effects of food composition: the effect on cessation of eating within a meal (satiation), and the effect on suppression or delaying of later hunger and food intake (satiety) (Blundell & King, 1996; Blundell *et al.*, 1996). Usually these studies have been carried out within part or all of a single day, although subjects may keep records of hunger into the next day. In medium-term studies, subjects are generally provided with some or all of their meals over a period of several days or a few weeks. The composition or quantity of food given in the experiment is invariably covertly manipulated, and usually consumed within the laboratory, where subjects may or may not be confined for the entire period of study. The main outcome variables in such studies are total and macronutrient intakes, and perhaps also overall total energy balance.

This body of research has considered major macronutrients directly, or indirectly through studies using macronutrient (fat and sugar) replacements in foods. Although the research has produced some general 'rules', there are within it also examples of individual study results having almost every conceivable interpretation. In part because of possible implications for commercial foods and food ingredients (e.g., non-nutritive sweeteners), this literature has generated considerable scientific debate. Previous reviews cite and describe specific experiments and differences in their design, findings, and interpretation (Rolls, 1991; Blundell & de Graaf, 1993; Bellisle & Perez, 1994; Blundell & Rogers, 1994; Blundell *et al.*, 1996; Rolls & Hammer, 1995; Anderson, 1995; Mela, 1996b), while a more general review of the outcomes of this work will be given here.

(a) Potential drawbacks of short- and medium-term laboratory studies

Although laboratory-based trials offer a high degree of control and sensitivity, several issues should be borne in mind in extrapolating from such studies to possible wider implications for dietary intakes and weight control under more natural conditions.

First, the methodologies used in most of these studies have been oriented toward addressing fundamental phenomena related to the physiological determinants and correlates of hunger, satiety, and regulation of energy intake. In many short-term studies, end points are motivational ratings (e.g., hunger or desire to eat), or perhaps consumption of a single test meal. The point is not to criticize or diminish the importance of such studies, but to emphasize that they typically were not really designed to characterize the actual dietary behaviour of consumers in natural situations, although they are often interpreted in that way. Biological signals related to satiety and regulation of energy balance are clearly important, but are only one of many contributors to the decision of what, when, and how much to eat (see Section 2.4). Even large behavioural effects seen under particular experimental situations may explain little of the variance in eating behaviour occurring under more realistic conditions.

Second, these studies are potentially sensitive to many details of experimental design, some of which are listed in Table 5.1. In particular, compensatory responses to the addition or concentration of macronutrients or sensory stimuli in foods or test stimuli may have quite different results from their removal or dilution. Other studies have used covert manipulations of test foods to achieve energy densities grossly differing from the traditional versions, or have narrowly limited the range or composition of foods with which intakes might be adjusted. The latter point is particularly crucial.

Third, most studies have been conducted over time periods and under conditions which would minimize learning about the post-ingestive effects and the recognition of learned satiety cues (Chapter 2) (Louis-

Table 5.1 Factors affecting responses to experimental manipulations in studies of appetite and feeding behaviour

o   Subject population
o   Antecedent diet
o   Setting: laboratory or free-living
o   Food composition
o   *Ad libitum* or fixed diet regimen
o   Opportunities to select foods of 'normal' composition
o   Amount of compensation required
o   Direction of compensation required
o   Time period of study
o   Subject beliefs or knowledge about manipulation

Sylvestre *et al.*, 1989). Similarly, shorter studies would not allow for the influences of any physiological responses which may develop over periods of longer than a few hours or days, including those (such as changes in BMR) which might influence energy balance through expenditure. Thus, there may be limited opportunity for involvement of processes which may be highly meaningful over periods of longer experience and duration. This is particularly of concern in studies which have shown marked undereating in response to energy dilution or, more typically, overeating when energy density is covertly raised.

Lastly, most studies have used covert experimental manipulation, and therefore knowledge or beliefs about the test foods and their energy or macronutrient content have not been a major focus of interest. Laboratory investigations which have particularly focused on information have suggested that individuals might respond counter-intuitively to information on fat content (e.g., inappropriately increasing fat or energy intakes) (Mattes, 1990; Caputo & Mattes, 1993; Shide & Rolls, 1995; Aaron *et al.*, 1995). Intriguing results were reported by Caputo & Mattes (1993), where subjects consuming identical mid-day meals (in the laboratory) increased their overall, freely chosen (outside the laboratory) dietary fat intakes during periods in which they were falsely told their experimental meals were reduced in fat. However, such contrary effects on eating behaviour have not been apparent in intervention trials using commercial reduced-fat or reduced-sugar products under realistic acquisition and consumption conditions (Gatenby *et al.*, 1995; 1997). Nevertheless, there remain important questions about how consumers respond to nutritional information and marketing claims, in terms of overall food selection and consumption patterns.

(b) Results of short- and medium-term laboratory studies

When individuals are presented with a buffet of mixed foods in a test situation, and allowed to eat *ad libitum* (to satiation), the energy consumed within the meal is often observed to be closely related to the energy density of foods provided. This is partly due to gastric distention and associated physiological signals (McHugh & Moran, 1991; Section 2.3.4), but as much or more reflects the fact that normal food intake is heavily guided by social norms and customary eating patterns (e.g., habitual numbers, volumes, or weights of particular food items consumed at a sitting). This is not a direct effect of food composition, since provision in a single test meal of a range of foods which are uniformly very high or very low in energy density, or covertly manipulated, may allow limited opportunity for either post-ingestive physiological signals to influence the size of the meal, or for a longer-term cognitive control over eating to develop. Because of these factors, there is a tendency to consume more energy when meals comprise foods of high energy density (in practice, high fat) (Blundell *et al.*, 1996; Poppitt & Prentice, 1996), and to eat less when familiar foods are manipulated in a way which reduces their energy content below normal. The potential for 'passive' (i.e., not actively stimulated) overconsumption of energy dense foods becomes potentially significant for energy balance if it is not counterbalanced by an equivalent later suppression of intake. Even under longer-term conditions, using a variable menu of normal foods as a vehicle for covert manipulations of energy density and/or macronutrient composition, subjects in experimental situations tend to eat relatively consistent weights of foods (Lissner *et al.*, 1987; Kendall *et al.*, 1991; Stubbs *et al.*, 1995, 1996), and this has also been seen under more free-living conditions (Lyon *et al.*, 1995).

Many short-term studies have focused on the suppressive effects of ingestion of foods and nutrients on hunger and later food intake (satiety). Experimentally, this is usually studied by giving subjects a fixed energy content preload of an experimental food or nutrient, followed by subsequent measurement of *ad libitum* intake of a buffet test meal comprising a range of food items. These types of studies have generated highly variable outcomes, depending upon the methodology used (Bellisle & Perez, 1994; Rolls & Hammer, 1995). Differences in outcomes appear to relate largely to 1) the absolute energy content or differences in energy content and composition (including minor constituents) of preloads, 2) the duration of the interval between preload and test meal (shorter intervals typically generating better compensation), and 3) type of test meal. In some cases studies have simply had too little power to resolve meaningful differences, leading to 'negative' findings (e.g., conclusion of an absence of difference). The potential difficulties of attempting to account for the differential outcomes of many specific methodological decisions are illustrated by observations of post-prandial hunger ratings being significantly influenced by flour particle sizes (Holt and Brand Miller, 1994) and by body posture (sitting vs lying down) (Horowitz *et al.*, 1993, Carney *et al.*, 1995).

Given these difficulties in interpreting the results of single studies, it is unfortunate that this type of work comprises such an overwhelming part of the literature on food composition and appetite control, and forms virtually the sole basis of many scientific reviews of the topic. Nevertheless, certain general conclusions may be drawn from this body of research.

First, there is a general tendency toward at least partial, and often quite good compensation for differences in the energy content of covertly manipulated meals or preloads. Energy intake tends to suppress later energy intake in a roughly dose-related manner. There is certainly some degree of inconsistency in the results of short-term studies: most show evidence of significant compensation, but many have concluded that there was no compensation at all over the period of observation; that is, preload energy differences had no effects on · subsequent intakes. However, in longer studies, good compensation for covert reductions in energy density within meals or snacks has been fairly consistently seen in studies where subjects are also allowed *ad libitum* access to a wide choice of foods while less complete compensation is often observed where subjects are relatively restricted to low energy density foods. This turns out to be an absolutely critical methodological issue, with potentially important practical implications. [The interested reader can refer to Bellisle & Perez (1994), Fricker *et al.* (1995), Poppitt & Prentice (1996), Blundell *et al.* (1996), and Rolls & Hammer (1995) for comprehensive lists of results and reviews of the many individual studies.] The results of several studies also suggest that the compensatory eating in response to covert reductions or dilution of energy may be more efficient and robust than responses to the concentration or supplementation of energy in foods and meals. However, there has rarely been complete control for variety, volumes, and acceptability of foods (and such control is both difficult and unrealistic). Furthermore, as noted by Poppitt & Prentice (1996), there may be differential threshold effects, whereby poorer compensation becomes much more likely when the concentration or dilution achieves certain degrees of change from 'baseline'.

Second, compensation for covertly manipulated preloads and meals is generally not strongly macronutrient-specific. That is, test meal or free-living intakes following preloads of differing macronutrient content have generally been found to take the form of a mixed diet of normal composition, and there is no clear evidence of selection for or against nutrients fed in higher or lower quantities (e.g., Rolls *et al.*, 1988b; 1992; Foltin *et al.*, 1990; 1992; Louis-Sylvestre *et al.*, 1994; Fricker, 1995). This result is an important outcome because of its potential implications for responses to specific macronutrient substitutes (e.g., Beaton *et al.*, 1992; Section 5.4.1). Thus, replacement of sugars with intense sweeteners may be predicted to generate a reduction in carbohydrate intake (as sugars), but (based upon non-specific compensatory eating) to a higher proportion of dietary energy being derived from fat. By similar logic, replacement of fat by fat substitutes should lead to a relative reduction in fat, and rise in carbohydrate intakes. In fact, though, the real responses to consumer use of products made with such substitutes is more complex (Mela, in press; 1997). In part, this is due to the way specific macronutrient-substituted foods may actually be used (e.g., reduced-sugar foods may largely be added into an existing diet, rather than substituting for or replacing sugar-containing items) (Mela, in press; 1997; Anderson & Leiter, 1996). Another factor, as noted previously, is that behavioural responses to real, commercial food products may be substantially influenced by the provision of label claims and information. It may also be worth noting that most studies have looked at manipulations primarily of fat or carbohydrate, and it is possible that specific selection for protein might occur more readily (Barkeling *et al.*, 1990; Gibson *et al.*, 1995).

Lastly, there appears to be a hierarchy in the satiating efficiency of macronutrients. Although some human studies have found no differences in intakes following isocaloric loads of different macronutrient composition (Geliebter, 1979; de Graaf *et al.*, 1992a) [a result which may be attributable to the use of liquid stimuli (Mattes, 1996)], the current general consensus of the literature and of researchers within this field is that calories from protein generate the strongest suppression of subsequent hunger and eating, followed by carbohydrates, and then by fat (Booth *et al.*, 1970; Hill & Blundell, 1986; Barkeling *et al.*, 1990; Rolls *et al.*, 1994; Holt *et al.*, 1995). These are very general rules applied to mixed diets, but it is clear that the source of protein or specific type of fat (e.g., Rolls *et al.*, 1988b; Stubbs & Harbron, 1996) or form of carbohydrate (see below) may have significant influences on short-term intakes, and these have not been fully explored in longer-term studies. Many of the relevant experiments also have not fully controlled for interactions with other meal components or volume effects. Nevertheless, a high satiety value for protein also emerges from analyses of free-living dietary intakes (de Castro, 1987). Additionally, this appears to be a general belief held by consumers (de Graaf *et al.*, 1992b), though subjects in that study also perceived sweet carbohydrates to have virtually no satiety value, a result which clearly conflicts with empirical studies (see below; Rogers *et al.*, 1988; Blundell & de Graaf, 1993; Rogers & Blundell, 1989b). Energy from alcohol appears to have very little suppressive effect on energy intakes from other sources (Tremblay & St-Pierre, 1996; Mattes, 1996; Foltin *et al.*, 1993), and Mattes (1996) has recently suggested that this may be in large part due to its consumption in beverage form.

The issue of sweet (sugars) vs non-sweet (starch) carbohydrates, and of sweetness in particular has been given considerable attention in short-term studies. Most of this literature shows that, as expected, nutritive high carbohydrate preloads – whether sugar or starch – suppress hunger, and generate a reduction in subsequent intakes roughly (if rather imperfectly) related to the preload calories ingested (e.g., Ho *et al.*, 1990; Rogers & Blundell, 1989a; 1989b; Rolls *et al.*, 1989; 1991; 1994; de Graaf *et al.*,

1993b; reviewed by Blundell *et al.*, 1994; Anderson, 1995), a result which is also supported by longer-term studies (Mattes, 1990; Foltin *et al.*, 1990; 1992; Caputo & Mattes, 1992). However, there are a number of experiments which have found differences in short-term satiety responses between starches and sugars (de Graaf *et al.*, 1993b; Rolls *et al.*, 1988b), among different starch sources (e.g., Hospers *et al.*, 1994; Holt & Brand Miller, 1995; Raben *et al.*, 1994b), and among different specific sugars (Spitzer & Rodin, 1987). Differential effects are commonly attributed to post-prandial physiological events (e.g., insulin release and glcyaemic responses). In addition, there has been particularly heated debate over the putative role of sweetness and sweeteners in (primarily short-term) appetite control. Some investigators have concluded that sweetness *per se* can stimulate hunger and eating (Tordoff, 1988; Blundell & Rogers, 1994), while others reject this general notion, and adopt a quite different view of much the same body of experimental data (Rolls, 1991; Drewnowski, 1995). There is also evidence that specific intense sweeteners may have additional bioactive properties unrelated to their sweetness (Rogers & Blundell, 1989b; Rogers *et al.*, 1990; 1995a). As noted above, in common with much of the literature on food composition and satiety, the debate in the overall issue of sweeteners has largely hinged upon methodological details and the interpretations placed on specific results. The scientific process also has not necessarily benefited from heavy involvement of vested commercial interests. Other types of research studies provide a somewhat more consistent view of the role of sugars and sweeteners in relation to obesity (Hill & Prentice, 1995; Anderson, 1995; below and Chapter 6).

Studies of the effects of fat content in particular have been reviewed by Blundell *et al.* (1996), who detailed the (mixed) evidence which generally supports the view of a relatively weaker satiety effect of energy from fat compared with carbohydrate. Differences between short-term studies comparing fat and carbohydrate may particularly relate to the time course of satiety responses, the volume and energy content of preloads, and perhaps also the subject population (Rolls & Hammer, 1995; Blundell *et al.*, 1996). A crucial point is probably energy density, which has been controlled in few studies. When subjects have been fed high-fat (high energy density) diets for extended periods of time, they clearly tend to overeat relative to baseline or high carbohydrate diets (Duncan *et al.*, 1983; Lissner *et al.*, 1987; Mattes *et al.*, 1988; Westerterp *et al.*, 1996c; Stubbs *et al.*, 1995; Tremblay *et al.*, 1989; 1991a). This effect is largely eliminated when energy density is experimentally controlled (Stubbs *et al.*, 1996; van Stratum *et al.*, 1978), indicating that effects are not primarily due to a direct effect of fat itself. [This is also observed in infants (Catt *et al.*, in press) and laboratory rats (Ramirez & Friedman, 1990; Warwick & Schiffman, 1992).] Given the fairly close relationship between energy density and fat content of normal foods and diets, it may be argued that parallel changes in these two factors have high ecological validity. Notably, though, changes in food technology have led to the increased development and marketing of foods quite markedly reduced in fat content but having little or no reduction in energy density.

There is mixed evidence regarding associations between obesity and post-prandial satiety, and design and interpretation of studies is complicated by several factors. Because total energy expenditure and intake would normally be greater for heavier than for lighter individuals (Section 3.3), it might be most appropriate to adjust preloads or analyse intakes of test meals in relation to normal intakes or estimated metabolic requirements. Even where this is done, differences may occur due to physical capacity and rates of gastric emptying. It may also be the case that lean–obese differences are more apparent for preloads of particular compositions, or that behavioural responses reflect particular psychological correlates of the obese sample. For example, Rolls *et al.* (1994) reported that, compared with lean unrestrained subjects, compensation for fat calories was less exact amongst subjects who were obese or who scored highly for eating restraint (see Chapter 8). Although data from that study suggest subjects did not readily differentiate the preloads, it is known that the post-prandial responses and eating behaviour of subjects can be markedly influenced by differences in the perceived caloric content of meals (Wooley *et al.*, 1972, Section 8.3.1). In contrast to the results of Rolls *et al.* (1994), French *et al.* (1993) found that obese subjects reported lower hunger than lean subjects, following both low- and high-fat preloads, though the obese subjects paradoxically indicated an earlier return of the desire to eat another meal. Other studies have found similar satiety responses amongst lean and obese subjects (Duncan *et al.*, 1983; Hill & Blundell, 1989), but there are also quite substantial laboratory trials which found weakened responsiveness of obese subjects to covert variations in the energy density of food (Campbell *et al.*, 1971).

5.1.2 Long-term and field trials

There is now a large number of recent studies which have examined diet and body weight relationships amongst non-obese subjects placed on extended (multi-week) *ad libitum* reduced-fat/high-carbohydrate diets comprised of normal foods. These studies have invariably found that this dietary change is accompanied by modest spontaneous reductions in energy intakes or body weight (Sheppard *et al.*, 1991; Kendall *et al.*, 1991; Retzlaff *et al.*, 1991; Sandström *et al.*, 1992; Gatenby *et al.*, 1995; Raben *et al.*, 1995; Schaefer *et al.*, 1995; Siggaard *et al.*, 1996) or fat mass (Lyon *et al.*, 1995). The specific fat reductions and control of or changes in other dietary constituents (e.g., NSP) have varied between these studies, and it is possible that subjects in free-living studies also modified their lifestyle in other ways during the trials. However, it is notable that spontaneous

decreases in total energy intake or body weight are also a common observation (at least initially) in more general clinical and experimental studies
in which free-living subjects have been advised to reduce the proportion
of energy derived from fat within *ad libitum* diets (e.g., Chlebowski *et al.*,
1993; Kasim *et al.*, 1993; Boyd *et al.*, 1990; Cole-Hamilton *et al.*, 1986; Lee-
Han *et al.*, 1988; National Diet–Heart Study Research Group, 1968;
Schectman *et al.*, 1990; Shintani *et al.*, 1991; Theusen *et al.*, 1986). There are
also several relevant studies which have specifically focused on *ad libitum*
very low fat diets as a method of weight loss amongst obese subjects
(Hammer *et al.*, 1989; Schlundt *et al.*, 1993a; Shah et al, 1994; Jeffery *et al.*,
1995), and all report significant weight losses on the low fat diets, equivalent in some cases to weight loss on energy restricted diets. Although
energy density of diets is rarely reported, it was not specifically controlled in any of the above studies, and can probably be safely assumed
to have been reduced concomitant with reductions in the proportion of
dietary fat.

Subjects in most of the studies cited above have had initial dietary
intakes in the typical western range of 35 to 40% of energy from fat, and
there appears to be a threshold or gradient effect for undereating in relation to changes in the fat content (and presumably energy density) of
diets. The reductions in relative fat intake in most of the studies have
generally been from initial intakes of about 40% down to 25 to 30% or less
of energy from fat, but a few have also included periods of exceptionally
low fat intakes (below 15% of energy). The spontaneous weight loss
occurring in non-obese individuals adopting moderately fat-reduced
diets tends to be modest, e.g., changes in fat intake from about 40% down
to 30% energy from fat typically has resulted in body weights stabilizing
at about a 1 to 3 kg reduction from baseline in the first few months (e.g.,
Figure 5.1). Somewhat greater weight loss responses have been observed
amongst initially fatter vs leaner subjects (Siggaard *et al.*, 1996; Raben *et
al.*, 1995) and, as noted, with very low-fat diets incorporated into weight
loss programmes. Lyon *et al.* (1995) have reported that loss of fat mass
amongst moderately obese subjects was highly correlated with a measure
of compliance with an *ad libitum* low fat (but only slightly lowered energy
density) diet, and other studies find greater weight loss occurring with
more marked reductions in fat intakes (e.g., Thuesen *et al.*, 1986). Subjects
who start with initial diets lower in percent energy from fat, and under-
take only small reductions in fat intakes, show relatively good maintenance of energy balance and no change in weight (Westerterp *et al.*, 1996c;
Gatenby *et al.*, 1997; Mela, 1997).

The time courses and durations of weight loss, maintenance or regain
amongst subjects on reduced-fat diets is not well established. In general,
adjustments of intakes back to 'baseline' may be quite slow, especially
where the diet composition is substantially and covertly altered.
Analyses of data from Kendall *et al.* (1991) have suggested that adjust-

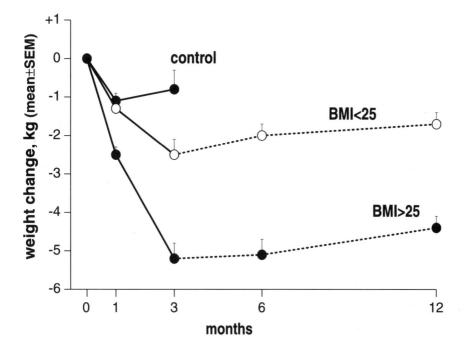

Figure 5.1 Spontaneous weight changes among normal weight and overweight subjects adopting *ad libitum* reduced-fat diets, compared with study controls. Mean fat intake of intervention groups were 39.0% of energy at baseline to 28.0% at week 12. Data and figure adapted from Siggaard *et al.* (1996) with permission.

ment to such diets may occur over about a 3 to 6 month period, with energy intakes slowly rising back toward initial values. Some longer-term studies have observed maintenance of modest mean reductions of body weight over periods of 1 to 2 years on reduced-fat diets (Siggaard *et al.*, 1996; Sheppard *et al.*, 1991; Retzlaff *et al.*, 1991; Kasim *et al.*, 1993; Chlewbowski *et al.*, 1993; Tuobro & Astrup, 1997), but in other cases any weight loss was largely or fully regained in a similar time frame (National Diet–Heart Study Research Group, 1968; Lee-Han *et al.*, 1988; Boyd *et al.*, 1990; Sandström *et al.*, 1992; Jeffery *et al.*, 1995). Inspection of the data from many of these studies reveals significant discrepancies between measured weight changes and subjects' self-reported dietary intakes (e.g. Boyd *et al.*, 1990; Gatenby *et al.*, 1997). Mis-reporting (Section 3.3.2) and, in particular, poor compliance with long-term dietary regimens may therefore underlie some of the apparent contradictions in long-term study results.

5.1.3   Energy density, dietary bulk and energy intake

The potential influence of energy density on intake and energy balance is apparent from the trials cited above, and has been most directly tested in the short-term trials of Stubbs *et al.* (1995; 1996). Those studies showed that differential changes in energy balance observed on high- and low-fat diets were largely eliminated when experimental diets were designed to have equivalent energy densities, and subjects ate similar quantities of the various diets, regardless of compositional differences (Figure 5.2). As noted, there is a strong tendency to eat a consistent weight of food against a background of modest changes in energy density, and adjustments to such changes are apparently very slow. However, there are few relevant data available from free-living subjects consuming 'normal', unmodified commercial foods.

The present relationship between fat content and energy density of diets (Poppitt & Prentice, 1996) implies that, unless specific experimental foods and diets are specially constructed (e.g., Stubbs *et al.*, 1996; Catt *et al.*, in press; Ramirez & Friedman, 1990), compensatory responses to changes in dietary fat levels would almost inevitably require changes in total food volume. However, calculation of actual energy density of total diets, while ostensibly simple, is complicated by decisions regarding the handling of water and other (especially non-caloric) beverages by individual investigators. (For example, water from soup or milk would usually be counted, but water in hot beverages less likely, and plain water often excluded.) Thus, reported or computed energy density values

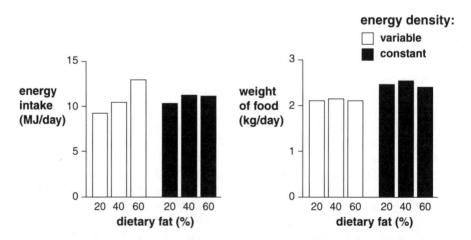

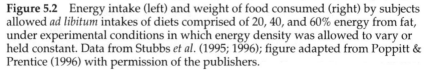

Figure 5.2   Energy intake (left) and weight of food consumed (right) by subjects allowed *ad libitum* intakes of diets comprised of 20, 40, and 60% energy from fat, under experimental conditions in which energy density was allowed to vary or held constant. Data from Stubbs *et al.* (1995; 1996); figure adapted from Poppitt & Prentice (1996) with permission of the publishers.

Table 5.2 Examples of reported or calculated energy densities of diets consumed in feeding trials investigating effects of energy density

Reference	Energy density groups (Energy density of diets, kcal/g)		
	Low	*Medium*	*High*
Duncan *et al.*, 1983	0.7	–	1.5
Lissner *et al.*, 1987	1.4	1.6	1.9
Kendall *et al.*, 1991	1.3	–	1.5
Stubbs *et al.*, 1995	1.1	1.3	1.7
Lyon *et al.*, 1995	0.75	–	0.9

between studies (e.g., Table 5.2) may not be directly comparable. Few studies provide data from which energy density can be determined and, when reported, its derivation may not be obvious. Nevertheless, it is apparent that an extreme situation is a 2-fold difference in energy density, while a more realistic outcome of substantial dietary change is likely to be ratio of about 1:1.5 in the energy density of low to high energy density diets.

The change from an initial diet composed of 40, 45, and 15% to one of 25, 60, and 15% of energy from fat, carbohydrate, and protein, respectively, would correspond to a 12.5% decrease in the caloric density of the diet on a dry weight basis. Making very rough assumptions that fat is unhydrated, while protein and carbohydrate are associated with 3 parts water, and that 1 part in 5 of the total diet weight is additional 'free' water, the overall energy density of the initial diet above would be reduced by from 1.7 to 1.2 kcal/g (7.1 to 5.0 kJ/g). This is within the range of the diets used in the experiments in Table 5.2. Thus, if food volume intake remains constant, this dictates a very substantial reduction of about 700 kcal (2.9 MJ) from a typical 2500 kcal/day (10.5 MJ/day) intake, similar to the outcomes observed by Lissner *et al.* (1987) and Stubbs *et al.* (1996).

Short and medium-term studies of caloric compensation indicate that humans can react quickly and accurately to differences of less than that magnitude occurring in provided meals, but probably **only** when a wide range of other normal foods (i.e., energy density not held constant) are freely available. In the example above, food volume intake on the low energy density diet would have to rise by about 600 g/day to maintain initial energy intakes. There is abundant evidence that lean individuals with very high energy needs, such as endurance athletes and manual labourers, can readily accommodate and sustain markedly elevated volumes of food (e.g., Jenson *et al.*, 1992), although this clearly requires overt changes in the size or frequency of meals. This level of intake is also well within normal day-to-day variation. Thus, the failure to alter intakes in line with changes in energy density is probably not due to any strict physical limitations on intake or capacity, but is consistent with the generally permissive response of the appetite control system under these conditions (Section 2.4). These data therefore support the view that energy intake in humans is not under tight physiological regulation (Kendall *et al.*, 1991), and that energy density can have significant 'passive' influences on intakes, at least over short- and medium-term periods.

Although cognitive factors (e.g., habitual, established meal patterns) may explain failures to adjust to changes in energy density within single meals, the factors which influence (lack of) adjustments to energy density within longer-term studies are less apparent. Specifically, one might expect rapid learning about the post-ingestive effects of the diet, and the development or re-establishment of conditioned satiety at appropriately higher or lower volume intakes. This, however, may only be possible under certain conditions, as suggested by data from Warwick & Schiffman (1991). They found that rats given diets in which flavours were inconsistently paired with rotating schedules of diets varying in energy density (high, medium, low) gained significantly more weight than controls. However, no differences from controls were observed amongst groups of animals which had specific flavours always paired with particular energy density diets (on the same rotating schedule), or receiving only the flavour variations (on a single medium energy density diet). These data suggest particular conditions under which learning and conditioned satiety may and may not take place, and suggest that results of human studies (e.g., Kendall *et al.*, 1991; Stubbs *et al.*, 1996) might in part reflect the difficulty for subjects of altering established responses to foods under conditions where menus consist of a range of changing items with variable sensory attributes.

While it is well-established that energy density of most diets reflects relative fat content, other compositional factors can significantly influence energy density and its relationships with intake in short-term studies. In particular, differences in the energy densities of many different foods are largely explained and readily manipulated by variation in the proportion of water they contain. Yet, not unexpectedly, experiments find no effect of water alone, nor of reducing energy by the simple addition of water to fixed rations, on physiological responses (e.g., gastric emptying) or satiety (Carbonnel *et al.*, 1994). Furthermore, conflicting data suggest that energy in fluids may be less satiating than in solid forms (Mattes, 1996). These lines of evidence suggest that low energy density (high volume) alone is not enough to produce the undereating and weight loss observed in many studies decribed above, but that the structural, osmotic and rheological properties of foods, and the matrix in which water and other bulk ingredients are bound or suspended may be important influences upon satiety and energy intake.

A considerable amount of related research has focused on the potential role of NSP and also resistant starches on satiety and energy intakes. In general, this work seems to show that addition of either non-caloric soluble (e.g., gums) or insoluble (e.g., cellulose) NSP to a preload or test meal tends to promote satiation and satiety, and clearly delays the return of hunger following a meal (see Burley & Blundell, 1995; Levine & Billington, 1994). Although there are a number of possible modes of action of NSP, it is commonly suggested that the primary effect on energy intake and postprandial satiety is mediated by effects of increased volume and distention of the gastrointestinal tract (French & Read, 1994). As with *ad libitum* reduced-fat diets, long-term consumption of high NSP regimens appears to be generally associated with a very modest spontaneous weight loss (Ali, 1982; Ryttig *et al.*, 1989; British Nutrition Foundation, 1990; Levine & Billington, 1994). The outcomes from this work therefore seem to be entirely consistent with data on other compositional changes which may affect energy density of the diet (or perhaps in this case, the ingesta). Further resolution of these issues will require greater focus on the structural and mechanical properties of foods and food colloids, both pre- and post-ingestion.

5.1.4 Macronutrient substitutes

Public concern with body weight management or other potential effects of excessive fat or sugar consumption have prompted massive industrial efforts in the development and marketing of intense sweeteners, bulk replacers, and fat replacement ingredients and technologies for macronutrient modification in foods. The range of materials used and proposed for use as sugar and fat replacers, and their different properties and applications, are discussed at length in the food science literature and other sources (e.g., Setser & Racette, 1992; Schiffman & Gatlin, 1993; Khan, 1993; Lucca & Tepper, 1994). Their potential implications for weight control in the general population ultimately depend upon the actual composition of the resulting food products, the degree of differences in composition from their traditionally formulated counterparts, and consumer food selection and usage behaviours which may have additional impacts on overall dietary outcomes.

(a) Fat and sugar substitute materials

Sugar (primarily sucrose) replacement in foods is primarily accomplished through use of intense sweeteners, bulk sweeteners, and non-sweet bulking agents. A range of different intense sweeteners, which may be tens to thousands of times sweeter than sucrose, are either not metabolized or appear in foods at concentrations so low as to make a negligible contribution to energy intakes. The main dietary source of intense sweetners is beverages, followed by use as 'tabletop' sweeteners, and lesser amounts in food applications such as yoghurts, jams, and prepared desserts. Bulk sweeteners primarily include a range of sugar alcohols which, as the name implies, are used in foods at levels roughly comparable to sucrose. Bulking agents, such as a range of different oligosaccharides (Crittenden & Playne, 1996) and polydextrose (Setser & Racette, 1992) may impart little sweetness to foods, but these and some of the sugar alcohols are used to produce a desired texture, with appropriate taste quality derived from use ·in combination with intense sweeteners. Sugar alcohols, oligosaccharides, and polydextrose may undergo variable degrees of bacterial fermentation in the large colon (Livesey *et al.*, 1993; Bornet, 1994; Gibson *et al.*, 1996), yielding a range of metabolizable by-products and making the physiological fuel values of such materials difficult to determine with precision.

Typical values for sugar alcohols are in the range of 2 to 3.5 kcal/g (8 to 15 kJ/g), and an 'official' single value of 10 kJ/g (2.4 kcal/g) is currently applied for labelling purposes in the European Union (Livesey, 1991; Van Es, 1991; Bornet, 1994). The physiological fuel values of polydextrose and oligosaccharides are generally found to be in the lower range of 1 to 2 kcal/g (4–8 kJ/g) (Ranhotra *et al.*, 1993; Achour *et al.*, 1994). Unpleasant gastrointestinal side-effects of high intakes of sugar alcohols and resistant oligosaccharides place limits on their broader use in the food supply or concentration in specific foods.

Some examples of current and proposed ingredients for fat replacement are listed in Table 5.3. These comprise a varied range of materials, which can substantially differ in potential applications and physiological effects; their functional, sensory and nutritional characteristics are discussed in detail in other sources (e.g., Iyengar & Gross, 1991; Khan, 1993; Lucca & Tepper, 1994; Mela, 1996c; in press). Carbohydrate- and protein-based fat replacement materials can be considered to be nutritionally well understood, and their digestion and metabolism raise few new issues or complications. While these materials suffer from very significant sensory and functional limitations as fat replacers, they are presently used in a range of foods, and are generally effective in delivering fat-like textures in many products with high water contents.

Ingredients in the other major category, the lipid-based materials, can have functional and sensory characteristics very similar to the fats they might replace, and therefore offer much broader scope for potential applications. Several of the lipid-based materials in Table 5.3 are completely resistant to hydrolysis in the gut, and are therefore excreted intact, with effectively zero metabolizable energy value. However, uncertainty about the long-term safety, and particularly nutritional and gastrointestinal side-effects, has been an obstacle to the wider approval and food use of non-absorbable lipids (Mela, 1996c; in press). At this writing, only one of these materials, a mix of hexa-, hepta-, and octa- fatty acid esters of

Table 5.3 Examples of current and proposed ingredients for fat replacement (from Mela, In press [a], with permission)

Carbohydrate and protein-based
Modified glucose polymers
Modified starches
   e.g., from tapioca, corn, potato, rice, oats
Non-starch polysaccharides
   e.g., pectins, gums, marine colloids, cellulose derivatives
Native proteins
   e.g., gelatin, maize protein, whey protein concentrate
Microparticulated proteins

Lipid-based
Fatty acid esters of sugars or sugar alcohols
   e.g., olestra
Other non-absorbed/poorly absorbed non-triglyceride lipids
   none currently approved
Structured lipids containing specific fatty acids
Medium-chain triglycerides

Emulsifiers and functional ingredients
   e.g., polyglycerol esters, mono- and diglycerides, actylates, lecithin

sucrose ('sucrose polyester', now assigned the generic name olestra), has been approved for very limited food use (only in the United States). Several other materials take advantage of the incomplete absorption of naturally occurring long-chain saturated fatty acids, and the lower caloric density of medium and short chain fatty acids. These are used to generate structured triglycerides with a reported energy density of approximately 5 kcal/g (20 kJ/g) (Peters *et al.*, 1991; Finley *et al.*, 1994).

(b) Reduced-sugar and reduced-fat foods: influences on dietary intakes

Other than any specific pharmacological effects of the ingredients themselves, fat and sugar substitutes can only impact on weight control through the effects that consumption of products containing them might have upon overall dietary intakes. Critical to this is whether consumption of reduced-sugar or reduced-fat foods actually generates changes in sucrose or fat intakes, or energy density of the diet.

Data from experimental studies (Mela, 1997; Gatenby *et al.*, 1997; Naismith & Rhodes, 1996) and theoretical considerations (Beaton *et al.*, 1992; Anderson & Leiter, 1996) suggest that replacement of sucrose with intense sweeteners should lead to a reduction in carbohydrate intake (as sugars), but perhaps also to a higher proportion of dietary energy being derived from fat. In a prospective intervention trial, we found that use of reduced-sugar foods led to a significant decline in sucrose intakes, and amongst initially high sucrose consumers this was accompanied by a significant increase in the proportion of energy from fat in their diets (Gatenby *et al.*, 1997; Mela, 1997). Furthermore, there is also considerable evidence that fat and sugar intakes tend to be negatively correlated within and between many populations (Section 6.3). However, the limited cross-sectional data indicate that individual or population use of sugar substitutes does not have any significant association with intakes of any macronutrients, including sugars (Mela, in press; Chen & Parham, 1991; Anderson & Leiter, 1996). This apparent discrepancy can be resolved by considering how reduced-sugar products are actually used.

Models predicting that intense sweetener use might result in lower carbohydrate and greater fat intake rest on the assumptions that 1) consumers actually replace sugar-sweetened products with the sugar substituted versions, and 2) that individuals exhibit caloric compensation which is not food- or macronutrient-specific. Most experimental feeding studies suggest that the latter is generally true [Section 5.1.1(b)]; but available information is consistent with the notion that, in practice, sugar-substituted foods are commonly added to pre-existing diets rather than specifically used in place of sugar-containing foods. Given this, and that much of sugar substitute use is in products with negligible macronutrient or energy content (e.g. 'diet' beverages and tabletop sweeteners), the impact of additional intense sweetener intakes on intakes of sugars or total energy or, indeed, intakes of any macronutrients (or micronutrients) might actually be very small. This view of consumer behaviour should be borne in mind in extrapolating from research studies based on the assumption or imposition of direct substitution.

None of the relevant studies on sugar substitutes has computed or reported implications for energy density, but this does not generally hold a close relationship with sucrose content of foods. Although reduced-sugar foods themselves are generally of lower energy density than their traditionally formulated counterparts, because of the issues raised in the preceding discussion it is not clear whether use of reduced-sugar foods would have a meaningful effect on overall energy density of the diet, or even whether any effects would be positive or negative. In the only long-term prospective study where free-living consumers directly purchased and used reduced-sugar foods, this led to a significant reduction in sucrose intakes, but no change in total energy intakes (relative to controls) or in body weight over a 10-week period (Gatenby *et al.*, 1997).

These data and others provide theoretical and empirical support for the view that use of non-nutritive sweeteners should not be expected to generate spontaneous weight loss. The potential role of these products within weight loss programmes is less certain, but there are few data which actually lend support to the specific restriction of sugar intakes as a part of weight loss strategies. Data from a 'pilot' study by Kanders *et al.* (1988) is often cited as evidence of the benefits of use of intense sweeteners in slimming, although the results are equivocal. Recent studies have apparently failed to identify any substantial benefit of sucrose restriction in weight loss diets (Surwit *et al.*, 1996; Raben *et al.*, 1996; West & de Looy, 1996), although there is little information on the long-term acceptability or compliance with diets containing sugars vs sugar substitutes. Much of the emphasis on sugar intakes and obesity seems to have developed from anecdote, but the issue has also been promoted and pursued in the scientific literature (see Geiselman & Novin, 1982). Given present knowledge of effects of food composition, there seems to be little convincing evidence specifically linking long-term consumption of carbohydrate in any form to the development of human obesity (and some evidence to the opposite). Nevertheless, established views still flourish in the academic literature; for example, 'researchers have firmly established that carbohydrates, especially the low-molecular-weight sweet sugars, contribute to obesity to the extent that they increase the palatability of foods in general and cause foods to be consumed in amounts greater than those needed for normal caloric maintenance' (Daniel & Whistler, 1994, page 342). Such a view is clearly not consistent with the metabolic, sensory, or epidemiological data presented in this book, or elsewhere (Hill & Prentice, 1995; Anderson, 1995).

Modelling studies indicate that marked reductions in fat intake could be achieved through use of a limited number of reduced-fat alternative products, at least amongst individuals who usually eat particular items with high frequency (Lyle *et al.*, 1991), although many different dietary approaches could be taken to reach the same effect (Smith-Schneider *et al.*, 1992). As with sugar substitutes, these models largely assume direct substitution for full-fat products by their reduced-fat alternatives.

Relevant prospective intervention studies of free-living consumers, focusing specifically on realistic consumption of commercial reduced-fat foods, generally indicate that their use should contribute to a reduction in the proportion of energy derived from fat (Gatenby *et al.*, 1995; Gatenby *et al.*, 1997; Westerterp *et al.*, 1996c; de Graaf *et al.*, in press). In these trials, subjects were not fixed into strict dietary or food selection regimens, and had the opportunity to simultaneously purchase and consume modified and traditional items of any composition *ad libitum*, and hence the potential to achieve any final level of relative macronutrient intake. This methodological approach contrasts with more controlled studies where subjects have been placed on regimens of covert and/or relatively fixed composition (such as Kendall *et al.*, 1991) or been assigned very clear and prescriptive dietary targets (e.g., for fat intake or weight loss). Marked reduction in relative fat content (and energy density) of the diet is generally associated with modest spontaneous weight loss (Section 5.1.2). However, in free-choice studies of consumers, it is apparent that changes in macronutrient intake amongst users of reduced-fat foods is largely restricted to those subjects with a starting fat intake above 35% of energy, with little change occurring amongst subjects with moderate or low initial fat intakes (de Graaf *et al.*, in press; Mela, 1997). It is likely that use of many reduced-fat products should generate reductions in overall diet energy density; however, because of the actual formulation of these products (specifically, replacement of fat by carbohydrate), energy density may differ little from the traditional full-fat versions.

Overall, given these data, and considering the effects of diet composition described elswhere in this Chapter, substitution for fat seems likely to be a helpful approach to the prevention of overweight, though only if it is in fact associated with meaningful reductions in fat intakes and energy density. On the other hand, the situation for simple substitution for sugar in foods is less clear, particularly if it is associated with compensatory increases in fat consumption, unless use of reduced-sugar foods can also be clearly shown to be associated with a reduced overall diet energy density. However, effectiveness of such products also rests on averting any physiologically or cognitively based behavioural responses which might prompt counteracting changes in food selection patterns and energy intakes. It should also be borne in mind that the apparent nutritional purposes of these products (reduced sucrose or reduced fat intakes) can be achieved by many different approaches, not necessarily requiring use of specifically modified food products (Kristal *et al.*, 1992; Smith-Schneider *et al.*, 1992; Mela, in press). Thus, the more important questions may relate to how or whether such products contribute to (or possibly obstruct) compliance, acceptance, and maintenance of desired dietary habits.

5.2   PALATABILITY, FOOD COMPOSITION AND ENERGY BALANCE

The theoretical and fundamental backgrounds to the issue of palatability and eating behaviour are examined in Chapter 2, and here we consider evidence relating palatability to the selection and intake of diets which may specifically contribute to overeating and obesity.

In both the lay and scientfic literature, it is widely assumed that 'palatability' (usually spoken of as a property of a food) is an important determinant of intake. This seems an intuitively attractive proposition. In consumer surveys, sensory properties are invariably rated as a primary determinant of food selections and brand choice. Furthermore, both experimental and anecdotal observation show that, when given a simple choice within a meal, individuals are more likely to select and consume more of foods which are better liked (more 'palatable'). And, in general, sweet and savoury high-fat, energy-dense foods are judged to be highly 'palatable'. However, these common sense facts are not evidence that there is a primary *independent* effect of palatability on intake. This implies the existence of unlearned attractions and behavioural responses. If palatability has independent behavioural effects, then it becomes important to identify whether these explain variance in human body weight status. There are a number of complexities to this issue, which influence the interpretation of experimental data.

Experimental results attributed to 'palatability' may often actually be fundamental effects of food composition. As noted in the preceding sections, there is increasing evidence from human studies that diets high in fat or energy density may be associated with overeating and weight gain. However, many short-term experiments have confounded palatability and composition, by comparing (usually) highly liked, energy-dense foods or diets to less liked foods or diets of lower energy density. Furthermore, it is possible that certain sensory qualities may stimulate intake by influences beyond palatability alone (e.g., Green & Blundell, 1996; Greenberg & Smith, 1996). Animal studies specifically attempting to dissect the influences of composition and palatability or flavour variety have led to mixed interpretations regarding the existence and relative contribution of the short-term independent effects of each factor (Treit *et al.*, 1983; Louis-Sylvestre *et al.*, 1984; Warwick & Schiffman, 1991; Naim & Kare, 1991; Friedman & Mattes, 1991; Section 2.3.3). Some of the discrepancies may be related to the ability of animals to use flavours as a reliable cue to energy density under certain conditions where food composition and flavour are varied (Warwick & Schiffman, 1991; Section 5.1.3).

Research into the basis of the apparently high sensory appeal of high-fat or energy-dense foods bears out the complexities involved in making these distinctions. As discussed in detail in Chapter 2, palatability of a food stimulus can clearly be altered by the nutritional or other physiological aftereffects with which it is associated. Several studies suggest that animals may express an ostensibly unlearned liking for fat-associated, 'greasy' textures at birth or soon thereafter (Ackerman *et al.*, 1992; Ackroff *et al.*, 1990; Elizalde & Sclafani, 1990a). However, these experiments have not excluded the very real possibility of associative learning occurring during the exposure to sensory characteristics of milk prior to weaning (see Mela & Catt, 1996). Warwick *et al.* (1990) have described lingering preferences for high vs low-fat diets amongst animals which had been fed low-fat diets following high-fat post-weaning diets. In human infants, Nysenbaum and Smart (1982) reported modest evidence suggesting more avid sucking for higher vs lower fat milks; however, no differences were observed by Woolridge *et al.* (1980) or in recent work from our own laboratory (Catt *et al.*, in press). There is other evidence from rats showing that acceptance and intake responses to the orosensory properties of fats (nutritive or non-nutritive) can be expressed independently of any apparent associated post-ingestive reinforcement (Carlisle & Stellar, 1969; Greenberg & Smith,1996; Lucas & Sclafani,1996a). These data strongly suggest that there is an unlearned component to the positive hedonic response to 'fatty' textures and, interestingly, also indicate that this generalized sensory response is heightened by food deprivation (Lucas & Sclafani, 1996a).

While there may be unlearned attractions to some fat-associated sensory (probably textural) quality, there is also good evidence from longer-term feeding experiments that rats come to greatly prefer and consume nutritive over non-nutritive fats (Hamilton, 1964; Carlisle & Stellar, 1969; Ackroff *et al.*, 1990). Studies on young children also confirm that human flavour preferences can be shifted by positive associations with higher-fat, more energy-dense food vehicles (Johnson *et al.*, 1991; Kern *et al.*, 1993). Several experiments suggest that odour volatiles (or perhaps specific free fatty acids or other breakdown products) may provide the sensory cue which allows differentiation of oil sources and learning to be expressed (Ramirez, 1992; Kinney & Antill, 1996; Mabayo *et al.*, 1996). The formation and duration of preferences for higher-fat stimuli and diets may, however, be considerably influenced by prior dietary experience (Lucas & Sclafani, 1996b; Warwick *et al.*, 1990; Tepper & Friedman, 1989; Reed & Friedman, 1990). In addition, although there have been few direct comparisons, it appears that isocaloric high-fat and high-carbohydrate stimuli have a similar capacity to induce development of learned flavour preferences in animals (Mehiel & Bolles, 1988; Tordoff *et al.*, 1987), suggesting that caloric density and provision of usable fuels for oxidation (Tordoff *et al.*, 1987), rather than fat *per se*, may be the critical reinforcing component of test media and foods (Section 2.3.3).

At a very practical level, there are logical arguments against a simple relationship amongst the hedonic value of foods, long-term energy intake, and obesity in humans. Differences in palatability do not appear to be a necessary prerequisite for changes in *ad libitum* energy intake when dietary energy density is varied. Duncan *et al.* (1983), Lissner *et al.* (1987), Kendall *et al.* (1991), and Stubbs *et al.* (1995) all found differences in energy intake and weight change on diets varying in fat and/or energy density, but also reported that hedonic ratings of the experimental diets were similar, suggesting that differences in palatability of the regimens did not meaningfully contribute to the outcomes. However, it is possible that different results might have been observed if palatability of the diets had been systematically manipulated, especially if particular diets were strongly unpleasant.

Vast differences in palatability of eaten foods are not generally experienced within the agro-economic climate of most western nations, where most consumers are surrounded by a world of readily accessible, highly 'palatable' items, and can choose to eat foods which they like, and avoid foods which they dislike. The general presence and intake of highly liked foods is not new, and is not necessarily a primary or sufficient cause for overconsumption. It would be extremely difficult to attribute recent increases in the prevalence of obesity in these societies to some concomitant recent improvement in the sensory quality or hedonic acceptability of the food supply. Indeed, while most people like most foods, they would not want to eat even their most favoured foods at every possible occasion. In support of this, data from the United States armed forces (Meiselman *et al.*, 1974) revealed that only 48 out of a list of 378 food items received less than a neutral mean score for liking. Furthermore, ratings of preferred frequency of consumption indicated that respondents would not wish to consume any of the top ranked 25 items (excluding beverages) as often as every other day. There are also a very large number of foods which are frequently consumed, and contribute a high proportion of energy intakes, despite the fact that they are not individually regarded as exceptionally highly liked. Basic criteria for the cultural recognition of an entity as 'food' (as opposed to just 'edible') would seem to imply that the item is eaten with some degree of frequency, and reasonably well-liked, by at least a significant portion of the population. This does not, however, exclude the possibility that there is a subset of the population for whom the availability of foods having a particular combination of sensory appeal and composition (e.g., high fat, energy dense) represents a situation within which underlying psychological, behavioural, and/or physiological conditions can be manifested in overeating (Chapters 8 and 9).

There is no clear evidence that obesity is specifically associated with a heightened responsiveness to 'palatable' foods, although it remains possible. Under a variety of choice situations, both lean and obese individuals will be more likely to consume foods which are better liked (more palatable). It has, however, been suggested that obese individuals may demonstrate greater responsiveness to the hedonic aspects of foods, with palatability having a particularly potent influence on consumption (Mela, 1996b; Spitzer & Rodin, 1981; Chapter 8). This may be true, but most of the relevant data have come from short-term studies and laboratory settings, and it has not been established whether sustained selection and consumption of more 'palatable' foods over a longer period continues to stimulate overconsumption, or whether data derived from single foods extends to meal combinations or entire diets eaten in normal surroundings. There is, to our knowledge, presently no study which has systematically tracked individuals' ratings for liking of all foods selected over a significant time period, in order to assess whether diets which consist of a greater volume or frequency of better liked foods is associated with greater energy intake or measures of adiposity.

The sensory components and hedonic value of foods may influence postprandial appetite; however, studies have found that consumption of more palatable meals or preloads may either enhance (Hill *et al.*, 1984; Rogers & Schutz, 1992) or suppress (Warwick *et al.*, 1993) subsequent feelings of hunger and also food intake at a later meal. Sensory stimulation and palatability clearly influence a spectrum of pre- and postprandial metabolic events, some of which are known to modulate hunger and nutrient utilization (Simon *et al.*, 1986; Teff & Engelman, 1996; Feldman & Richardson, 1986). Notably, cephalic phase insulin release has been shown to be better related to differences in dietary restraint (Chapter 8) than to obesity (Simon *et al.*, 1986) or to differences in the palatability of the food stimulus (Teff & Engelman, 1996). While palatability does not apparently have any significant effect on postprandial energy expenditure (Westrate *et al.*, 1990), there seems to be justification to continue to examine the effects of palatability in one eating occasion on later appetite control, and its relationships with diet, cognitive restraint and weight control. Some care may be required to avoid artifactual effects of food manipulations; e.g., Westerterp-Plantenga *et al.* (1992) found that TEF was raised upon first experience with an unfamiliar food (an effect ascribed to enhanced sympathetic nervous system activity).

These arguments support the view, detailed in Chapter 2, that ingestion may be positively stimulated by palatability, but that palatability is in turn often a learned response to the post-ingestive nutritional or physiological consequences of ingestion. When palatability is controlled, high-fat, energy-dense diets still appear to exert strong and lasting independent effects upon intakes. The position then becomes circular: palatable foods produce high energy intakes in part because they tend to be highly energy dense, and energy-dense foods produce high energy intakes in part because they are highly palatable. In the real world palatability is not controlled, and learned (and perhaps also inborn) preferences can contribute to a high palatability of energy-dense foods and diets, the composition of which allows for passive intake of high amounts of energy.

5.3   POST-PRANDIAL INFLUENCES OF FOOD COMPOSITION

In addition (or related) to differences in their influences on processes of satiation and satiety, changes in the macronutrient mix may prompt different post-prandial responses which could be implicated in weight control. These experiments generally use diets in which composition is varied at fixed energy contents. As in other work, the primary manipulation has been the ratios of fat and carbohydrates. While we acknowledge that changes in food composition will have a wide range of effects on blood and tissue biochemical measures, the discussion here will focus exclusively on aspects of energy balance.

Although differences in TEF have been demonstrated in studies feeding pure macronutrients or meals with extremes of macronutrient content, it does not appear that TEF is much affected by the composition of foods within 'normal' ranges (Westerterp-Plantenga *et al.*, 1997). Several short-term studies show that, although nutrient utilization is markedly influenced by wide variations in diet composition, macronutrient composition does not appear to significantly influence energy balance on isoenergetic diets fed at or below weight maintenance levels (Verboeket-van de Venne *et al.*, 1994; Abbott *et al.*, 1990; Hill *et al.*, 1991b; Hurni *et al.*, 1981; Lean & James, 1988). However, these studies also consistently indicated that, while RQ and FQ (Section 3.4.1) were similar on higher-fat diets, FQ exceeded RQ on the high-carbohydrate diets. This would indicate the latter diets led to a negative fat balance (fat intakes below fat oxidation), a situation which would over time result in weight loss. The apparent discrepancy between these data and the data on energy expenditure seems most likely to reflect the time course over which suppression of fat oxidation develops on a high carbohydrate diet (Horton *et al.*, 1995). The data on energy balance are supported by longer-term studies (below).

With the notable exception of one trial (Prewitt *et al.*, 1991), long-term trials confirm that isoenergetic diets varying in fat and carbohydrate differ little in their effects on energy balance or body weight when fed at weight maintenance levels (Roust *et al.*, 1994; Rumpler *et al.*, 1991) or as part of hypocaloric, weight loss regimens (Peterson & Jovanovic-Peterson, 1995; Golay *et al.*, 1996a; 1996b; Leibel *et al.*, 1992; Rumpler *et al.*, 1991). This parallels the result found when subjects were allowed to eat *ad libitum* from diets of differing composition but the same energy density, since intakes of these diets were approximately equivalent (Stubbs *et al.*, 1996). The responses of lean and obese individuals to long-term diet manipulations within the normal range (27 vs 40% energy from fat) also appear to be similar (Roust *et al.*, 1994). However, Thomas *et al.* (1992) suggested that lean individuals may adjust RQ to shifts in FQ more quickly, and that this might improve resistance to weight gain on high-fat diets. The 'nutrient utilization' hypothesis (Section 3.4.2) also provides a mechanism whereby high-fat diets may be more problematic for weight control in susceptible individuals.

In contrast to these other studies, Prewitt *et al.* (1991) reported that maintenance of body weight required substantially higher energy intakes from a 20% fat diet than from a 37% fat diet. However, this study used free-living subjects who may have altered their physical activity or, more likely, not eaten all of the food provided for them on the low-fat diet. The latter possibility would be consistent with data on the effects of *ad libitum* reduced fat, low energy density diets on food intake and satiety (Section 5.1). Long-term changes in the proportion of fat in the diet do not apparently have any effects on physical activity and energy expenditure (Verboeket-van de Venne *et al.*,1996; Westerterp *et al.*, 1996b).

When macronutrients are fed in excess of requirements, differences between fat and carbohydrate could theoretically become more apparent. It is well known that energy from fat is more efficiently converted to storage fat than energy from other macronutrients (Danforth, 1985; Donato, 1987). The reasons for this largely lie in the established differences in metabolic efficiency of formation of depot fat from these substrates; viz., the greater cost of *de novo* lipogenesis from non-fat substrates compared

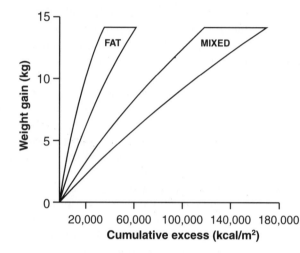

Figure 5.3   Apparent differences in rates of weight gain relative to caloric excess, during intentional overfeeding of different groups of men with a mixed or a high-fat diet. Note that only the high-fat diet group was in a research unit with restricted access to activity, smoking, and caffeine. Figure from Danforth (1985) with permission.

with the re-esterification of dietary fatty acids. Simply stated, it is considerably more efficient to re-form body fat from dietary fat than to synthesize it from something else. Studies of prolonged overfeeding on different diets apparently seem to show evidence of this effect (Danforth, 1985); however, the result shown in Figure 5.3 almost certainly exaggerates this effect, for reasons described below.

While humans clearly have the capacity to convert carbohydrate to fat, the evidence from a large number of biochemical and metabolic studies indicates that this occurs to only a very limited extent under the usual physiological and dietary conditions of western diets (Acheson *et al.* 1982; 1984; Björntorp & Sjöström, 1978; Hellerstein *et al.*, 1991; Hellerstein, 1996; Hoffman *et al.*, 1980; Passmore & Swindells, 1963; Sandhofer *et al.*, 1969; Weiss *et al.*, 1986). High rates of *de novo* lipogenesis from carbohydrate can occur, but apparently only with prolonged consumption of high carbohydrate loads in excess of energy expenditure (Acheson *et al.*, 1988; Pasquet *et al.*, 1992). The historical inclusion of *de novo* lipogenesis as a common and significant feature of human energy metabolism probably stems from misapplication of animal data. There is evidence that, compared with humans, the enzymatic machinery in laboratory animals maintains a much greater potential for high rates of lipogenesis (Zelewski & Swierczynki, 1990), and most biochemical studies have relied upon animals fed commercial laboratory pellets or semi-synthetic diets extremely low in fat, hence maximizing lipogenic activity.

This low level of fat synthesis from carbohydrate has been incorrectly interpreted as indicating that it may be difficult to induce fat deposition on a high-carbohydrate, low-fat diet (Mela, 1996a). This fails to take account of the fact that high-carbohydrate diets markedly suppress fat oxidation (Section 3.4.1). Thus, the well-controlled overfeeding study of Horton *et al.* (1995) showed that, with time, excess intakes given as fat or carbohydrate eventually produced similar rates of net fat storage. In the case of carbohydrate overfeeding, this was due largely to suppression of fat oxidation (plus storage of dietary fat), rather than lipogenesis. Notably, though, there was a 7–14-day time period required for the two diets to achieve these similar effects. In the interim period, fat oxidation was not fully inhibited by the high carbohydrate load, and fat storage was higher with fat overfeeding. These authors therefore suggested that, whereas there may be no difference with sustained diets, periodic bouts of excessive fat intakes might be more likely to produce fat deposition and weight gain than similar excesses comprised largely of carbohydrate.

In light of current understanding of carbohydrate–fat relationships, results such as those shown in Figure 5.3 are anomalous, and in this example are apparently due to other differences in the protocols other than diet, such as access to physical activity. Such a marked difference in efficiency of weight gain is likely to occur only with a significant level of lipogenesis, and this seems to require excessive consumption of a regimen quite exceptionally (for western diets) low in fat content.

5.4 SUMMARY

Food composition may have both behavioural and physiological influences on energy balance, which could reflect direct effects on hunger and satiation, relationships with palatability and the desire to eat, and post-prandial influences on energy metabolism.

In the short term, a very large number of compositional and subject characteristics have been shown to influence appetite. However, observations in the short and the long term also can be highly dependent upon the methodology applied. In general, some degree of compensatory eating occurs in response to covert reductions or supplementation of energy in foods and meals, but the response is imperfect, especially to supplementation. It also appears that energy from fat may not suppress hunger or delay eating to the same extent as energy from other macronutrients. There is mixed evidence regarding the likelihood of 'defects' in the responses of obese individuals in such tests.

Over the longer term, when provided in the context of an unlimited diet of varied composition, changes in the composition of a limited number of foods (e.g., casual use of reduced-fat or reduced-sugar products) seem to influence the macronutrient composition of the diet, but may be expected to have only small impact upon spontaneous energy intakes. However, the effects are dependent upon the magnitude of change: significant changes in the composition of the total diet, particularly its energy density, appear to have more substantial and lasting effects on energy intakes. Individuals placed on long-term, *ad libitum* low-fat (low energy density) diets consistently show modest, spontaneous weight losses, and it seems likely that such diets would also exert a protective effect against weight gain.

These data generally support the view that energy intake in humans is not under tight physiological regulation, and indicate that energy density can have significant 'passive' influences on intakes, at least over short- and medium-term periods. However, little work has been carried out on structural and mechanical properties of foods which may interact with nutrient content to influence hunger and satiation.

Changes in intakes on different diets may be commonly attributed to 'palatability', and it is possible that obesity is associated with a heightened responsiveness to palatable foods. However, palatability cannot be readily separated from diet composition, which can be shown both to influence energy intake independent of palatability, and to be a determinant of palatability itself.

When energy intake is held constant, short-and long-term trials confirm that diet composition has (perhaps surprisingly) very little effect on energy balance or body weight. There may be certain situations (e.g., irregular patterns of consumption) and individuals in which higher fat consumption tends to promote greater fat deposition relative to similar energy intakes of carbohydrate. However, obligate or total energy expenditures do not appear to differ except between extremes of composition. If energy expenditure does not differ in relation to composition, then any long-term effects on energy balance can **only** be attributable to influences on intake.

It therefore seems that the primary influence of food composition is its effects upon eating behaviour.

CHAPTER SIX

Sensory responses, food preferences and macronutrient selection

It is commonly suggested that the liking for selected sensory qualities and food types may be heightened in overweight and obese individuals, and that this may be a factor contributing to or sustaining excessive energy intakes. Historically, almost all of this research has been directed toward sweet taste preferences, as a result of supposed associations between sweet foods, sugar intake, and overeating, but more recent work has focused on fats. Research examining preferences and choices have applied a wide range of methods, with a variety of different possible outcome measures (Table 6.1).

Table 6.1 Examples of measurement variables in assessments of sensory and food preferences

Test items
    Simple controlled stimuli
    Complex real or model foods
Context
    Sensory evaluation (laboratory) test
    Home trial
    Actual purchase situation
Hedonic ratings
    Tasting
    Questionnaire
Preferred frequency of consumption ratings
    Tasting
    Questionnaire
Behavioural data
    Purchase information or records
    Diet history or records
Food groupings
    Nutritional criteria
    Sensory characteristics
    Source or degree of preparation required
    Typical use/culinary role

6.1   OBESITY, SENSORY PERCEPTION AND SENSORY PREFERENCES

Several *caveats* should be borne in mind in interpreting the results of sensory studies, with particular relevance to overweight subjects. There is always a potential for cognitive bias; i.e., subjects reporting what they wished they felt or what they believe to be the most appropriate response. This may, for example, lead obese subjects to be less inclined to report a liking for obviously sweet stimuli. There may also be confusion between liking (sensory preference) and desire or motivation to consume a stimulus (cf. Section 2.3.5). Thus, subjects may assign lower ratings to stimuli which they like, but which they would not want to eat for unrelated reasons (e.g., because of concerns regarding weight gain). Cause and effect are not clear: most studies have examined subjects already overweight or obese, and even objectively verified preferences or behaviours could be an outcome of current status, dissimilar to those preceding or coincident with periods of active weight gain. Lastly, the implications of sensory preferences for food selection or overeating are not obvious. While common experience suggests that sensory factors exert a role in human food selection, there is a lack of more objective measurement of the function of sensory and other factors in this process, and numerous reasons why experimentally derived sensory and dietary intake data generally fail to bear out close associations (Shepherd & Farleigh, 1989).

6.1.1   General sensory and hedonic responses

Obesity does not appear to be associated with differences in perceptual sensitivity to the organoleptic characteristics of foods. In particular, there is relatively good agreement that obese and lean individuals do not differ in their sensitivity to or perceptions of intensity of sweetness in foods or beverages (Drewnowski *et al.*, 1985; Frijters & Rasmussen-Conrad, 1982; Grinker, 1978; Grinker *et al.*, 1972; Rodin, 1975a; Rodin *et al.*, 1976; Thompson *et al.*, 1976; Thompson *et al.*, 1977; Witherly *et al.*, 1980). Most studies have also found no difference in the sweet taste preferences of lean and obese subjects (Drewnowski *et al.*, 1985; Frijters & Rasmussen-Conrad, 1982; Grinker *et al.*, 1972; Pangborn & Simone, 1958; Rodin, 1975; Thompson *et al.*, 1977; Witherly *et al.*, 1980). This also includes studies of newborn babies of obese and non-obese mothers (Grinker *et al.*, 1986). However, there are occasional reports of both increased (Cabanac, 1971; Rodin *et al.*, 1976) and decreased (Grinker *et al.*, 1972; Johnson *et al.*, 1979) liking for sweet taste among overweight individuals, and more complex assessment methods have pointed to possible effects of recent or long-term weight loss on sweet taste preferences (e.g., Rodin *et al.*, 1976; Rodin, 1980; Kleifield & Lowe, 1990).

Far less information is available regarding perceptions and hedonic responses in relation to other taste, aroma, or textural qualities, or to the complex qualities of real foods. Malcolm *et al.* (1980) reported no differences between lean and obese subjects for taste sensitivity or liking of sweet, sour, salty, or bitter stimuli, and Thompson *et al.* (1977) found no differences for the perceived intensity or liking of a food-related aroma (benzaldehyde). Drewnowski *et al.* (1982) reported no consistent lean vs obese differences in flavour perception or preferences for a range of commercially available sweetened soft drinks. However, Witherly *et al.* (1980) noted that, relative to normal weight subjects, obese subjects tended to be less capable of discriminating viscosity, assigned higher intensity scores for viscosity of a test beverage, and appeared to prefer a lower viscosity. This latter finding contrasts with more recent data on sensory responsiveness to fats (described below), and further work on texture perception and preferences seems warranted.

6.1.2 Sensory responsiveness to fat-containing stimuli

The most recent work on sensory perception and preferences in the obese has focused on perceptions and acceptance of fats in foods. Obese and lean subjects have not been found to differ in their perceptions of fat content or creaminess of a range of sweetened milk and·cream samples (Drewnowski *et al.*, 1985) or model oil-in-water emulsions (Mela *et al.*, 1994). However, Drewnowski and colleagues (Drewnowski & Greenwood, 1983; Drewnowski *et al.*, 1985) showed that fat could greatly enhance liking for a sweetened, milk-based test vehicle and, in particular, raised the notion that sugar might represent an important vehicle for sensory acceptance of fat in the diet. In a widely cited study, Drewnowski *et al.* (1985) presented evidence that obese and recently reduced, formerly obese individuals show enhanced preferences for higher fat levels in this test food system, and suggested that liking and consumption of sweet, high-fat foods might be a particular feature in the development or maintenance of obesity. In contrast, Pangborn *et al.* (1985) found relative body weight unrelated to preferences for plain or chocolate flavoured milks of differing fat content. Subsequent studies by Drewnowski and colleagues (Drewnowski *et al.*, 1991; Drewnowski & Holden-Wiltse, 1992) have generally confirmed their initial findings, and suggested that a greater preference for sweet, high-fat stimuli is particularly associated with a history of weight cycling.

The work of Drewnowski and colleagues (1985; 1991; 1992b; Drewnowski & Holden-Wiltse, 1992) has focused almost exclusively on fat–sugar combinations, and their results are often interpreted as suggesting that these are of particular concern in relation to food preferences and control of eating. However, we (Mela & Sacchetti, 1991) found a positive relationship, in subjects of normal weight for height, between percent body fat and the preferred fat content of a test battery comprised of both sweet and savoury foods, supporting the possibility that a more general-ized liking for fat-associated qualities, or fat–savoury combinations might be linked to a prediposition for obesity. This view is also in agree-ment with other ideas relating to heightened responsiveness to palatabil-ity in general (Section 8.2). It is also supported by the results of Kanarek and colleagues, who found that liking for a higher fat content in a test food (popcorn) was increased by higher salt content, amongst restrained, but not unrestrained women (Kanarek *et al.*, 1995), while measures of restraint did not relate to consistent differences in response to fat content of a sweet–fat combination (Frye *et al.*, 1994). However, Warwick & Schiffman (1990) reported no clear evidence for a greater fat preference amongst overweight subjects, for either fat–sugar·or fat–salt mixtures, although these data are weakened by the fact that the latter stimuli (salt added to milk or cream) were generally disliked. Fisher and Birch (1995) assessed young children's liking for fat-associated sensory qualities using a test battery comprising savoury high-fat and a mix of sweet and savoury low-fat items, and found significant positive correlations of fat preferences with measures of both child and parent fatness, and the child's fat intake.

One consistent finding seems to be that subjects who are **predisposed** to obesity all show heightened hedonic responses to fat-containing stim-uli: the children of fatter parents (Fisher & Birch, 1995), people who feel they need to restrain their eating for weight control (Kanarek *et al.* 1995), non-obese subjects at the high end of body fatness (Mela & Sacchetti, 1991), and those who are already obese or have previously been obese (Drewnowski *et al.*, 1985).

If predisposition for obesity is characterized by heightened sensory responsiveness to fats (and fat intakes, Section 6.2.3), the fundamental basis for this remains obscure. Liking for fat-associated sensory qualities in general may be acquired and sustained through experience, by the post-ingestive, psychobiological effects of fats contributing to an associa-tive conditioning process (Sections 2.3.3 and 5.2; Mela, 1995). It is con-ceivable that fat-containing foods might have greater reinforcing psychobiological effects for certain individuals or under certain condi-tions, therefore becoming more potent stimuli for the acquisition and maintenance of conditioned preferences, and increased liking. Physiologically, this might be mediated through variations in the stimu-lation or function of neural mechanisms involved in the acquisition or expression of hedonic responses in general. We (Mela, 1996b) have specu-lated on the possibility of a single or integrated underlying mechanism, causing both a preference for a high fat intake as well as predisposing individuals to gain weight on such a diet. However, at present there is no empirical evidence for this.

6.2 OBESITY, FOOD PREFERENCES AND SELECTIONS

There are surprisingly few published studies comparing either the stated food preferences or reported sources of nutrients consumed by lean and obese individuals. This information would appear to be central to addressing issues regarding whether specific foods or food groups are particularly linked with overeating. There are, however, a number of obstacles to conducting and interpreting research on acceptance or consumption of specific food groups. The primary difficulty is categorization of food items. Foods can and have been placed together based upon nutrient profile (high fat, low energy density, etc.), sensory characteristics (e.g., sweet, savoury), source or site of preparation (processed vs home-prepared), assumed role in cuisine ('snacks' vs 'meals'), or various combinations of these. These many different categorization schemes are clearly incompatible with each other, and specific schemes often seem contrived and illogical. Many studies lack a clear rationale for the categorizations used, and these different procedures do not facilitate development of a coherent summary of their results.

Table 6.2 provides an attempt at such a summary, and illustrates these problems, as well as the inconsistent outcomes of the research. The interpretation of the results of individual studies is also problematic. As with dietary intake data, the self-report data are highly suspect, and causality is clearly difficult to establish because obese individuals may select, or claim to select or avoid certain foods as a result of their present weight status.

In perhaps the most sophisticated field study, Coates *et al.* (1978) randomly selected and visited 65 suburban homes, collecting anthropometric data on family members and categorizing stored food by a defined system based on both energy density (kcal per serving) and overlapping descriptive categories. This approach is particularly interesting, because it ostensibly presents an accurate snapshot of actual food selections without bias due to self-reporting. In general, they found little evidence of any consistent relationships between degree of family or parental overweight and presence of foods in particular categories. However, degree of overweight in fathers was positively correlated with the number of (in their words) 'junk' (high fat/high sugar, ready to eat) and dessert items, and negatively correlated with low calorie foods.

A field study by Gates *et al.* (1975) also warrants mention, because it is both frequently cited and notably flawed. The investigators classified cafeteria foods into 2 groups: 'the protective foods that supply needed nutrients' (milk, meat and eggs, legumes, non-starchy vegetables, fruits, juices), and those 'relatively high in calories in proportion to their nutrient content' (virtually everything else, from bread and pasta to snack foods and sweets). Cafeteria patrons identified as obese in appearance were noted to consume a greater proportion of foods from the latter category than did non-obese patrons. The food categories used in this

Table 6.2 Examples of results of studies comparing self-reported preferences or intakes of specific foods and food groups of obese and non-obese subjects. Subjects were all adults unless stated otherwise. FFQ = Food Frequency Questionnaire used to assess intakes

Reference and measure	No. food groups	Differences, obese relative to non-obese: Direction of response and foods	
Meiselman, 1977	8		
Preferred frequency		↑	Entrées
Hedonic		↑	Entrées
Coates *et al.*, 1978	7		
Stored food		↑ (father)	Desserts 'junk' foods
		↓ (family)	'Processed' foods
Meiselman & Wyant, 1981	12		
Hedonic		↑	Carbonated beverages
Kulesza, 1982	17		
FFQ		No differences observed	
Baeke *et al.*, 1983	10		
2-day intake (correlation)		↓ (♀)	Fats & oils
		↓ (♀)	Sugars
		↓ (♂)	Fruit & veg
Pangborn *et al.*, 1985	9		
FFQ		↑	Meats
		↓	Avocado, olive
Roland-Cachera & Bellisle, 1986	17		
FFQ (age 7 to 12)		↑	Meats
		?	Eggs
Jacobsen & Thelle, 1987	12		
FFQ (correlation)		↑ and ↓	Many at low correlation (r < 0.1)
		↑	Low fat milk
		↓	Bread
Ortega *et al.*, 1995	13		
Weighed intake		↑	Fish
(age 15 to 17)		↓	Non-alcoholic beverages, Miscellaneous foods
Correlations with BMI:		↑	Fish, eggs
		↓	Fruit
Parker *et al.*, 1997 FFQ	7	None related to subsequent 4 yr weight change	

study were so broad and of such questionable rationale that it is difficult to draw any firm conclusions about consumption of specific foods or food groups. Furthermore, the procedures left open a substantial margin for unintentional bias on the part of the investigators. Nevertheless, the study has been used to support the view that certain types of foods and sweets are specifically preferred or overeaten by obese individuals (e.g., Drewnowski *et al.*, 1985).

Dietary intakes studies have generally revealed few if any consistent differences in specific food selection patterns associated with obesity. Morgan *et al.* (1983) analysed intakes of sugar and snacks (foods eaten between 'meals') from a large marketing study of 5 to 18 year olds, and found no consistent associations of weight status with eating behaviour. Kulesza (1982) reported no difference in consumption of 17 food groups by lean and obese Polish women. Baeke *et al.* (1983) found that percent body fat among Dutch men was negatively associated with proportion of energy derived from fruits and vegetables, and intakes of both sugar/sugar-rich products and fats and oils were negatively associated with fatness in females. However, there is a strong likelihood that the latter results reflect under-reporting, as total energy intake also declined with weight status in females (see Section 3.3). Pangborn *et al.* (1985) found that only self-reported consumption of meat was significantly greater among overweight than normal weight subjects.

In a summary of their studies of (United States) armed forces personnel, Meiselman (1977) reported that underweight subjects assigned higher hedonic and preferred frequency ratings to desserts, whereas overweight respondents tended to assign higher hedonic and preferred frequency ratings to entrées, particularly meats. In further analyses of this database, Meiselman and Wyant (1981) found that overweight subjects tended to show a greater preference for meats and entrées compared with average or underweight subjects, who showed a greater preference for fruits. Discriminant analysis suggested that preferences of lean individuals were best predicted by sweet dessert categories, while carbonated beverages, meats and sandwiches predicted preferences of obese subjects. However, the authors note that their results may partly reflect a sexual dichotomy, in that males are over-represented in the overweight group, and the preferences of males and females tended to correspond to the respective preferences of overweight and average weight subjects.

Possible gender differences in food preferences are also apparent in the work of Drewnowski *et al.* (1992b), who collected and analysed data on food preferences from a large population of obese individuals. They reported that the males indicated greater preferences for low-carbohydrate, high-fat or fat-plus-protein combinations (e.g., meats), while females preferred more fat-plus-carbohydrate combinations and sweet items (e.g., cakes, ice cream). However, the gender differences reported in that work are not consistently split along these lines, and the preferences expressed by both groups show many similarities. In general, foods with a high fat content (as opposed to high carbohydrate or sugar alone) tended to dominate responses in this obese population. Unfortunately, in the absence of corresponding responses from normal weight individuals, it is not clear whether the expressed preferences are actually specific to obesity, or characterize the general population. Casual inspection of the results suggests that most of the foods rated as highly liked by the obese subjects are also more widely popular (cf. Meiselman & Wyant, 1981). Drewnowski (1985) applied a novel, multidimensional scaling approach to assessing preferences of normal weight and obese subjects. Although the range of foods was rather limited, the results suggest greater liking for clusters of foods characterized as 'healthy' (milk, eggs, peanut butter, fruits and vegetables) and as energy-dense 'snacks' (ice cream, candy, carbonated beverages), by normal weight and obese subjects, respectively. However, dietary analyses focusing specifically on fat–sugar combinations have not found an association between BMI and intakes of sweet biscuits (cookies), cakes or confectionery (New & Grubb, 1996).

Although there is a lack of clear evidence (positive or negative) regarding whether foods high in 'extrinsic' (added) sugars or fat–sugar combinations are specifically linked to variance in weight status or overall macronutrient intakes, the view that these foods hold special and damaging roles in diet and weight control is widely held. Emmett & Heaton (1995) proposed that added sugars act as a particularly important vehicle for fat, a feature of this view being that sweetness promotes greater fat intake 'by making the fat more palatable' (Emmett & Heaton, 1995, page 1537). This was based largely on absolute intakes of fat and sugars from a limited dietary intake data set, and their interpretation has been criticized for the failure to correct for energy intakes. Larger eaters (whether due to obesity, physical activity, or normal body size) tend to eat more of everything, and it would not be remarkable to find that needs above average may be partially fulfilled by foods high in added sugars. In addition, the available evidence from sensory and preference studies outlined above suggest that a dominant role. for salted, savoury (rather than sugared, sweet) fat sources must be considered plausible. This view also gains support from analyses of data from a study where we asked subjects to assign predominant taste characteristics to foods as eaten and recorded, which revealed that fat intakes correlated positively with measures of consumption of foods characterized as 'salty', but negatively with intakes of 'sweet' foods (Figure 6.1) (unpublished analyses of data from Mela, 1989). Furthermore, the vast majority of dietary fat in the UK, like most western nations, is contributed by meat and meat products, spreading fats, dairy products, and other foods which are low in carbohydrate and generally unsweetened (Ministry of Agriculture, Fisheries and Food, 1995; Gregory *et al.*, 1990). Lastly, epidemiological data support a link between fat intakes, but not sugar, with obesity (see below). Nevertheless, relationships amongst sugar (and salt) and fat intakes, sensory preferences, and weight status, would be clarified by improved identification of the sources of variance in fat intakes, and by work linking actual food choices and individual consumer characteristics with subjective (sensory) and objective (nutrient composition) information on specific foods.

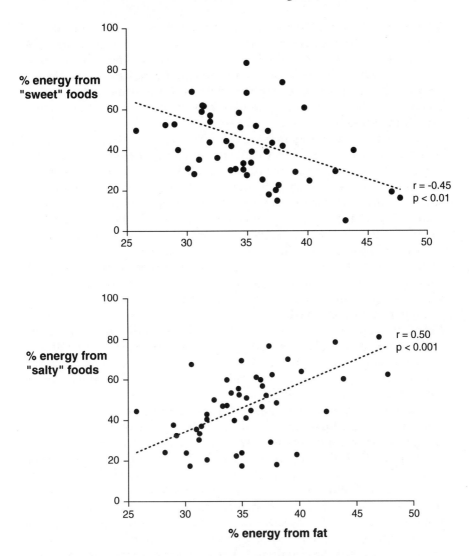

Figure 6.1 Relationships between dietary percent of energy from fat, and percent of energy derived from foods self-described as predominantly 'sweet' (top) or 'salty' (bottom) in 7-day diet records. n = 47 young men; unpublished data from Mela (1989).

6.3 MACRONUTRIENT INTAKES AND WEIGHT STATUS

In addition to the established problems of collecting valid dietary intake data (Section 3.3.2 and above), there are other difficulties in analyses and interpretation. For example, few studies in the obesity literature have controlled for dietary and lifestyle variables known to be significantly interrelated. This is particularly problematic, because a rise in the percentage of total energy intake derived from one macronutrient **must** correspond to reductions in the relative contribution of others. In addition, in common with other behavioural research, most studies have examined subjects already overweight or obese; thus, observed behaviours could be an outcome of current status, and dissimilar to those preceding or coincident with periods of active weight gain.

Intakes of fat and sugars have been the clear focus of much of the research on relationships between diet and weight status. Despite the noted problems with assessing dietary intakes, results from a large number of studies over the past 25 years document relatively consistent (if weak) positive associations between percent energy from fat and fatness (Table 6.3; reviewed by Lissner & Heitmann, 1995). Tucker & Kano (1995) found that the relationship between percent dietary fat and percent body fat was significant, even after controlling for other relevant lifestyle and dietary variables. This supports the view from other types of research (Chapter 5) that fat intakes may be exerting an independent influence on weight status (although this may reflect high energy density, which was not reported or controlled). Energy density is not commonly reported, although it can be relatively safely assumed that a diet high in percent energy from fat would signify a diet high in energy density. Westerterp *et al.* (1996a) found that, relative to lean controls, obese women ate a diet which was higher in fat and was shifted toward a higher proportion of foods high in energy density.

Longitudinal studies have generated mixed results regarding relationships between fat intakes at one time point and subsequent changes in weight or body composition (Klesges *et al.*, 1992; Colditz *et al.*, 1990; Parker *et al.*, 1997; Rolland-Cachera *et al.*, 1995; Eck *et al.*, 1995). However, there may be differences in susceptibility to high-fat diets due to genetic (Section 4.2.4; Heitmann *et al.*, 1995) or lifestyle (Simoes *et al.*, 1995; Lissner *et al.*, 1996) factors, and the short time frame of the studies could mask responsiveness to high fat intakes amongst a subsection of the population.

The apparent epidemiological links between fat intakes and measures of fatness also extend to children. Eck *et al.* (1995) reported that 3 to 5 year old children 'at risk' of obesity (having an overweight parent) had higher relative fat intakes at baseline, and greater 1 year weight gains than controls (neither parent overweight), suggesting that this pattern of intake might be established early in life. Other studies have found fat intakes of young children and adolescents were related to measures of fatness of these subjects (Obarzanek *et al.*, 1994; Ortega *et al.*, 1995; Maffeis *et al.*, 1996; Gazzaniga & Burns, 1993; Fisher & Birch, 1995), and also of their parents (Nguyen *et al.*, 1996; Fisher & Birch, 1995).

Where total carbohydrate or starch intakes have been reported, they are usually found to be negatively related to fatness (Gazzaniga & Burns, 1993; Ortega *et al.*, 1995; Tucker & Kano, 1992; Eck *et al.*, 1992; Dreon *et al.*,

Table 6.3 Relationships between measures of fatness (%BF = percent body fat; BMI = Body Mass Index; Wt/Ht = weight/height ratio) and dietary percent energy from fat. Cross-sectional studies, all n > 75 ; + = positive association, − = negative association, ns = no significant relationship. Modified and updated from Lissner & Heitmann (1995). Subjects were all adults unless otherwise stated

Reference	Subjects	Measure of fatness	Association
Lee & Lawler, 1983	122 ♂	Wt/Ht	ns
Fehily *et al.*, 1984	493 ♂	BMI	ns
Lissner, 1987	9286 ♂, ♀	%BF	+
Dreon *et al.*, 1988	155 ♂	BMI, %BF	+
Romieu *et al.*, 1988	141 ♀	BMI	+
Tremblay *et al.*, 1989	133 ♂	%BF	+
George *et al.*, 1990	679 ♂, ♀	BMI	+
	360 ♂, ♀	%BF	ns
Miller *et al.*, 1990	216 ♂, ♀	%BF	+
Colditz *et al.*, 1990	32K ♀	BMI	+
Eck *et al.*, 1992a	6572♂, ♀	BMI	ns (♂)
			− (♀)
Tucker & Kano, 1992	205 ♀	BMI	+
Slattery *et al.*, 1992	5115 ♂, ♀	BMI, skinfolds	ns
Klesges *et al.*, 1992	294 ♂, ♀	BMI	+
Miller *et al.*, 1994b	78 ♂, ♀	%BF	+
Lissner & Lindroos, 1994	412 ♀	BMI	ns
Obarzanek *et al* , 1994	2379 ♀ (age 9–10)	BMI	ns (black ♀)
			+ (white ♀)
Nelson & Tucker, 1996	203 ♂	Skinfolds	+
Maffeis *et al.*, 1996	82 ♂, ♀ (age 7–11)	%BF	+

1988; Tremblay *et al.*, 1989; Miller *et al.*, 1990; 1994; Nelson & Tucker, 1996; Westerterp *et al.*, 1996a), although few studies have corrected for fat intakes or energy density, which are invariably lower with rising carbohydrate content of diets. Hence, the apparent 'protective' effect of carbohydrate in these analyses could be secondary to the effects of these other dietary characteristics. Total protein intakes (as percent of energy) have generally been found to be unrelated to fatness in cross-sectional and longitudinal studies (Tucker & Kano, 1992; Miller *et al.*, 1990; Dreon *et al.*, 1988; Nelson & Tucker, 1996, Tremblay *et al.*, 1989; Gazzaniga & Burns, 1993; Maffeis *et al.*, 1996; Westerterp *et al.*, 1996a; Parker *et al.*, 1997), but positive relationships have been reported in a small number of cases (Lee & Lawson, 1983; Fehily *et al.*, 1984; Ortega *et al.*, 1995; Rolland-Cachera *et al.*, 1995).

A large number of studies have considered relationships between sugars intakes and measures of weight status. Measures of 'total' sugars (or 'simple carbohydrates') include sugars from all sources (including fruits),

Table 6.4 Relationships between measures of fatness (%BF, percent body fat; BMI, Body Mass Index BW, body weight; Wt/Ht weight/height ratio) and measures of sugars intakes. Cross-sectional studies, all n > 75; − = negative association, ns = no significant relationship. Subjects were all adults unless otherwise stated

Reference	Sugars type	Subjects	Measure of fatness	Association
Garn et al., 1980	Added sugars	4907 ♂, ♀ (8–11 y)	Skinfolds	ns
Lee & Lawler, 1983	Sucrose	122 ♂	Wt/Ht	ns
Fehily et al., 1984	Sucrose	493 ♂	BMI	−
Dreon et al., 1988	Sucrose	155 ♂	BMI	−
			%BF	ns
Miller et al, 1990	Total sugars	107♂	%BF	ns (♂)
		109 ♀		− (♀)
Lewis et al., 1992	Added sugars	10995 ♂, ♀ (4–18 y)	BW	ns
		17047♂, ♀	BW	−
Tucker & Kano, 1992	% energy from 'Sweets'	205 ♀	BMI	ns
Gibson, 1993	Total sugars	1744 ♂, ♀ (10–15 y)	BMI	−
Miller et al., 1994b	Total sugars	78 ♂, ♀	%BF	ns
	Added sugars (as % total)			+
Bolton-Smith & Woodward, 1994	Total sugars	11626 ♂, ♀	BMI	−
	'Extrinsic' sugars			−
	'Intrinsic' sugars			ns
Bolton-Smith & Woodward, 1995	Total sugars	10359 ♂, ♀	BMI	−
	'Extrinsic' sugars			−
	'Intrinsic' sugars			−
Gibson, 1996	'Extrinsic' sugars	2197 ♂, ♀	BMI	−
Nelson & Tucker, 1996	'Simple carbohydrates'	203 ♂	Skinfolds	ns

and are clearly the appropriate measures for analyses of mono- and di-saccharides as nutrients or biochemical entities. Other analyses concentrate on sucrose, 'added' or 'extrinsic' sugars, and therefore attempt to focus more finely on the sugars associated with classes of foods which may be of particular interest. Notably, however, even when these distinctions are made, there is only one cross-sectional study which has found any measure of sugars intake positively related to fatness, and other analyses have either found no relationship or a negative relationship with intakes of total or specific categories of sugars (Table 6.4).

The data on sugars in relation to diet and body weight must be interpreted with particular caution, however, due in part to the very consistent 'sugar–fat seesaw' effect (McColl, 1988). Proportions of fat and sugar are invariably found to be negatively correlated within and between many populations (e.g., Gibney, 1990; 1995; Lewis *et al.*, 1992; Gibson, 1993; Baghurst *et al.*, 1994). Surprisingly, none of the studies relating sugars intakes with weight status have controlled for fat intake, leaving open the possibility that the common observation of a negative correlation is largely an artifact of the relationship between the macronutrients in most diets. The use of ratios (e.g., fat:sugar) in analyses would tend to exaggerate this effect. Another concern is that, because major sources of sugars in the diet are much more readily apparent than fat content (which may be extremely difficult to gauge in many foods), and acceptable substitutes for sugars are widely available, avoidance (under-reporting or under-eating) of sugars within diet records may be more common than for fats. Obese subjects might also be actively reducing their sugar intakes as part of efforts to maintain or lose weight. However, consumption of specific intense sweeteners has been found to be positively (Parker *et al.*, 1997) and negatively (Serra-Majem *et al.*, 1996) correlated with weight gain and BMI, respectively. Despite these *caveats*, the relationship between sugars and body weight – even if it is secondary to other aspects of diet composition – is consistent with other views of the general role of carbohydrate in weight control (Chapter 5).

6.4 SUMMARY

Data on sensory responses, food preferences, and macronutrient intakes must be interpreted with caution, but appear to present a somewhat consistent picture. It is unlikely that obesity is associated with or caused by differences in sensory function, as assessed by the sensitivity to, or perceived intensity of, organoleptic qualities of foods. Preferences for specific 'basic' taste and flavour characteristics in foods also do not seem to be related to weight status; however, while the evidence for this is strong for sweetness, there are few data on specific textures or volatile flavours. In contrast, many studies carried out since the mid-1980s have shown that predisposition for fatness may be related to heightened liking for sensory attributes associated with fats in foods. The fundamental basis for this preference and its quantitative contribution to dietary intakes and weight gain are not known.

Many difficulties are encountered in attempts to characterize specific food and food group preferences and selections, and studies attempting to relate these to weight status have had ambiguous results. There is no clear evidence that consumption of any particular food or food groups stands out as being specifically associated with the development or maintenance of obesity. Cross-sectional data on food and nutrient intakes do not bear out a special role for sweetness or sweet–fat combinations; however, further research should be directed toward assessing the food sources and attributes which may specifically explain observed variance in diet and body composition.

Despite known difficulties in gaining valid records of habitual intakes, cross-sectional data on macronutrient intakes reveal modest but consistently significant positive relationships between measures of fatness and percent energy from fat (which may also reflect energy density). While longitudinal data are less consistent, weak relationships may be due to non-homogeneous populations; specifically, the presence of subgroups differing in their susceptibility to dietary influences on body composition. Relative carbohydrate intakes have usually been found to be negatively related, and protein intakes unrelated to body composition. Intakes of total and specific food sources of sugars are generally split between those showing a negative association and those finding no association with fatness. Regrettably, few dietary intake studies have carried out the appropriate multivariate analyses which would help to identify whether these observed relationships are independent of other dietary or lifestyle factors.

CHAPTER SEVEN

Patterns of food intake

A large body of human and laboratory animal research has focused on rates of eating within meals, and on the broader temporal and circadian patterns of spacing and size of eating events over time. As much or more than other topics of behavioural and nutritional research on eating and obesity, this area has suffered from serious problems with confounding variables and, particularly, in the identification or interpretation of cause and effect.

As introduced in Section 2.1, **meals** (no quotation marks) is a generic term referring to any identifiable bout or episode of eating, whereas the term **'meals'** (quotation marks) will refer to bouts of eating or eating occasions which are in some way specifically defined or differentiated from others (the most common alternative being 'snacks').

7.1 MICROSTRUCTURE OF EATING

Studies of the microstructure of eating have concentrated on specific measures of behaviour occurring within a single meal, such as the rate and dynamics of ingestion, bite size, and chewing characteristics. There is a long history of attempts to use these parameters and others to characterize the existence of an 'obese eating style' (see Spitzer & Rodin, 1981; Rodin *et al.*, 1989). Although characteristic individual patterns may be identified, it has proven difficult to show that they are consistently related to obesity *per se*, and virtually impossible to distinguish cause and effect.

In experimental situations, better liked meals or foods generate larger, longer meals, with an accelerated rate of eating (Hill & McCutcheon, 1975; Bellisle & Le Magnen, 1981; Bellisle *et al.*, 1984; Hill & McCutcheon, 1984; Westerterp-Platenga *et al.*, 1991). Hill and McCutcheon (1975) suggested that a more rapid eating style could be associated with the development of obesity, because food intake might be occurring at a rate which outpaces the normal development of satiation and inhibition of eating. However, behaviour in such situations may clearly be dominated by or interact with underlying factors such as state of hunger, eating restraint, and responsiveness to palatability (Chapter 8). Furthermore, any interpretation of this research must control for the confounding effect of body size, which (apart from obesity) is also associated with faster eating (Hill & McCutcheon, 1984; Barkeling *et al.*, 1995). That is, larger (taller, heavier) individuals tend to eat more quickly. This is not surprising, considering both anatomical capacities and social constraints. Other studies have reported conflicting results as to the existence of differences in eating rates between obese and non-obese subjects (see Rodin *et al.*, 1989; Westerterp-Platenga *et al.*, 1991). In more sophisticated analyses of eating rates, Westerterp-Platenga *et al.* (1991; 1992) reported that both high restraint and obesity were associated with linear cumulative intakes (a lack of slowing) over an extended meal, while normal-weight, low restraint subjects tended to decelerate their eating during the same period. This might arise partly because obese and restrained individuals curtail their meal before physiological satiation cues begin to slow their eating (cf. Section 2.3.4), in an attempt to restrict their food intake. However, measures of ingestion rates were not found to relate to measures of total intake and, in general, significant or consistent implications of the microstructure of eating for satiety mechanisms and overall control of intake have not been clearly demonstrated. Nevertheless, given the recent interest in the 'passive' overconsumption of high-fat, energy-dense meals (Blundell *et al.*, 1995), the possible interactions of diet composition, rates of eating and satiation may warrant further exploration.

7.2   EATING FREQUENCY AND OBESITY

Studies in the 1950s and 1960s suggested that animals force fed or limited to consumption of larger, less frequent meals ('gorging') tended to show an increase in body fat and a decrease in body protein relative to animals allowed to consume smaller amounts of food at regular intervals ('nibbling') (reviewed by Cohn *et al.*, 1965; Leveille, 1970; Leveille & Romsos, 1974; Adams & Morgan, 1981; Le Magnen, 1983). Numerous anatomical and physiological adaptations were reported to occur in response to decreases in eating frequency, and generally viewed as accommodating the intake, assimilation, and storage of large food intakes within short time periods. However, studies which equalized energy intakes during high and low frequency feeding regimes did not demonstrate such clear effects on body weight or composition (Hill *et al.*, 1988; Sivapalan and Tobin, 1986), and the earlier studies have been criticized for the techniques used to alter eating frequency and the applicability of the rat as a model for this behaviour. In addition, it was observed that 'gorging' patterns of eating may arise as a consequence rather than a cause of obesity (Rogers & Blundell, 1984; Rogers, 1988).

Paralleling the animal work was a series of epidemiological and human feeding studies which seemed to indicate that eating less frequently could be associated with increases in several chronic disease risk factors, including obesity (see Fábry, 1970). The prospective trials and metabolic studies which ensued have continued to generate interest in the physiological and anthropometric correlates and outcomes of different eating patterns.

7.2.1 Defining and interpreting eating patterns

Relatively few studies have described human eating simply in terms of overall frequency or clearly defined bouts, and the majority have instead applied the colloquial terms, 'meals' and 'snacks', or 'snacking'. Unfortunately, identification of the potential implications of eating patterns in free-living people is obscured rather than facilitated by this classification practice. Physiologically, a single eating occasion might be characterized by its energy content, the time since the preceding (or to the next) feeding occasion, or some combination of these. These may be further qualified by taking account of the body size or habitual energy intake of individual subjects. These quantitative, nutritionally relevant definitions do not necessarily coincide with individual or cultural perceptions of 'meals' and 'snacks', which more often invoke considerations of time of day, the specific types or numbers of food items (regardless of nutrient composition), the perceived quantity of food, the social situation, or the structure of the eating event. Time bands have often been used to designate eating occasions as being 'meals' (e.g., eaten between 0600 and 0930; 1200 and 1400, and 1700 and 2000) or 'snacks' (eaten outside those times); however, this applies culturally specific definitions, and may force data into an artificial, investigator-led framework. Subjective definitions are also problematic: clearly, what is a 'meal' to one person might be a 'snack' to another, or even to the same person on another day. Thus, self-reports of 'meals' and 'snacks' can reflect significant individual biases, as well as being ambiguous and inconsistent. Yet, it is often assumed that 'meal' has an established and equivalent meaning to all people. As an example, 'snacks' have been operationally defined as 'any foods, excluding beverages, eaten at a time other than a meal' (Cross *et al.*, 1994, p. 1400), with no definition of a 'meal' given.

In addition to the problems of 'meal'–'snack' nomenclature, there is confusion caused by references to so-called 'snack foods' (usually referring to a range of ready-to-eat, manufactured products, typically high in energy and low in micronutrient density), which may or may not coincide with the foods that are actually eaten as 'snacks' (which can include almost anything). Certainly, many foods such as fruits, yogurts, and sandwiches are commonly eaten as 'snacks', yet are not usually perceived as or implied by the term 'snack food'. Depending upon the subject group and definition for 'snacks', these eating occasions have been found to be lower (Summerbell *et al.*, 1995), higher (Ruxton *et al.*, 1996) or similar (unpublished data from Gatenby *et al.*, 1994) in fat content in comparison with foods eaten in 'meals'. Composition can be easily influenced by the definition applied; e.g., in the example above (Cross *et al.*, 1994), exclusion of beverages from being a 'snack' food could have considerable effect on measures of nutrients such as sugars (in soft drinks and hot beverages) and calcium (from milk) in 'snacks'.

There is also a major problem of cause and effect in trying to relate patterns of 'meals' and 'snacks', or any measure of eating frequency to weight status. Overweight, restrained or dieting subjects may choose to alter eating patterns as part of their personal strategy for restraining intake in the hope of achieving weight reduction (Crawley & Summerbell, 1997; Bellisle *et al.*, 1995; Hawkins, 1979), or may (unwittingly) change their criteria for what constitutes a 'meal'. The criteria for a 'meal' have been shown to influence apparent relationships of eating patterns with intakes (McBride *et al.*, 1990). Individuals with higher levels of physical activity may eat more frequently. Butterworth *et al.* (1994) reported that marathon runners achieved a relatively high energy intake by eating frequently, rather than by consuming larger meals. These runners rarely missed 'main meals' and also frequently consumed 'snacks' (as defined by time of day). These results are supported by other studies on the eating patterns of athletes (Kirsch & von Ameln, 1981; Lindeman, 1990), and increased eating frequency has also been observed subjects adopting a quite modest increase in daily exercise (Durrant *et al.*, 1982) . Active subjects may therefore confound the interpretation of epidemiological studies, by tending toward higher energy intakes (but lower fatness) in association with more frequent eating.

Lastly, but importantly, the questionable validity of diet records, particularly from obese or restrained eaters (Section 3.3.2), severely clouds interpretation of epidemiological research results on eating frequency, and this point is repeatedly highlighted in the discussion which follows. The specific method of diet recording may also influence results; e.g., we have observed that reported numbers of self-defined 'snacks' and 'meals' differed between subjects recording weighed vs estimated food portion sizes (Gatenby *et al.*, 1994).

7.2.2 Epidemiological studies of eating frequency and 'snacking'

There are now a very large number of epidemiological studies evaluating the associations between measures of adiposity and meal patterning in free-living consumers. Many of the cross-sectional epidemiological studies present limited information on dietary intakes and, as discussed throughout this Chapter and elsewhere (Section 3.3.2), there are serious doubts about the validity of the self-reported dietary and frequency data.

Earlier literature is interpreted as supporting a relationship between fatness and low eating frequency. Perhaps the most widely known data on relationships between eating frequency and obesity were generated by Fábry and colleagues in Czechoslovakia during the 1960s and early 1970s (Fábry *et al.*, 1964; Hejda & Fábry, 1964; Fábry & Tepperman, 1970).

In their original publications (Hejda & Fábry, 1964; Fábry et al., 1964), they reported significant negative relationships between the numbers of self-reported 'meals' (excluding 'snacks') and fatness in groups of middle-aged and older men. However, it is notable that the group with the lowest reported frequency of eating (associated with greater fatness) also recorded the lowest energy intake (Hejda & Fábry, 1964), suggesting that under-reporting might have substantially influenced the reported relationships. These results on eating frequency were supported by Metzner *et al.* (1977), who assessed intakes of over 2000 men and women by 24 hour dietary recall. Subjects were classified into one of 8 eating frequency groups, by defining a 'meal' as an intake greater than 40 kcal with a gap of at least 30 minutes between it and the next eating event. Relationships between 'adiposity index' and 'meal' frequency were corrected for energy intakes per unit body weight, and lower levels of adiposity were found in those groups of subjects who ate most frequently. Actual energy intakes were not reported. Kulesza (1982) also found a link between eating frequency and adiposity in a study of obese and lean women. These groups were said to differ for several specific eating and 'meal' pattern measures. In particular, most of the obese subjects reported eating only 2 to 3 'meals' per day, whereas more than 80% of the lean subjects consumed 4 'meals' daily (although no 'meal' definitions were reported). There were no significant differences in the energy intakes of these groups. Ries (1973) reported data from a survey in which dietary histories were used to determine energy and nutrient intakes of 253 normal-weight and 916 overweight subjects. Reported energy intake increased non-significantly with increasing adiposity, and mean reported eating frequencies were 4 times per day for the normal-weight subjects and 3.7 and 3.6 for the overweight men and women, respectively (no statistical comparison reported).

In contrast to the older literature, the majority of more recent studies have failed to identify significant relationships between measures of eating frequency and weight status. Hawkins (1979) investigated the self-defined 'meal' and 'snack' frequencies of 240 normal-weight and overweight undergraduate students. Four-day food records showed little association between overweight and eating frequencies (energy, nutrient and physical activity data were not recorded). Dreon *et al.* (1988) found no associations amongst measures of energy intake (from 7-day records), BMI, and eating frequency (as determined by eating occurring within 7 designated 'meal' or 'snack' time bands) amongst sedentary obese men. As with other studies, the absence of a relationship between energy intake and weight or BMI is suspicious, although the group were all obese, and other sensible relationships with diet composition were observed. In a study of obese women, Basdevant *et al.* (1993) defined 'snacks' as eating occurring 'between the usual times for meals', and 'snackers' as individuals who consumed at least 15% of their daily intake in these occasions. Mean BMI did not differ between 'snackers' vs 'non-snackers', but self-reported energy intakes were much lower in the the the 'non-snackers', who also reported having lost more weight in the preceding 2 months. These results are consistent with substantial under-reporting of eating frequency in this group, although no data were presented on body weights. We (Gatenby *et al.*, 1994) found no significant associations between measures of fatness and numbers of eating occasions, either as total eating frequency or self-defined as 'meals' or 'snacks'. The total number of eating occasions was positively associated with energy intake in females, which suggests that more active women were eating more frequently.

In one of the only attempts to conduct a long-term longitudinal analyses of eating frequency, Kant *et al.* (1995b) examined baseline and 8 to 10 year follow-up data on eating frequency and body weights in relation to 24-hour recall data from the first US National Health and Nutrition Examination Survey. Baseline eating frequency was inversely related to baseline BMI, but not to BMI at follow-up. However, low reported eating frequency (from diet recalls) at baseline was also paradoxically associated with both low energy intakes and high weight gain; while high weight gain was associated with **high** eating frequency (from a questionnaire) at follow-up. It is apparent that the original data set suffers from widespread and gross under-reporting (see original report by Braitman *et al.*, 1985), and Kant *et al.* (1995b) largely attribute their anomalous results to problems in the self-report data. They conclude that eating frequency did not have an independent association with weight gain.

Edelstein *et al.* (1992) found no relationships between eating frequency and BMI from a food frequency questionnaire and survey of over 800 subjects, although limited response options (1 to 2, 3, or 4 'meals and/or snacks' per day) may have considerably reduced observed variance in the population. Notably, though, the data suggest that lifestyle characteristics of frequent eaters might be quite different from those eating infrequently. Less frequent eaters were significantly younger, more likely to smoke, drank more alcohol and had lower intakes of total energy and fat. Notably, 'Type A' behaviour (characterized by time-driven conduct, a strong orientation towards work responsibilities or task completion and easily provoked hostility) has been associated with the consumption of small, frequent 'meals' (Gallacher *et al.*, 1988). It is clearly unwise to assume that groups classified by eating frequency differ only in respect of the number of daily eating events. Other lifestyle factors such as smoking may also confound relationship between eating habits and obesity.

The majority of studies of children have also not supported a relationship of fatness and eating freqency. Kaufman *et al.* (1975) assessed the eating habits of 480 teenagers (13 to 14 years old) using a diet history, and found that the obesity was associated with fewer reported 'main meals' and no difference in the number of 'snacks'. Although the investigators suggest that the lower energy intakes reported by the obese group are a consequence of the strong motivation of these children to prevent obesity by dietary means, under-reporting seems a more plausible explanation. Ruxton *et al.* (1996) reported that high vs low consumption of 'snacks' (defined by time of day) was not associated with energy intakes or weight status of 7 to 8 year old children. Similarly, in an extensive analysis of 'snack' consumption and meal patterns of a large group of 5 to 18 year olds, Morgan *et al.* (1983) also found no consistent relationships of these measures with fatness. Unfortunately, neither of these publications presents data with which to judge the validity of the diet records. In their overall analysis of diet records from over 700 teenagers, Crawley & Summerbell (1997) observed a significant negative correlation between BMI and reported eating frequency. Although removal of possible under-reporters (PAL < 1.35) did not affect the correlation, it was apparent that the relationship observed in the total sample was dependent upon the inclusion of a small number of boys who were overweight and dieting and girls who considered themselves overweight.

7.2.3 Prospective trials of eating frequency and energy balance

There have been numerous studies in which subjects have been placed on fixed or *ad libitum* patterns of meal size and frequency, and these are summarized in Table 7.1. Weight change was not the major focus of all of these studies, though most employed a hypocaloric diet. In most cases diets were provided for the subjects, while in others they were free-living (and potentially less compliant with the protocol). Given the weak evidence for direct effects of eating frequency on energy metabolism (see Section 7.2.4), those studies where food intake was actually controlled by the experimenters would seem less likely to find any effects of eating frequency.

Few of the prospective studies have examined free-living subjects allowed to select their own food intakes. In the longest trial, unlikely ever to be repeated, the meal frequencies of students aged 6 to 16 in 3 boarding schools were altered for an entire year (Fábry *et al.*, 1966). While one school maintained the initial frequency of 5 meals per day, this was changed to 3 and 7 meals per day at the others, with comparable meal items and total amounts available. Older children (aged 11 to 16 years) eating 3 meals per day exhibited significantly greater increments in measures of fat deposition and weight relative to height. However, while total food consumption was said to be similar at all 3 sites, individual amounts and types of food eaten and physical activity undertaken by the children were not recorded. The results appear intriguing, but other differences in practices between study sites remains a possible alternative explanation for these apparent effects of eating frequency.

Debry *et al.* (1978) observed greater weight loss on 7 vs 3 meals per

Table 7.1 Experimental manipulations of eating frequency: Effects on body weight and fatness (Modified from Burley *et al.*, 1994)

Reference	Protocol	Duration	Subjects, design	Outcome
Fábry *et al.*, 1966	3, or 5 or 7 meals/d Free-living	1 year	226 ♀ and ♂ aged 6–16 Between-subjects design	Significant increased skinfold thickness in older children only on 3 meals/day
Bortz *et al.*, 1966	1, 3 or 9 times/d 600 kcal formula diet	3–4 weeks each pattern	6 obese ♀ Within-subjects design	No effect of eating frequency
Swindells *et al.*, 1968	2, 3 or 9 times/d Fixed 2457 kcal/d	6 days each pattern	6 non-obese ♀ Within-subjects design	No effect of eating frequency
Finkelstein & Fryer, 1971	3 or 6 times/d Fixed 1700 kcal/d Fixed 1400 kcal/d	30 days each pattern	8 overweight ♀ Between-subjects design	No effect of eating frequency
Young *et al.*, 1971	1, 3 or 6 times/d Fixed 1800 kcal/d	35 days each pattern	11 moderately obese ♂ Within-subjects design	No effect of eating frequency
Young *et al.*, 1972	1 or 6 times/d Fixed 2800 kcal/d	5 weeks each pattern	10 non-obese ♂ Within-subjects design	No effect of eating frequency
Debry *et al.*, 1973	3 or 7 times/d 1200–1800 kcal/d Free-living	1 month each pattern	119 obese ♂ Within-subjects design	Weight loss greater on 7 times/d

Reference	Protocol	Duration	Subjects / Design	Result
Durrant et al., 1978	75% of energy needs as 1 or 5 times/d, or fixed at 770 kcal/d	1 week each pattern	19 overweight ♀ Within-subjects design	No effect of eating frequency
Garrow et al., 1981	1, 3 or 5 times/d Fixed 800 kcal/d	1 week each pattern	38 overweight ♀ Within-subjects design	No effect of eating frequency
Dallosso et al., 1982	2 or 6 times/d Fixed 42 kcal/kg	2 weeks each pattern	8 non-obese ♂ Within-subjects design	0.8 kg weight gain on 2 times/d; none on 6
Arnold et al., 1993	3 or 9 times/d Usual diet Free-living	2 weeks each pattern	19 non-obese ♂ and ♀ Within-subjects design	No effect of eating frequency
Verboeket-van de Venne & Westerterp, 1993	2 or 3–5 times/d 1000 kcal/d Free-living	4 weeks	14 mod. obese ♀ Between-subjects design	No effect of eating frequency
Verboeket-van de Venne et al., 1993	2 or 7 times/d Fixed at average daily requirement; Free living	1 week each pattern	10 ♂ Within-subjects design	No effect of eating frequency

day, over a fairly long study period involving a high number of subjects and a within-subjects design. Many other studies may have lacked this level of power. Verboeket-van de Venne and Westerterp (1993) had a low number of subjects and a between-subjects design, and tested only a very marginal difference in 2 eating frequencies, both of which were well below reported 'habitual' eating frequency before the study. Arnold *et al.* (1993) found no effects of eating frequency on body weights of non-obese subjects consuming their usual foods, but a change of weight in this population would probably require longer than the two weeks duration of that study. Verboeket-van de Venne *et al.* (1993) also saw no differences in weight status among subjects consuming a fixed energy balance diet (determined from baseline records) in 2 or 7 meals per day . Although the study periods were only 1 week each, the investigators applied a number of sophisticated techniques to examine energy metabolism and body composition. The small gain in body weight after two weeks of 'gorging' reported by Dallosso *et al.* (1982) may be interesting. Despite careful assessment of energy expenditure and a similar prescription of physical activity between conditions, the authors concluded that the gain in body weight had occurred in response to small decreases in spontaneous physical activity which remained undetected by the experimental techniques used (see Section 7.2.4).

The literature is somewhat contradictory regarding the effects of eating frequency on weight gain during **overfeeding**. In two studies of the effects of overfeeding, greater weight gain was achieved when a surplus intake was consumed as only one or two meals daily (Miller & Mumford, 1973; Mahler 1972) as compared with a pattern of 17 meals or an hourly supplement. However, Nunes & Canham (1963) found no differences in weight gain in 11 young men fed either 9 or 3 times daily.

Taken together with the results described in Section 7.2.4, these prospective trials indicate that differences in the frequency of eating of the same diet probably have little or no influence on energy balance, at least when total energy intake is fixed. Certainly variation within the 'normal' range of eating frequencies seems unlikely to have any meaningful effects. Nevertheless, the data on free-living subjects suggest possible benefits to weight control of avoiding extremely low eating frequencies.

These studies have generally focused on evenly distributed and regular bouts of eating. It is possible that appetite control may be particularly poorly responsive to extra eating events inserted between regular 'meals' (Booth, 1988), although empirical evidence to support this view is lacking. Booth (1988) has proposed that eating between 'meals' may be implicated in poor weight control, and suggests that caloric 'snacks' may fail to elicit appropriate satiety and compensatory response in subsequent 'meals', thereby contributing specifically to overeating and obesity. He has furthermore proposed that elimination of caloric 'snacks' may be a

Table 7.2 Studies investigating effects of eating frequency on the thermic effect of food (TEF) (from Burley *et al.*, 1994)

Reference	Eating pattern (no. eating occasions)	Duration of study and TEF measurement	Subjects	Outcome
Belko & Barbieri, 1987	2 *vs.* 4 2 in 5 h 4 in 7.5 h	1 day study 10 h measurement	12 ♂	No effect of eating patterns
Kinabo & Durnin, 1990	1 *vs.* 2	1 day study 6 h measurement	8 ♀: high carb./low fat 10 ♀: low carb./high fat	No effect of eating patterns or diet
Molnar, 1990	I *vs.* 3 over 4.5 h	1 day study 5 h measurement	5 obese ♂ and ♀ children	TEF higher with 1 meal *vs.* 3
Tai *et al.*, 1991	1 *vs.* 6 over 3 h	1 day study 5 h measurement	7 ♀	TEF higher with 1 meal *vs.* 6
LeBlanc *et al.*, 1993	I *vs.* 4 over 160 mm	1 day study 4 h measurement	6 ♂ and ♀	TEF higher with 4 meals *vs.* 1
Verboeket-van de Venne & Westerterp, 1993	2 *vs.* 3–5 13 h	4 weeks on a hypocaloric diet 15.5 h measurement	14 mod. obese ♀	No effect of eating patterns
Verboeket-van de Venne *et al.*, 1993	2 *vs.* 7 13 h	1 week habituation 15.5 h measurement	10 ♂	No effect of eating patterns

critical element to the success of weight loss strategies. These views make for compelling arguments, but have yet to be seriously evaluated, and the practical implications are unknown. In contrast, Westerterp-Plantenga *et al.* (1994) suggest that improved short-term compensatory eating responses might **arise** from habitual 'snacking'. They reported that habitual 'nibblers' (classified by eating frequency) made up the reduction in energy content of a 'light' lunch within 5 hours, while compensation by habitual 'gorgers' was not seen within 48 hours (responses to excess energy loads were not studied).

The likelihood of certain eating patterns predisposing to or protecting against excessive energy intakes may be resolved with better understanding of the temporal nature of appetite control between meals in free-living subjects on *ad libitum* diets. In particular, there is a need for experimental work to determine the effects of variability in eating frequency, and the timing of insertion of extra eating events ('snacks'), and their composition, on long-term energy balance in different subject populations.

7.2.4 Eating frequency and energy metabolism

In numerous human and animal experimental feeding studies, division of fixed or *ad libitum* daily food intakes into smaller, more frequent episodes has been associated with flatter glucose tolerance test responses, lower insulin concentrations, and improved lipid profiles, compared with less frequent eating. Although in many cases comparisons were between extremes of low and high frequencies, it is apparent that feeding patterns can have significant physiological effects.

With regard to energy balance and obesity, effects on nutrient partitioning and thermogenesis have been of particular interest. Although long-term 'gorging' in rats was found to increase the activity of enzymes involved in lipogenesis, this may not be relevant to human energy metabolism on western diets (Section 5.3). There are few data to support the contention that lipogenesis is enhanced with infrequent eating in human beings. Knittle (1966) reported a difference in the diurnal pattern of lipogenesis following 4 to 6 weeks of 1 or 6 daily eating episodes, but did not find evidence for 'superlipogenesis' on the less frequent eating regimen. More recently , Jones *et al.* (1995) found no effects of 3 vs 6 meals per day on lipogenesis, using highly sensitive measurement techniques.

Considerable effort has been focused on possible effects of eating frequency on components of energy expenditure, particularly TEF. This research has tested the possibility that TEF might respond non-linearly to energy intake, with some degree of stimulation attributable to the act of eating itself. A summary of the studies which have investigated TEF and eating frequency is presented in Table 7.2, which shows that these have most often found no significant effects of meal patterns. However, it may be premature to state this as a firm conclusion because the study designs have varied in so many respects, including subjects, frequencies and spreads of food intake over time, size of eating occasions relative to total daily energy intake, food compositions, and the duration of measurement of the thermic response. Nevertheless, as noted in Section 3.2.1, TEF may be the most difficult to measure and least reproducible component of energy expenditure, and variation in thermogenic effect of food may account for only very small differences in daily energy expenditure between obese and lean individuals (Ravussin and Swinburn, 1993).

Studies which have looked at total energy expenditure and nutrient utilization have generally not demonstrated any significant differences in response to eating frequency (Swindells *et al.*, 1968; Garrow *et al.*, 1981; Dallosso *et al.*, 1982; Verboeket-van de Venne & Westerterp, 1993; Verboeket-van de Venne *et al.*, 1993; Taylor & Garrow, 1996). Overall, therefore, it appears that any effects of eating frequency on TEE are probably trivial relative to other factors affecting energy balance. Tai *et al.* (1991) calculated that the 'savings' in energy expenditure generated by consuming one large meal per day vs the same amount of energy as 6 daily meals, would amount to a maximum of 48 kcal (200 kJ) per day. It is, however, possible that a 'gorging' pattern of eating may be associated with a reduced level of physical activity in free-living situations (Dallosso *et al.*, 1982), though this has not been seen in calorimeter studies (Taylor & Garrow, 1996). Changes in spontaneous physical activity have been reported in 'gorging' rats, and thought to contribute to the apparent enhancement of feed efficiency on these regimens (Fábry *et al.*, 1963; Leveille & O'Hea, 1967). In addition, Young *et al.* (1972) reported extreme sleepiness in six out of ten study participants who were consuming one large meal per day.

7.3   CIRCADIAN DISTRIBUTION OF EATING

In 1970, Fábry and Tepperman commented on the changes in lifestyle in highly industrialized countries which have led to the shift in energy intake towards the evening hours. These authors suggested that the frequency of eating interacts with the timing of food intake to encourage the development of obesity. However, the literature on the relationship between the circadian distribution of energy intake and measures of adiposity is somewhat mixed. Many studies have observed that obese individuals consume a smaller proportion of reported energy intakes in the form of breakfast, and a higher proportion during the evening, compared with lean subjects (Beaudoin & Mayer, 1953; Machinot *et al.*, 1975; Baeke *et al.*, 1983; Bellisle *et al.*, 1988; Fricker *et al.*, 1990). On the other hand, others have failed to find any association of weight status with the distribution of energy intake across the day (Durrant *et al.*, 1982; Maxfield and

Konishi, 1966; Dreon *et al.*, 1988; unpublished data from Gatenby *et al.*, 1994). In the largest and most quantitative study, Kant *et al.* (1995a) found no associations between BMI and extent of eating occurring in the evening (using either 1700 or 2000 hours as the cutoff) in extensive analyses of 4-day intake records from over 1800 subjects.

It is possible that a relationship between fatness and circadian patterns of eating could occur secondary to influences of time of day on typical food intakes. Breakfast is reported to be the 'meal' most often skipped by people who are attempting to control or reduce body weight, including children and adolescents (Chao & Smit Vanderkooy, 1989). This eating occasion in many western cultures is found to be associated with a higher carbohydrate intake (due primarily to customary consumption of breads, fruit and fruit juice, cereals and porridge). Thus, fat intake tends to be concentrated toward later periods of the day, and skipping of the morning meal could predispose individuals to consumption of a diet higher in fat (Ballard-Barbash *et al.*, 1994), which may be associated with overeating and obesity independently of meal patterns (Chapter 5).

There have been few prospective studies in which specific comparisons have been made between diets given in the morning vs the evening. Experiments on healthy non-obese subjects, which were only published as brief reports, involved administration of daily food intake as one meal, consumed either in the morning or evening (Hirsch *et al.*, 1975; Jacobs *et al.*, 1975). In each case, weight loss occurred in the morning meal condition, and weights remained stable or were slightly elevated in the alternative eating pattern. Unfortunately, no data are provided with regard to total energy or macronutrient intakes. The effect of shifting energy intake away from the late evening towards the first half of the day has also been tested in overweight and obese subjects (Armstrong *et al.*, 1981). In this study 59 subjects were allocated either to a behaviour modification group, or a 'meal-reversal' group in which the majority of food intake was concentrated into the first half of the day. Weight loss after eight weeks was significantly greater in the overweight, but not obese subjects who were following the 'meal-reversal' program. A further study, however, failed to find any difference in weight loss when 10 obese subjects were fed a very low calorie diet for 18 days at either 1000 or 1800 hours (Sensi & Capani, 1987). Most recently, Keim *et al.* (1997) have presented results which suggest that shifting intakes toward larger evening meals might offer improved protection of fat-free mass but somewhat less total weight loss in weight reduction diets. They cite a number of possible physiological effects which contribute to this outcome.

Overall, evidence for a causal link between the circadian distribution of energy intake and obesity appears weak, when diet composition is taken into account. However, it is conceivable that the outcomes of weight loss diets might be influenced by concentrating eating into different periods of the day.

7.4 SUMMARY

Despite a very large and occasionally exciting body of animal and human research results, the bulk of evidence now clearly indicates that overall frequency and distribution of energy intakes within and across the day probably have no substantial independent influence on energy metabolism, and are unlikely to be an important causal factor in obesity. The human epidemiological research in this area, which spurred much of the initial interest, appears to be greatly flawed, due to weaknesses of both the data and their interpretation. The research in this area also continues to be beset by inappropriate terminology and weak quantitative methods.

Although work on eating patterns has not generated the benefits for weight control suggested by early studies on the topic, there are related issues which merit further consideration. In particular, there has been little work on variability or irregularity of eating within and across days, or the temporal relationships between food intake and appetite, and their possible effects on physiological and cognitive weight control (Section 8.6). It is possible that the apparent associations between weight status and eating patterns do exist in certain populations, but these relationships are most likely to be a result of weight concern and other lifestyle factors, or perhaps due to influences of eating patterns on diet composition. These phenomena may also be of interest in themselves.

CHAPTER EIGHT

Externality, dietary restraint and the cognitive control of eating

8.1 EXTERNAL CUE CONTROL OF EATING AND THE NEED FOR RESTRAINT

In Chapter 2 we concluded that there is no precise physiological control over energy intake in relation to expenditure, and that external food-related cues can exert a strong influence on appetite. In the context of an environment where energy expenditure is low and food abundant, these features of the appetite control system predispose the individual to overeating and obesity. One of the ways that this tendency can be counteracted is by the deliberate control of food intake (Section 1.3.2). In the present Chapter we discuss dieting and dietary restraint in more detail. There is now a large body of research on this aspect of human eating behaviour. Paradoxically, however, many of these studies have implicated dieting as **undermining** eating control. Dieting is also a significant psychological stressor; for example, it is associated with depression and an impairment of cognitive performance (Goodwin *et al.*, 1990; Cowen *et al.*, 1992; Green & Rogers, 1995). Nevertheless, the cognitive control of food intake undoubtedly plays a critical role in the avoidance of weight gain and treatment of obesity.

8.2 SOME BACKGROUND AND THE EXTERNALITY THEORY OF OBESITY

In the late 1960s Schachter and his colleagues began a series of highly original and influential studies on human eating behaviour which led to the proposal of the so-called externality theory of human obesity (Schachter, 1971b; Schachter & Rodin, 1974). This drew parallels between the behaviour of rats made obese by ventromedial lesions of the hypothalamus and the behaviour of obese people. Compared with their lean counterparts, both obese rats and people were supposedly less willing to work to obtain food, less sensitive to a food preload (i.e., they showed poor caloric compensation), but were influenced more by the sight and 'taste' (i.e., palatability) of food (see also Section 6.1). So, for example, the amount of milkshake consumed by obese human subjects was found to be relatively more affected by a manipulation of the palatability of the milkshake. In a procedure disguised as a taste test, obese subjects consumed more of a palatable milkshake and also less of a less palatable milkshake than did lean subjects (Decke, quoted in Schachter, 1971a). Such results were interpreted as showing that the obese are more reactive or more 'driven' by external cues (and perhaps also emotional arousal, section 9.2), but are less sensitive to internal hunger and satiation cues than lean individuals. Furthermore, this was argued to be a prominent factor in the aetiology of obesity. High external responsiveness (perhaps due to an underlying hypothalamic defect) would, in the face of a highly palatable and available food supply, encourage overeating and hence the development of obesity.

These ideas were subsequently tested in a variety of further studies which, while confirming many of the original results, also indicated that the relationship between externality and overweight is more complex than originally proposed (Rodin, 1975b; Spitzer & Rodin, 1981). Nonetheless, Spitzer and Rodin (1981) were able to conclude from their comprehensive review of studies on human eating behaviour that 'palatability is the most consistent variable influencing amount eaten and **producing over-weight–normal differences in amount eaten**' (page 293, our emphasis). Furthermore, in an important but rarely cited study, Rodin and Slochower (1976) demonstrated that pre-test differences in generalized external responsiveness (i.e., responsiveness to both food and non-food stimuli) predicted weight change in a population placed in a novel environment. This change included both weight gains and losses among the subjects (children attending summer camp) which were assumed to be related to how the food offered at camp compared with the quality and availability of food at home. Since these findings were obtained from a sample of subjects who had no history of overweight, they suggest that externality is not simply a consequence, or indeed a correlate, of obesity. The possibility that the trait of externality predisposes to obesity therefore remains a plausible hypothesis (cf. Sections 5.2 and 6.1). Unfortunately, however, this concept has since been largely ignored in favour of related ideas concerning dietary restraint and the effects of dieting.

8.3 WEIGHT CONCERN, DIETING AND OVEREATING

8.3.1 Restraint and disinhibition

Following on directly from Schachter's influential research, a further significant advance in the study of human food intake and body weight control was the recognition of the important influence of voluntary dietary restriction on human eating behaviour. This was initially highlighted by Nisbett (1972), who proposed that the obese–normal differences in eating behaviour identified by Schachter and colleagues (1971b) were due to the greater hunger of obese individuals.' This difference in hunger was assumed to arise because of a higher prevalence of dieting in the obese population. Nisbett suggested that the obese have a high set-point for weight (or more realistically a high body fat set-point; but see section 1.3.2), but because of societal and medical pressures many tend to maintain a weight below this set-point. Paradoxically, therefore, obesity and overweight were supposed to be associated with chronic hunger.

Such a view clearly rejects the notion that eating behaviour is determined solely by physiological and sensory cues and the related sensations of hunger and satiation. Instead, it proposes that it is commonplace to resist the operation of these factors. This self-imposed resistance or restraint is motivated by the desire to suppress weight. The desire to lose weight or maintain a low weight by 'dieting' is, however, not confined to overweight and obese people. Indeed, there are many dieters whose weight is statistically normal or below normal (Dwyer *et al.*, 1970; Grunewald, 1985; Jeffery *et al.*, 1984; Nylander, 1971; Hill *et al.*, 1992). Nisbett's hypothesis, therefore, suggests an examination of the eating behaviour of people classified according to their degree of **dietary restraint and dieting** rather than body weight. This was first carried out in a series of studies which used the Restraint Scale and the Revised Restraint Scale (RRS) developed by Herman & Polivy (Polivy *et al.*, 1978). This self-report questionnaire assesses concern with dieting and weight, and short-term weight fluctuation (Table 8.1).

In what soon became a widely quoted study, Herman and Mack (1975) gave subjects preloads of either two glasses of milkshake, one glass, or none, and then required them to rate the taste of various ice creams. These ice creams were provided in large quantities, and the subjects were told that once they had completed the taste ratings they could eat 'more if they wished'. Whereas the intake of ice cream was inversely related to the size of the preload in unrestrained subjects, restrained subjects responded in a so-called 'counterregulatory' fashion, that is their intake of ice cream increased as the size of the preload increased (Figure 8.1). A similar result was obtained by manipulating subjects' beliefs about the calorie content of the preload consumed, while keeping its actual calorie content constant. Restrained subjects (as defined by the RRS) ate much more following a preload identified as high in calories than when exactly the same preload was identified as low in calories. Unrestrained subjects, on the other hand, showed a non-significant trend towards a lower intake in the 'told high-calorie' condition (Spencer & Fremouw, 1979; see also Polivy, 1976). These results have been interpreted in terms of a process of **disinhibition**. The preload, by forcing the perceived intake of calories above a critical threshold (or 'diet boundary', see section 8.3.2), causes normally

Table 8.1   The Revised Restraint Scale. In much of the research using this questionnaire individuals displaying a high score are designated as 'restrained eaters' or 'dieters' and those displaying a low score as 'unrestrained eaters' or 'nondieters'. The classification is, however, somewhat arbitrary, because usually subjects are divided into groups of restrained and unrestrained eaters based on a median split of their scores. Furthermore, as explained in the text, other questionnaires developed subsequently define restrained eating more narrowly. From Herman (1978), with permission

---

1. How often are you dieting?

    Never; rarely; sometimes; often; always. (Scored 0–4)

2. What is the maximum amount of weight (in pounds) that you have ever lost within one month?

    0–4; 5–9; 10–14; 15–19; 20+. (Scored 0–4)

3. What is your maximum weight gain in one week?

    0–1; 1.1–2; 2.1–3; 3.1–5; 5.1+. (Scored 0–4)

4. In a typical week, how much does your weight fluctuate?

    0–1; 1.1–2; 2.1–3; 3.1–5; 5.1+. (Scored 0–4)

5. Would a weight fluctuation of 5lb affect the way you live your life?

    Not at all; slightly; moderately; very much. (Scored 0–3)

6. Do you eat sensibly in front of others and splurge alone?

    Never; rarely; often; always. (Scored 0–3)

7. Do you give too much time and thought to food?

    Never; rarely; often; always. (Scored 0–3)

8. Do you have feelings of guilt after overeating?

    Never; rarely; often; always. (Scored 0–3)

9. How conscious are you of what you are eating?

    Not at all; slightly; moderately; extremely. (Scored 0–3)

10. How many pounds over your desired weight were you at your maximum weight?

    0–1; 1–5; 6–10; 11–20; 21+. (Scored 0–4)

---

restrained eaters to suspend their self-imposed restraint, thereby releasing their underlying desire to eat (due to hunger, emotional or other reasons) (Herman, 1978; Herman & Mack, 1975; Herman & Polivy, 1984). The pattern of thinking which was identified with such behaviour can be characterized as follows: 'My diet has been broken (by the requirement of the experiment to consume the preload), I might as well go ahead and enjoy myself/stop feeling hungry (eat a lot of the test foods), I can always

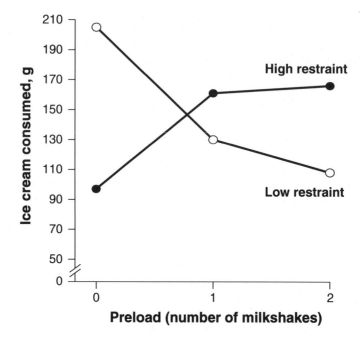

Figure 8.1   Responses of restrained and unrestrained eaters to preloading. Restraint measured using the Restraint Scale subsequently modifed slightly as the RRS (Table 8.1). Data from Herman and Mack (1975) with permission.

start my diet again tomorrow.' This, in turn, has sometimes been called (by Herman and Polivy, 1984) the 'what-the-hell effect'!

In addition to food preloads, emotional events (induction of anxiety and depressed mood), the consumption of alcohol, the behaviour of others and even anticipated future overeating have been shown to precipitate breakdown of dietary restraint in restrained eaters (Baucom & Aiken, 1981; Herman, 1978; Herman & Polivy, 1975; Ruderman, 1985). These, together with the results of a large number of other subsequent studies, provided good support for the 'disinhibition hypothesis' (Ruderman, 1986), which assumes that disinhibitors of eating in restrained eaters can be cognitive (e.g., 'I've blown my diet'), emotional and pharmacological (alcohol). More generally, this research has confirmed a major role for cognition in the short-term regulation of food intake.

8.3.2   The boundary model of eating regulation

The disinhibition hypothesis in relation to restrained eating was elaborated formally by Herman and Polivy (1984) in their 'boundary model' of the control of eating (Figure 8.2). This model proposes that physiological influences operate to maintain food intake within a certain range, with aversive effects of hunger keeping consumption above some minimum level and aversive effects of satiety keeping it below some maximum level. The area between these 'hunger' and 'satiety' boundaries is called the zone of 'biological indifference', and it is within this range that cognitive, emotional and other psychological factors are hypothesized to have their greatest influence on food intake. Furthermore, the model assumes that restrained eaters differ from unrestrained eaters in having a lower hunger boundary and a higher satiety boundary, and also in having a third boundary, the self-imposed 'diet boundary', located between their hunger and satiety boundaries. The diet boundary is viewed as entirely cognitive and represents the restrained eater's self-imposed quota of calories for a given occasion, and crucially is lower than the physiologically determined satiety boundary. In other words, referring to the model shown in Figure 2.2, the diet boundary is reached before the negative feedback effects of eating outweigh the positive feedback effects. Why restrained eaters should have a widened zone of biological indifference is not very clear, although it was suggested (Herman & Polivy, 1984) that this occurs because of restrained eaters' history of repeated dieting and overeating resulting in them habituating to extreme sensations of hunger and satiety.

In any case, these two features of the model, the diet boundary and the wider zone of biological indifference, are essential to the model's account of the behaviour of restrained and unrestrained eaters, and in particular its explanation of the effects of preloading. Assuming that unrestrained eaters are moderately hungry at the start of the experiment, they can eat a substantial amount in the 'taste test' before meeting their satiety boundary (dashed line in Figure 8.2A). When preloaded, they are closer to their satiety boundary at the beginning of the taste test, and are therefore not able to eat as much in that test (full line in Figure 8.2A). In contrast, restrained eaters eat only a little when not preloaded, keeping below their diet boundary (dashed line in Figure 8.2B). Preloading, however, is likely to breach the diet boundary, consequently removing inhibitions on eating until the elevated satiety boundary is reached (full line in Figure 8.2B). In addition, emotional stress is thought to increase eating in restrained eaters by reducing the salience or importance of the diet boundary, so that under stress or during depression eating proceeds as if the diet boundary had been removed.

Figure 8.2 also shows how the eating patterns of binge eaters (bulimics) and restricting anorexics (see section 8.6) are described by the model. During a binge, binge eaters transgress both their diet boundary and their satiety boundary, eating more than the disinhibited restrained eater. Thus the binge eater is not constrained by the unpleasant effects of satiety, but instead stops eating only on the point of reaching physical capacity. In contrast, restricting anorexics are presumed to have a lower diet boundary than restrained eaters, and be willing to tolerate the discomfort

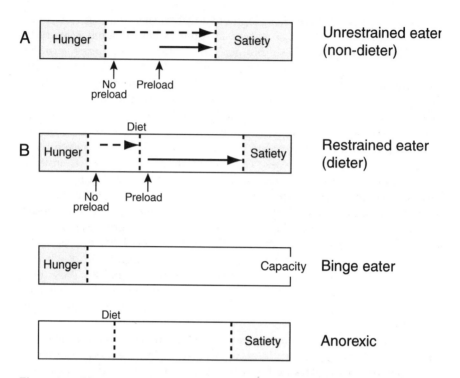

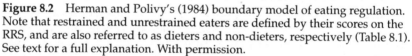

Figure 8.2   Herman and Polivy's (1984) boundary model of eating regulation. Note that restrained and unrestrained eaters are defined by their scores on the RRS, and are also referred to as dieters and non-dieters, respectively (Table 8.1). See text for a full explanation. With permission.

of being close to or below their hunger boundary (which is already lower than that of unrestrained eaters).

The boundary model is a description, rather than an explanation, of restrained, anorexic and binge eating behaviour. Nevertheless, in describing the interaction of physiological and cognitive controls on eating it provides a good framework for discussing the findings of a large body of research on dietary restraint and appetite regulation. A notable feature of the model is that it allows social factors, palatability, food variety and other 'non-physiological' influences to have a strong impact on food intake, even in unrestrained or 'normal' eaters. This of course is entirely consistent with much of the evidence reviewed in earlier chapters of this book (cf. section 2.4).

8.3.3   Processes underlying disinhibited eating

The explanation for disinhibited eating in restrained eaters in terms of a temporary abandonment of restraint following a failure to stay within the self-imposed rules for eating is very plausible. It does, though, suggest a simplistic all-or-nothing (or none-or-all!) cognitive style which might seem to underestimate the sophistication of many restrained eaters and dieters, who will presumably have experienced and had the opportunity to learn from previous instances of disinhibited eating. In fact, surprisingly little is known about the thinking of restrained eaters, or their emotional responses, in this situation.

One clear finding, though, is that disinhibited eating can occur even when no preload has been consumed and in the absence of the direct manipulation of mood. Several studies, for example, have shown that exposure to the sight and smell of palatable foods without eating, and even exposure to pictures of food, can provoke the subsequent disinhibition of eating in restrained subjects (Collins, 1978; Robinson *et al.*, 1983; Rogers & Hill, 1989; Jansen & van den Hout, 1991; Fedoroff *et al.*, 1997). A further similarity with the effects of preloading was that unrestrained subjects ate less when previously exposed to food stimuli (Rogers & Hill, 1989). More recently, exactly parallel results were obtained for restrained versus unrestrained women given a 'taste-test task' after viewing television advertisements containing either stereotypical images of slim, attractive women or control advertisements (Seddon & Berry, 1996). These results cannot, of course, be explained easily by the boundary model, since the restrained eater's diet boundary is not transgressed merely by looking at food, or looking at images of culturally idealised women.

A somewhat different account of the processes underlying disinhibited eating proposes that it is the emotional distress caused by the consumption of 'forbidden foods' which undermines the restrained eater's ability to maintain restraint (Herman & Polivy, 1988). Increased anxiety might also explain, for example, the effect of being confronted, but not preloaded, with palatable high-calorie foods (Rogers & Hill, 1989). In a preloading study, Ogden and Greville (1993) confirmed the expected increase in anxiety in restrained eaters following consumption of a high-calorie preload; however, they also found that accompanying the anxiety, these subjects experienced marked increases in feelings of rebelliousness and defiance, and a desire to challenge the limitations set by their restraint. In other words, the restrained eaters responded to preloading with an 'active state of mind' (see also Ogden & Wardle, 1991), rather than passively abandoning their dietary goal, as suggested by Herman and Polivy (1984) when they used the term 'what-the-hell effect'.

Yet another proposal is that disinhibited eating occurs because 'restrained eaters are particularly responsive to environmental cues concerning appropriate food intake' (Lowe, 1993, page 109). Here the critical effect of preloading and a variety of other factors which provoke disinhibited eating is supposed to concern the information which these manipulations convey to the restrained eater about the amount of eating expected in such situations. This is very close to the concept of externality

(Lowe, 1993), bringing the argument almost full circle back to the origins of restraint theory (section 8.3.1).

8.4   RESTRAINT, AND SUCCESSFUL AND UNSUCCESSFUL DIETING

8.4.1   Restraint without disinhibition

In the above discussion on dietary restraint and disinhibited eating we have followed Herman and Polivy and their colleagues in referring to subjects scoring high and low on the RRS as, respectively, restrained and unrestrained eaters. Herman & Polivy have also used the terms dieters and nondieters interchangeably with restrained and unrestrained eaters (e.g., Herman, 1978 ; Herman & Polivy, 1984). Subsequent research, however, has shown that these descriptions require redefining.

The significance of the RRS is its ability to identify individuals with different eating patterns, and particularly eating in response to preloading and manipulations of, for example, mood. The items making up the RRS (Table 8.1), though, are concerned principally with dieting and weight fluctuation, and these subscales have been confirmed by factor analysis (e.g., Ruderman, 1993). None of the questions appears to capture very directly the notion of restraint as self-imposed resistance to eating (Herman, 1978). In contrast, two questionnaires developed after the RRS claim to identify a separate restraint factor.

The first of these questionnaires is the Three Factor Eating Questionnaire (TFEQ, Stunkard & Messick, 1985) which, as its name suggests, identifies three factors named 'Cognitive Restraint of Eating', 'Disinhibition' and 'Hunger'. It consists of 51 items, such as 'When I have eaten my quota of calories, I am usually good about not eating any more' (Restraint); 'I usually eat too much at social occasions, like parties and picnics' (Disinhibition); 'I often feel so hungry that I have to eat something' (Hunger).

A similarly narrow definition of restraint is found in the 33-item Dutch Eating Behaviour Questionnaire (DEBQ, van Strien *et al.*, 1986). Example items for the restraint scale are: 'If you put on weight, do you eat less than you usually do?', 'Do you eat less at mealtimes than you would like to eat?' and 'Do you watch exactly what you eat?' In addition to measuring 'Restrained Eating', the DEBQ includes two further scales, 'Emotional Eating' (e.g., 'Do you have a desire to eat when you are irritated?') and 'External Eating' (e.g., 'If the food tastes good to you, do you eat more than usual?' and 'Do you eat more than usual when you see others eating?').

There is some overlap between the RRS and the restrained eating scales of the TFEQ and the DEBQ. For example, several items from the RRS are included in the TFEQ, and all but one of these loads on the restraint factor (e.g., 'Would a weight fluctuation of 5 lb affect the way

you live your life?' and 'How conscious are you of what you are eating?').
Nonetheless, the TFEQ and the DEBQ restrained eating scales differ substantially from the RRS in that they have few items on overeating and
weight fluctuations, and they emphasize cognitive and behavioural
strategies for limiting food and energy intake (Lowe, 1993). Crucially,
they also appear to identify restrained eaters who are less susceptible to
disinhibited eating in laboratory tests (reviewed by Lowe, 1993; but see
section 8.4.3). This has led to the suggestion that the RRS tends to identify
unsuccessful dieters, whereas the TFEQ and DEBQ restraint scales largely
identify successful dieters (Heatherton *et al.*, 1988). Empirical support for
this was provided by the results of a study which investigated the interrelationships between scores on these three scales, self-reported food
intake, various measures of disordered eating and figure consciousness
(Laessle *et al.*, 1989a). A high score on the RRS was found to be associated
with weight fluctuation, and with disinhibited eating as measured by the
Eating Disorders Inventory bulimia scale (Garner *et al.*, 1983) and the
TFEQ disinhibition scale. High scores on the TFEQ and DEBQ restraint
scales, on the other hand, were associated with low self-reported energy
intake, but not with bulimic (binge eating) tendencies or weight fluctuation (see also Wardle, 1987; van Strien, 1996). Figure consciousness was
positively correlated with RRS scores as well as with TFEQ and DEBQ
restraint scale scores. These results are further supported by those of an
earlier study which found that RRS concern for dieting scores, but not
RRS weight fluctuation scores, were significantly correlated with DEBQ
restraint (Wardle, 1986). In other words, the behaviour predicted by the
RRS differs markedly from that predicted by the TEFQ and DEBQ
restraint scales (see section 8.6 for further discussion).

8.4.2   Restraint, dieting and weight suppression

Yet a further elaboration of the relationships among restraint, dieting and
weight fluctuation is presented by Lowe (1993), who identifies three critical variables which can predict or influence the eating behaviour of
restrained eaters. Ordered in terms of successful eating and weight control, these factors are (from least to most successful): 'Frequency of
Dieting and Overeating', 'Current Dieting' and 'Weight Suppression'.
The first variable is supposed to be the best predictor, and indeed a cause,
of proneness to disinhibited eating. In other words, it is argued that
increased food intake induced by preloading, mood manipulations or
exposure to food cues is more closely related to the individual's history
of dieting, bouts of overeating, and consequently weight fluctuation, than
their current state of eating restraint (as measured by the TFEQ or
DEBQ). This would be consistent with the finding that high scores on the
RRS scale predict disinhibited eating, if it is assumed that the weight
fluctuation factor on this scale indicates weight losses and gains which

have resulted from previous cycles of dietary restriction and dieting failure (overeating). Lowe (1993) proposes that the mechanism underlying the effect of past dieting–overeating cycles is that they distort the restrained eater's 'ability to perceive (or generate)' internal depletion and repletion cues. This is the similar to the 'boundary model' (Figure 8.2) but, whereas Herman and Polivy (1984) argue that disinhibited eating occurs because of the breakdown of the cognitive control of eating, Lowe essentially proposes that this is due to heightened externality in these frequent dieters/overeaters (Section 8.2).

Lowe's (1993) second variable, 'Current Dieting', refers to individuals who report that they are currently dieting to lose weight. Most if not all current dieters are found to have high scores on retrained eating scales, but at any one time only a minority of restrained eaters report that they are currently dieting (Lowe *et al.*, 1991, Rogers & Green, 1993). The significance of current dieting may be related to both the cognitive and biological aspects of dieting. Compared with restrained non-dieters, current dieters are more likely to be in negative energy balance, show greater dissatisfaction with their body weight and shape, and may be more preoccupied with thoughts of food and eating (Green & Rogers, 1993; 1995; Hickford *et al.*, 1997). Crucially, current dieters also appear to be **less** vulnerable to preloading and other manipulations which typically disinhibit eating in restrained non-dieters, but they tend to eat more in situations where eating control in not obviously challenged (reviewed by Lowe, 1993). For example, Lowe *et al.* (1991) found that current dieters ate less ice cream than restrained eaters (as defined by the RRS) following preloading, but that they increased their intake and ate more than restrained and unrestrained eaters when not given a preload. While this unexpected finding is not easily explained, Lowe (1993) suggests that, paradoxically, preloading may help current dieters to resist urges to eat because it increases the salience of their dietary goals, whereas their guard may be down when there appears to be no immediate threat (e.g., when the 'taste test' is not preceded by a preload).

Lowe (1993) also argues that these different responses of restrained non-dieters and current dieters can account for the different behaviour patterns predicted by the RRS compared with the TFEQ and DEBQ restraint scales. Rather than simply measuring successful and unsuccessful dieting (section 8.4.1), he assumes that the TFEQ and DEBQ select a greater proportion of current (i.e., not easily disinhibited) dieters than the RRS. This is because the TFEQ and DEBQ restraint scales have a strong bias towards items describing actual dieting behaviours.

The third variable discussed by Lowe (1993) is weight suppression or weight reduction. Weight suppressors are individuals who, like current dieters, are assumed to have undergone previous cycles of dieting, weight loss and weight gain, but who have for a lengthy period of time to the present achieved sustained eating and weight control. When preloaded with a milkshake, weight suppressors, irrespective of their level of dietary restraint (RRS), ate significantly less ice cream than non-suppressors (Lowe & Kleifield, 1988). Weight suppression was defined as the difference between a subject's heaviest weight ever and his or her current weight, and it was found that the subjects in the weight suppressor group had been at or close to their lower weight for an average of 20 months. These subjects were also somewhat less hungry, both before and after preloading. It was concluded that 'weight suppressors … were for the most part successful dieters who showed several signs of having adapted to the lower weights they were maintaining' (Lowe & Kleifield, 1988, page 159).

8.4.3 Rigid and flexible control of eating: another dimension of restraint?

As indicated above, there is agreement that the RRS is more likely than the TFEQ restraint scale (and the DEBQ restraint scale) to identify individuals prone to disinhibited eating. Nonetheless, under some circumstances, such as exposure to the sight and smell of palatable food, high TFEQ restraint has been found to predict increased 'taste test' food intake, an ability it shares with the TFEQ disinhibition scale but not the TFEQ hunger scale (Rogers & Hill, 1989). This is not surprising, since in general population scores on the TEFQ restraint and disinhibition scales tend to be (weakly) positively correlated (Stunkard & Messick, 1985; Hill *et al.*, 1991a). Other studies have found that disinhibited eating occurs only in subjects scoring high on both TFEQ restraint and disinhibition scales, and furthermore that there are certain items from the TFEQ restraint scale that are more typically related to high scores on the disinhibition scale (Westenhoefer, 1991; Westenhoefer *et al.*, 1994). Westenhoefer (1991) has argued that these items can be viewed as forming a 'rigid control of eating' subscale of the TFEQ restraint scale, compared with a majority of the remaining items, which identify a 'flexible control of eating' subscale. Subsequently, he developed a rigid and flexible control of eating questionnaire comprising 18 TFEQ restraint items plus 14 new items (see Westenhoefer *et al.*, 1994), and suggested that rigid control increases susceptibility to eating difficulties, whereas flexible control is a 'less problematic strategy of long-term weight control' (page 27).

This idea would be consistent with the possibility that an individual adopting an all-or-nothing approach to dieting will be particularly prone to bouts of disinhibited eating. In terms of the boundary model (section 8.3.2), individuals imposing a rigid diet boundary will presumably be more likely to feel that they have 'blown' their diet following a preload than would individuals who have a flexible diet boundary, which on certain occasions is adjusted upwards to accommodate greater consumption without being breached (Westenhoefer, 1991). This aspect of the distinction between rigid and flexible control of eating is illustrated by the following items from Westenhoefer's questionnaire: 'While losing weight I try to stick to a plan', 'I alternate between times when I am strictly dieting and times when I do not pay much attention to what and how much I eat' (Rigid subscale), and 'If I have eaten a little bit more during one meal, I compensate for that at the next meal' (Flexible subscale). However, other items such as 'How often are you dieting in a conscious effort to control your weight' (Rigid subscale) do not refer explicitly to a cognitive strategy, and in general it is unclear to what extent the Rigid subscale measures a particular strategy for gaining control of eating, or the consequences of the failure to maintain control. If it is the latter, then rigid control is more like RRS 'restraint' and Lowe's (1993) 'Frequency of Dieting and Overeating' variable, both of which are strongly predictive of proneness to disinhibited eating (sections 8.2.1 and 8.2.4).

In fact, Westenhoefer *et al.* (1994) found that the rigid control of eating scale failed to predict disinhibited eating after a milkshake preload; however, this was also the case for the RRS, perhaps indicating methodological differences between this and earlier studies. One explanation is that, in contrast to North American subjects, European subjects, as tested by Westenhoefer, generally do not perceive milkshakes to be a 'diet-breaking' food (Ogden & Wardle, 1991).

8.5   EFFECTS OF DIETARY RESTRAINT AND DIETING ON EATING IN EVERYDAY LIFE

8.5.1   Daily food intake in restrained eaters

The research described above has investigated the effects of dietary restraint on eating behaviour in laboratory settings. There is, in contrast, relatively little information available on everyday food intake and eating patterns of restrained eaters. This is much more difficult to study accurately because it relies on self-recording of food intake which is subject to under-reporting. The general problem of under-reporting is well known, but is exaggerated in certain groups such as the obese, and may also be expected to be greater in restrained eaters who by definition show increased concern with food and eating (Hill *et al.*, 1995; Section 3.3.2).

It is perhaps not surprising, therefore, that restraint measured both by the TFEQ and the DEBQ has been found in several studies to be negatively related to energy intake recorded in food diaries (reviewed by de Castro, 1995). One study (Green *et al.*, 1994), furthermore, found that current dieters reported the lowest intake, followed by highly restrained non-dieters, with low-to-medium restrained eaters recording the highest intakes (restraint measured by DEBQ). These intakes represented, respectively, 71%, 86% and 101% of the subjects' Estimated Average

Requirements for energy (Department of Health, 1991). There is also good agreement that the apparently reduced energy intake in restrained eaters is due mainly to lower reported intakes of energy-dense items of high-fat and high-carbohydrate content (Laessle *et al.*, 1989b; de Castro, 1995).

The extent to which these findings can be accounted for by under-reporting is difficult to ascertain; however, there is some evidence to suggest that restrained eaters do actually eat significantly less than unrestrained eaters. First, total daily energy expenditure measured using the doubly-labelled water method has been reported to be lower in restrained (TFEQ) subjects (Tuschl *et al.*, 1990; Platte *et al.*, 1996), although the large difference found in the first of these two studies was probably due to a higher level of physical activity in the restrained compared with the unrestrained eaters (Section 3.3.1). Second, scores on the RRS have generally been found not to be significantly related to food intake (reviewed by de Castro, 1995). If the lower intakes due to restraint measured by the TFEQ and DEBQ were the result of an under-reporting bias, then a similar finding would be predicted for the RRS, since the RRS also reflects a concern with food and dieting. In fact, individuals scoring high on the RRS may fail to reduce their intake because the RRS tends to measure relatively unsuccessful eating and weight control (section 8.4.1). Thus in contrast to food intake, body weight is more strongly (positively) related to RRS scores than to TFEQ and DEBQ restraint (de Castro, 1995), although even for these latter measures restrained eaters tend to be slightly heavier (e.g., Rogers & Green, 1993; Tuschl *et al.*, 1990).

These findings show that the relationships between energy intake, energy expenditure, body weight and restrained eating are complex and difficult to disentangle. One possibility, however, is that individuals with relatively low energy requirements, perhaps due to inactivity or current or past dieting attempts (e.g., Heshka *et al.*, 1990; but see Platte *et al.*, 1996), are forced to adopt a restrained eating style in order to avoid excessive weight gain (cf. de Castro, 1995).

8.5.2 Role of dietary restraint and dieting in the aetiology of binge eating and bulimia

The primary symptom of bulimia or bulimia nervosa is binge eating, that is, the 'rapid consumption of a large amount of food in a discrete period of time' accompanied by the feeling that the eating is 'out of control' (American Psychiatric Association, 1994). Often, extremely large amounts of food [> 3,000 kcal (> 12.5 MJ)] are consumed during bulimic episodes, with most items being energy-dense high-fat, high-carbohydrate foods (Mizes, 1985; Hetherington *et al.*, 1994; van der Ster Wallin *et al.*, 1994). Binging is also usually followed by purging; for example, self-induced vomiting, abuse of laxatives or compulsive exercise, that is aimed at avoiding weight gain. The highest incidence of bulimia occurs in young women. Although a majority of these women with bulimia are of normal weight, binge eating also occurs in obese people and in patients with anorexia nervosa (Wardle & Beinart, 1981).

The finding of disinhibited eating in 'restrained eaters' in laboratory experiments has led to the claim that restrained eating plays a direct role in the aetiology of binge eating and bulimia nervosa (Polivy & Herman, 1985; Wardle & Beinart, 1981; Tuschl, 1990). For example, in Herman and Polivy's (1984) boundary model of eating (Figure 8.2), binging in bulimia nervosa is viewed as a progression from disinhibited eating in restrained eaters. This progression in generally assumed to involve a variety of 'psychophysiological' adaptations, including a reduction in the strength of conditioned satiety and modification of other learned aspects of appetite control (Chapter 2 and section 8.6), which allow, or even drive, the increasingly excessive bouts of eating characteristic of the bulimic patient (e.g., Herman & Polivy, 1988; Tuschl, 1990).

The pivotal role of 'dietary restraint and dieting' in the development of abnormal eating is also supported by the observation that chronic dieting 'invariably' precedes the onset of bulimia nervosa (Herman & Polivy, 1988). This does not mean, however, that restrained eating necessarily leads to binging or disordered appetite control. In fact, as we have already noted (section 8.4.1), restraint measured by the TFEQ and the DEBQ does not appear to be associated with binging, and in restrictive anorexia nervosa highly restrained eating is maintained apparently without any occurrences of binge eating (Wardle, 1990; Garner, 1993).

8.6   SOME FURTHER CONSEQUENCES OF DIETARY RESTRAINT: HUNGER AND EATING VARIABILITY

In this section we give an overview of the findings predicted by the RRS, the TFEQ and the DEBQ, and attempt to identify the principal factors which underlie the effects of dietary restraint on eating and weight control. As we have noted above, there are certain fundamental differences between these questionnaires. Table 8.2 shows that high scores on the RRS identify individuals whose weight tends to fluctuate, and who are prone to disinhibited eating and binge eating. In contrast, individuals scoring highly on the TFEQ and DEBQ restraint scales are likely to show a fairly stable pattern of eating and weight control, and appear to be able to maintain a low food intake even when challenged with food preloads and other potential disinhibitors of eating. There is, nonetheless, overlap between the TFEQ and DEBQ restraint scales and the RRS; for example, DEBQ restraint is significantly correlated with the RRS concern for dieting subscale (Wardle, 1986; Section 8.4.1). Also, individuals who score highly on both the TFEQ restraint and disinhibition scales are more prone to disinhibited eating than individuals scoring highly on either one or the other of these scales (Westenhoefer *et al.*, 1994), showing that restraint on its own is a relatively imperfect predictor of behaviour.

Actually, these various questionnaire scales and subscales mainly comprise items which describe past eating and overeating behaviour or weight fluctuation. Therefore the extent to which they reliably predict such behaviour will, assuming they are completed accurately (see Wardle, 1986), depend on the likelihood that the behaviour will be repeated in the future. Originally it was claimed that the RRS measured restrained eating or dieting, and that this behaviour had a negative impact on dietary control (e.g., Herman, 1978). It is now clear, however, that restrained eating is often associated with successful dietary control.

Table 8.2 Relationships of 'restrained eating' with some eating behaviour and body weight variables. Behaviour predicted by the RRS differs from that predicted by the TFEQ and DEBQ restraint scales (see text for details and references): >, more likely; >>, much more likely; >>>, very much more likely; for high versus low scorers on the different measures of restrained eating. RRS = Revised Restraint Scale (Herman & Mack, 1975; Polivy *et al.*, 1978); TFEQ-R = Restraint scale of the Three Factor Eating Questionnaire (Stunkard & Messick, 1985); DEBQ-R = Restraint scale of the Dutch Eating Behaviour Questionnaire (van Strien *et al.*, 1986)

	RRS	*TFEQ-R and DEBQ-R*
Disinhibition of eating in laboratory tests	>>>	>
Binge eating	>>>	>
Self-reported dietary energy intake	Low correlation	Negative correlation
Body weight	Positive correlation	Low correlation
Weight fluctuation	>>>	>
All-or-nothing approach to dieting	>>>	>
Frequency of dieting	>>>	>>
Currently dieting	>>	>>>
Hunger	Positive correlation	Low correlation
Salivation to sight and smell of food	Positive correlation	Low correlation
Eating variability	>>>	>
'Successful' dieting	No	Yes

The RRS predicts unsuccessful dieting, including disinhibited eating and weight fluctuation, because this is what it mainly describes (Tables 8.1 and 8.2).

One possible explanation for this predictability of successful versus unsuccessful dietary control is that these outcomes are due to certain self-perpetuating patterns of eating behaviour. Such a view is discussed by Lowe (1993), who describes several psychological and biological effects of dieting which could contribute, on the one hand, to the maintenance of weight suppression, and on the other hand to cycles of food restriction and overeating.

Perhaps the most critical of these observations is that hunger, or more generally appetite, tends to be diminished in weight suppressors but is increased in individuals having a highly variable eating pattern. This is demonstrated by the results of a study which investigated salivary responses as a function of two extreme styles of 'dietary restraint', namely strict and unrelenting dieting exemplified by a group of anorexic patients, and variable dieting exemplified by a group of bulimic patients (LeGoff et al., 1988). The anorexic patients were underweight and were classified as restricting anorexics (anorexic patients with bulimic symptoms were excluded from the study). All subjects were asked to identify various food odours (e.g., taco-flavoured corn chips, cinnamon bun and chocolate) and non-food odours (e.g., pencil shavings, clothing detergent and tobacco) with their eyes closed. Compared with age-matched control subjects, anticipatory salivation to the food odours, but not to the non-food odours, was exaggerated among the bulimics and reduced among the anorexics. The anorexics also reported lower levels of hunger. Other studies confirm this finding of reduced hunger in anorexics and, furthermore, show that restricting anorexics tend to report lower levels of hunger than anorexics with bulimic symptoms, but similar low body weights (e.g., Robinson, 1989; Halmi & Sunday, 1991; 1996; Hetherington & Rolls, 1991; Geracioti et al., 1992).

Two further results reported by LeGoff et al. (1988) are also very revealing. First, when the anorexic and bulimic patients' food intake patterns were to a large extent normalized after 60 days of intensive in-patient treatment, the differences in salivation and hunger responses disappeared or were markedly reduced. Second, an analysis which pooled data from all of the anorexic, bulimic and control subjects showed a strong positive correlation between 'caloric variability' and food-induced salivation. It was also found that caloric variability accounted for a greater proportion of the variance in salivary response than did body weight. Caloric variability was defined as the 'variability of the caloric content of meals', and was measured from food diaries completed for one week prior to the experimental tests conducted before and after the 60-day treatment programme.

LeGoff et al. (1988) conclude that these different appetite responses are a direct consequence of the different eating patterns adopted by restricting anorexic and bulimic patients. The explanation for the reduced anticipatory salivation and hunger associated with the unrelenting anorexic style of dietary restriction is that these conditioned responses have been extinguished, because typically little or nothing is consumed on occasions when food-related stimuli are present (Herman *et al.*, 1981; LeGoff *et al.*, 1988). This implies that, despite their undernourished weight, the presence of food and food-related stimuli will have a relatively weak (stimulatory) effect on appetite for such individuals. Paradoxically, therefore, they may experience reduced rather than enhanced appetite as dieting progresses, which will then contribute to further restriction of eating. This conclusion is consistent with the view that external stimuli conditioned to eating play a major role in the control of appetite, and also with the results of studies on the effects of weight-reducing diets showing that, although hunger and food-induced salivation are increased following short-term food deprivation, after longer-term food restriction these responses are more likely to be diminished (Section 2.2.4; Durrant 1981). In contrast, appetite may be enhanced in bulimic individuals, particularly in situations where overeating has occurred in the past, again with the result that the behaviour tends to become self-perpetuating (e.g., Jansen *et al.*, 1992).

Although anorexia and bulimia are characterized by highly pathological patterns of eating behaviour, in less extreme forms such patterns are probably typical of the behaviour of restrained eaters and dieters. This was acknowledged by Herman and his colleagues when they used the terms 'dieting drone' and 'fence-sitter dieter' to refer to dieters who tend either towards the anorexic or bulimic pattern of eating (Herman *et al.*, 1981). We suggest that these different eating or dieting styles also tend to be selected predominantly by, respectively, the DEBQ and TFEQ restraint scales versus the RRS (Table 8.2). Supporting this is the apparent absence of increased hunger in subjects scoring high on the TFEQ and DEBQ restraint scales, as demonstrated by the finding that scores on these scales show almost a zero correlation with scores on the TFEQ hunger scale (Hill *et al.*, 1991a). There are also telling similarities between the results of studies on food-stimulated salivation in restrained eaters and the findings reported by LeGoff *et al.* (1988) for anorexic and bulimic subjects (but see also Section 9.4.2). Klajner *et al.* (1981), for example, reported that the sight and smell of palatable food caused a three-fold greater increase in salivation in restrained eaters compared with unrestrained eaters as classified by the RRS. A similar finding was reported by LeGoff and Spigelman (1987). In contrast, food-induced salivation was found not to be significantly related to TFEQ-restraint (Rogers & Hill, 1989), or proportionally increased only slightly in TFEQ restrained eaters (Tepper, 1992). Further results showed that, within the same study, food-induced salivation was significantly and positively correlated with the subjects'

RRS scores, but not with their TEFQ-restraint scores (Sahakian *et al.*, 1981). Finally, although the RRS has also been reported as failing to identify significant differences in food-induced salivation (Wooley & Wooley, 1981), in that study the subjects were attending a fitness camp and were tested whilst undergoing a 'strictly-controlled 900 kcal [3.8 MJ] per day diet'. This, therefore, further confirms the tendency for appetite to be reduced during sustained food restriction.

8.7   DIETING, RESTRAINT AND OBESITY

As originally proposed, restraint theory predicted that many of the anomalies in the eating behaviour of obese individuals (Section 8.2), are due to their chronic dieting. However, it was reported that obese subjects failed to display the counterregulatory eating pattern associated with high levels of restraint (RRS). This was the case both for the group of obese subjects as a whole and, crucially, for obese restrained eaters (Ruderman & Wilson, 1979). In a more recent study, preloading did cause obese subjects to markedly increase their food intake (McCann *et al.*, 1992). This may have been expected, because as a group they were fairly highly restrained; but in fact the degree of overeating was found to be unrelated to their RRS scores. Instead a significant predictor of the subjects' counterregulatory eating was their history of binge eating. Thus the strong relationship between past and present patterns of eating is also observed for obese individuals, adding further force to the argument that these patterns are self-perpetuating and play a major role in undermining the cognitive control of food intake (Lowe, 1993; Section 8.6).

As well as demonstrating reasons for the breakdown of eating restraint, there is a need to focus on the features of dieting which are associated with **successful** eating and weight control. Rather than view dieting only negatively, it should be possible, for instance, to identify the actual cognitive and behavioural strategies used by the many dieters and restrained eaters who are able to achieve weight loss and subsequently maintain long-term weight stability (cf. Blair *et al.*, 1989). These are only hinted at by the questions comprising the TEFQ and DEBQ. Unfortunately, such an approach is generally lacking in current research on human eating behaviour.

8.8   SUMMARY

The externality theory of obesity proposed that the obese are more reactive to external food-related cues and also less sensitive to internal hunger and satiation cues than lean individuals. It was further argued that this is a critical factor in the aetiology of obesity: high external responsiveness predisposes individuals living in environments where food is abundant and highly palatable to overeat and therefore to gain excessive weight. These ideas were supported by the results of a series of very original studies begun in the late 1960s; however, externality has subsequently been largely ignored in favour of ideas concerning the effects of dieting and dietary restraint. It was suggested that the poor control of eating displayed by obese subjects in laboratory tests, such as overeating palatable foods and failing to adjust their intake in compensation for food 'preloads', is linked to dieting rather than externality. Classifying individuals according to their degree of dietary restraint measured by the Revised Restraint Scale (RRS) was found to predict a very striking phenomenon: highly restrained subjects actually ate more instead of less following a food preload. This 'counterregulatory' behaviour was interpreted in terms of a process of disinhibition. The preload, by forcing the perceived intake of calories above a critical threshold or 'diet boundary', causes normally restrained eaters to suspend their self-imposed restraint, thereby releasing their underlying desire to eat. Other disinhibitors of eating in restrained eaters, including emotional events, the consumption of alcohol, the behaviour of others and even anticipated future overeating, have also been identified. Partly on the basis of these results it was argued that restrained eating plays a direct role in the aetiology of binge eating and bulimia nervosa.

Psychometric analysis of the questions making up the RRS has shown that these measure principally 'concern with dieting' and 'weight fluctuation'. In later research two other questionnaires, the Three Factor Eating Questionnaire (TFEQ) and the Dutch Eating Behaviour Questionnaire (DEBQ), were developed with items which relate more directly to restrained eating and the conscious restriction of food intake. Crucially, individuals scoring high on the TFEQ and DEBQ were found to be relatively less susceptible to disinhibited eating, leading to the suggestion that the RRS tends to identify unsuccessful dieters, whereas the TFEQ and DEBQ restraint scales largely identify successful dieters. An explanation for this predictability of successful versus unsuccessful dietary control is that these outcomes are due to certain self-perpetuating patterns of eating behaviour. Thus, hunger tends to be diminished during strict, unbroken dieting, but increased in individuals having a highly variable eating pattern (such as occurs when eating is frequently disinhibited).

Dieting and restrained eating are motivated by concern to achieve a culturally and personally acceptable weight. However, dieting can be easily disrupted, with the consequence that eating and weight control is undermined. A significant challenge for future research on human eating behaviour is to identify more effective cognitive and behavioural strategies for managing dietary control.

CHAPTER NINE

Mood, food craving and food 'addiction' as causes of overeating

9.1 FOOD, MOOD AND APPETITE

It is not hard to find examples of effects of eating and drinking on mood – feelings of contentment and sleepiness often follow a large lunch, a cup of strong coffee is alerting, and eating chocolate may relieve tension, or cause the dieter to feel guilty. Some of these influences are related to individuals' attitudes towards particular foods, whereas other effects are mediated by specific physiological actions of dietary constituents (e.g., Rogers, 1995). In turn, mood and emotion have been implicated as having an impact on food choice and food intake, and several of these hypotheses suggest a link between the mood effects of food and 'food craving'.

9.2 EMOTIONALITY, THE PSYCHOSOMATIC THEORY OF OBESITY, AND BINGE EATING

Stated simply, the psychosomatic view of obesity is that obesity is due to overeating that occurs in response to emotional stimuli. While the most common response to arousal states, such as anger, fear and anxiety, is the loss of appetite, it is argued that some individuals react by eating excessively. Furthermore, eating then modifies the emotional state, for instance by reducing anxiety. Overeating is thus a learned behaviour which can be viewed either as a coping response, or as resulting from a confusion of internal cues associated with activation and stress and 'natural' hunger cues (Kaplan & Kaplan, 1957; Bruch, 1961; Robbins & Fray, 1980). These and related ideas have been investigated extensively and have received some empirical support. For example, individuals who are overweight are more likely to report eating when depressed or anxious (Plutchik, 1976). Also, both experimentally induced and naturally occurring anxiety have been shown to lead to overeating in the obese, whereas the same manipulations inhibited eating in lean subjects (Slochower, 1983).

There is also a relatively high prevalence of depression and anxiety among obese patients who report binge eating (Specker *et al.*, 1994). Binge eating or bulimia (see Section 8.5.2) tends to begin during a time of personal stress. In addition, many reports indicate that it is very common for actual bulimic episodes to be preceded by dysphoric mood states, and that mood is improved during binging (e.g., Mizes, 1985; Cooper & Bowskill, 1986; Hetherington *et al.*, 1994). For example, Cooper & Bowskill (1986) found a strong association between deterioration of mood and the onset of self-reported episodes of overeating in patients with bulimia, and also in women students who were highly restrained eaters and were on a diet. These observations have led to the suggestion that binging behaviour is negatively reinforced by the emotional relief (e.g., Mizes, 1985).

Nevertheless, whether or not such a mechanism does operate in bulimia and other examples of mood- and stress-associated eating, on its own this would seem to be insufficient to account for the very intense and excessive character of bulimic eating behaviour. Furthermore, after binging, bulimics frequently experience a rapid deterioration in mood, including guilt, self-disgust, fear of weight gain and depression, although purging can reduce these negative emotional states [thus purging may also be negatively reinforced (Mizes, 1985)]. It is also difficult to establish the exact causal relationships between the different features of the psychopathology of bulimia. For example, some authors have suggested that the overeating and depression, as well as other symptoms which coincide in bulimia such as substance abuse and impulsive behaviour, share a common pathology, but that they are not necessarily functionally interdependent. The link is thought to be a deficit in brain serotonergic activity (Rosenthal & Hefferman, 1986; Weltzin *et al.*, 1995; Section 9.3).

A specific difficulty with much of the research testing the psychosomatic theory of obesity is that it has failed to take into account the possible interaction between effects related to obesity and the effects of dieting and dietary restraint (Chapter 8). Thus, for example, current dieting appears to be a better predictor of the amount eaten when depressed than is obesity (Baucom & Aiken, 1981). These relationships can also be studied by examining the intercorrelations between the three sub-scales of the Dutch Eating Behaviour Questionnaire (van Strien *et al.*, 1986; Section 8.4.1) which measure restrained eating, emotional eating and external eating. A consistent finding is a small but positive correlation between emotional eating and restraint, a higher positive correlation between emotional eating and externality, and a non-significant correlation between restraint and externality (van Strien *et al.*, 1986; Wardle, 1987; Hill *et al.*, 1991a; Rogers & Green, 1993). Thus externality and dietary restraint tend to have separate influences on (over)eating behaviour, while emotional eating may be due, at least sometimes, to the disinhibition of restraint (Section 8.3).

A third idea relating eating and emotion is that eating occurs due to largely non-specific effects of the emotional stress (Robbins & Fray, 1980). From their extensive review of the literature these authors concluded that 'eating is induced by stress, but the eating does not act to reduce that stress ... The activating effects of stress produce increased attention to external stimuli, many of which are likely to be food-related. These stimuli elicit eating and also metabolic changes in anticipation of food. These metabolic changes provide further activation, which augments the eating response' (page 127). Earlier in the review they say 'The obese ... respond by turning to food, and, once attracted, home in in a spiral, like a moth towards a lamp' (page 123). In other words, this argues that the arousal accompanying emotional states increases responsiveness to salient external cues (cf. Section 8.2), which for obese people, and perhaps also for restrained eaters, are very likely to be foods and food-related cues. Their desire to eat is then further increased due to physiological events (e.g., cephalic phase insulin release; Section 2.2.3) triggered by exposure to these cues.

9.3   SEROTONIN, MOOD AND 'CRAVING' FOR CARBOHYDRATES

9.3.1   Meal composition effects on brain serotonin and mood

The carbohydrate cravers were significantly less depressed after snacking, whereas noncravers experienced fatigue and sleepiness. These findings suggest that carbohydrate cravers may eat snacks high in carbohydrates in order to restore flagging vitality, much as some people will pour another cup of coffee when they feel that their energy level or attention span is flagging.

(Wurtman & Wurtman, 1989, page 53)

The most prominent and extensively tested idea concerning effects of food on mood is the hypothesis proposed by R. J. Wurtman and colleagues linking carbohydrate and protein intake, brain serotonergic (5-hydroxytryptamine, 5-HT) function, and mood and behaviour. This was based on the results of studies mainly carried out on rats (e.g., Fernstrom & Wurtman, 1971a; 1971b; 1972; reviewed by Wurtman *et al.*, 1981). In outline the hypothesis is as follows. Consumption of a high carbohydrate meal increases the ratio of the plasma concentrations of the amino acid tryptophan relative to the sum of the other 'large neutral amino acids' (e.g., tyrosine, phenylalanine, leucine, isoleucine and valine) (abbreviated as Trp:ΣLNAA). This occurs because insulin released in response to the carbohydrate load facilitates the uptake of most amino acids, but not tryptophan, into peripheral tissues such as muscle. Uniquely for amino acids, tryptophan is bound to albumin in the blood stream, and the affinity of albumin for tryptophan actually increases in response to insulin as free fatty acids (FFA) are stripped off the circulating albumin (due to the effect of insulin on the removal of FFA from the circulation). Tryptophan is the precursor of the neurotransmitter serotonin and, since tryptophan and the other large neutral amino acids compete for entry into the brain and the rate-limiting enzyme for serotonin production (tryptophan hydroxylase) is not fully saturated with substrate under normal conditions, an increase in plasma Trp:ΣLNAA concentration leads to an increase in brain serotonin synthesis and, in turn, to increased serotonergic neurotransmission. In contrast, consumption of a meal high in protein is expected to have the opposite effect, primarily because most dietary proteins contain relatively very little tryptophan (Wurtman *et al.*, 1981).

The behavioural consequences which have been predicted to follow from these diet-induced changes in neurotransmission include altered food choice and food intake, and changes in pain sensitivity, aggressiveness, mood, and alertness (Spring *et al.*, 1987; Wurtman & Wurtman, 1989). The evidence for such effects, though, is mixed. Several studies found differences in the effects of high carbohydrate and high protein meals in the predicted direction of greater drowsiness, sleepiness and calmness after carbohydrate (Spring *et al.*, 1987), but these were not consistent across all subject groups, and a majority of mood and performance measures were unaffected by meal composition. Also, more recent studies (Deijen *et al.*, 1989; Christensen & Redig, 1993) failed to show any definite carbohydrate versus protein effects on mood, despite confirmation in the latter study of significant effects on Trp:ΣLNAA concentrations. Pivonka and Grunewald (1990) found that a sugar-sweetened drink increased sleepiness and decreased alertness compared with the effects of the same drink sweetened with aspartame or the same volume of water. These differences emerged about 30 minutes after the drinks were consumed. However, other similar studies have not revealed such clear results (e.g., Brody & Wolitzky, 1983), and these experiments did not test the effects of protein or other nutrient loads.

In addition to these effects of meal composition on alertness, Wurtman and Wurtman (1989) have developed a further hypothesis which proposes that carbohydrates can relieve depression. The hypothesis relates specifically to three 'disorders', carbohydrate-craving obesity (CCO), premenstrual syndrome (PMS) and seasonal affective disorder (SAD), the characteristics of which include depressed mood and supposedly a craving for and increased intake of high carbohydrate foods. Together with evidence implicating deficient serotonergic function in the aetiology of depression (e.g., Cowen *et al.*, 1992; Møller, 1992; Maes & Meltzer, 1995), this has led to the suggestion that the increase in carbohydrate intake constitutes self-medication to relieve the depression. In turn, in CCO the sustained increase in carbohydrate (and fat) intake causes obesity. In other words, CCO is 'a disease of mood, in which appetite control is sacrificed to affective state' (Wurtman & Wurtman, 1992, page 152).

The prediction is, therefore, that consumption of a high-carbohydrate, low-protein meal should have different effects in depressed and non-depressed individuals. Relatively few studies have tested this directly, although carbohydrate has been found consistently to be significantly less sedating in CCO, SAD and PMS subjects compared with controls (Lieberman *et al.*, 1986b; Rosenthal *et al.*, 1989; Wurtman *et al.*, 1989). Lieberman *et al.* (1986b) also demonstrated the predicted effects on depressed mood in CCO. In PMS subjects a carbohydrate meal was found to markedly improve several aspects of mood, including tension, anger, depression and confusion, all of which were unaffected in control subjects (Wurtman *et al.*, 1989). Both these latter studies, however, failed to establish whether the effects on mood were specific to carbohydrate, because responses to other meals (e.g., high in fat or protein) were not tested.

In a study of spontaneous meal patterns, de Castro (1987) found a significant negative correlation between self-reported depression and the proportion of carbohydrate (% of energy) consumed over a 9-day period. In addition, depression was positively correlated with proportionate protein intake, and feelings of energy were positively correlated with proportionate carbohydrate intake. These relationships, however, were not apparent in an analysis of meal to meal mood and food intake. Nor is the direction of the effects as predicted by Wurtman and colleagues, since the subjects were not depressed to begin with. High-carbohydrate, low-protein intake is supposed to increase somnolence, but not affect depression, in nondepressed individuals.

Finally, the effects of tryptophan itself on mood and behaviour are of interest because this can provide a test of the limits of the diet-serotonin hypothesis. Various studies have confirmed that oral administration of tryptophan alone (acute doses of 1.5 to 5 g) or in combination with carbohydrate has substantial effects on plasma Trp:ΣLNAA concentrations, and induces feelings of drowsiness and fatigue, decreases sleep latency, and reduces appetite including rated hunger and actual food intake (reviewed by Young, 1986; Spring *et al.*, 1987; Hill & Blundell, 1988; Steinberg *et al.*, 1992). Daily intakes of tryptophan from dietary sources are typically in the range of 1 to 1.5 g (Young, 1986). Tryptophan in larger pharmacological doses can also be an effective antidepressant, both when given alone and in combination with other treatments. Mild or moderately depressed people appear to benefit most from treatment with tryptophan, although it is less potent than standard antidepressant drugs (Young, 1986). This would be consistent with the view that a deficit in serotonergic activity is important as a vulnerability factor, but is not the proximate cause of depression (Maes & Meltzer, 1995). Tryptophan has also been found to improve depressive symptoms in SAD and PMS (McGrath *et al.*, 1989; Steinberg *et al.*, 1986), although it appears not to have been tested in CCO. Another research strategy has been to measure the effects of administering amino acid mixtures devoid of tryptophan. The results have shown that a lowering of mood following tryptophan depletion is most likely to occur in individuals with high baseline depression scores or who have a family history of depression (Young *et al.*, 1985; and reviewed by Young, 1991; 1993; Benkelfat *et al.*, 1994). Taken together, these studies of tryptophan and tryptophan depletion add significantly to the evidence indicating a role for serotonin in the aetiology of depression. However, as the next section shows, the pharmacological manipulation of tryptophan intakes is not evidence for an influence on mood of the tryptophan or macronutrient contents of typical diets.

9.3.2 Further evidence for and against carbohydrate craving as a cause of obesity

The CCO hypothesis proposes that dysphoric mood is associated with carbohydrate craving. This then is supposed to lead to increased carbohydrate intake, which in turn augments brain serotonergic activity and thereby ameliorates the depression (Wurtman & Wurtman, 1989). Some support for this comes from results reviewed in the previous section showing improvements in mood following the consumption of high-carbohydrate meals. Serotonergic mediation of these effects has also been tested. Wurtman *et al.* (1987) compared the responses of obese 'carbohydrate cravers' and obese noncarbohydrate cravers to the drug d-fenfluramine (which increases serotonergic neurotransmission). Measured against placebo treatment, d-fenfluramine had a more immediate and larger effect on the frequency of snacking and high-carbohydrate 'snack' intake in the carbohydrate cravers, although there was also a significant reduction in 'snacking' in the noncarbohydrate cravers during the third and final month on d-fenfluramine. These results were interpreted as being consistent with the proposal that d-fenfluramine decreases hunger for carbohydrates in the carbohydrate craver by mimicking the effects of carbohydrate consumption on serotonergic functioning. However, although d-fenfluramine also reduced intake at 'main meals' in the carbohydrate cravers (but not in noncarbohydrate cravers), this was due to a similar reduction in the intakes of all three macronutrients. In addition, d-fenfluramine did not appear to be superior to placebo in its effects on mood. [On the other hand, d-fenfluramine has been found to be effective in the treatment of depression in SAD and PMS (O'Rourke *et al.*, 1989; Brzezinski *et al.*, 1990), and in the latter of these studies the improvement in mood was accompanied by a suppression of premenstrual increases in carbohydrate and fat intake.]

An aspect of the mood, carbohydrate-craving and serotonin hypothesis which has not been widely discussed is the mechanism by which depressed mood is supposed to give rise to carbohydrate craving. One suggestion is that the depressed individual recognizes the beneficial effects of carbohydrates and accordingly deliberately increases carbohydrate intake in order to improve his or her mood (Wurtman, 1988). Wurtman and Wurtman (1989) have also proposed that the increased carbohydrate consumption may occur because the normal feedback regulation of carbohydrate and protein intake is disrupted in CCO (and in SAD and PMS). Normally, it is argued, consumption of carbohydrate would be expected to increase brain serotonin activity and inhibit further carbohydrate intake. In depression, when brain serotonin levels are low this response is reduced and the desire to eat carbohydrates persists. Other variants of these ideas have also been suggested (e.g., Møller, 1992), but none of them appears to have been tested directly. A further possibility is that appetite for carbohydrates is amplified because of an increased liking for high-carbohydrate foods reinforced by their effects on mood (Rogers *et al.*, 1992; Section 2.3.3). A similar suggestion was made to account for the observation that the carbohydrate to fat ratio normally chosen by subjects at either breakfast or lunch tended to correspond with the macronutrient composition favouring optimal post-meal alertness (Lloyd *et al.*, 1994; 1996; Rogers, 1995). These latter effects were apparent within 15 minutes of eating; however, changes in mood due to an effect of carbohydrate on brain serotonin, if they occur, will have a longer onset (see below) making it less likely that they will support strong conditioned preferences.

A critical test of the carbohydrate-serotonin hypothesis is to measure the effects of meal composition on physiological variables. As predicted, studies on human subjects have shown statistically significant differences in plasma Trp:ΣLNAA concentrations following 'meals' with a very a high carbohydrate versus high protein content (e.g., Ashley *et al.*, 1985; Lieberman *et al.*, 1986a; Teff *et al.*, 1989a; Christensen & Redig, 1993). Similar effects have been confirmed in SAD and obese subjects (Rosenthal *et al.*, 1989; Pijl *et al.*, 1993). The practical significance of these results, however, is uncertain. In particular, it appears that the magnitude of the effects is probably too small to produce functionally significant changes in brain serotonergic activity (Ashley *et al.*, 1985; Leathwood, 1987; Young, 1991). The actual changes observed were, for example, small increases in Trp:ΣLNAA plasma concentrations following high starch and high sugar meals and a larger decrease in the ratio after high protein meals. Differences in Trp:ΣLNAA concentrations did not reach their maximum until 2 to 3 hours after these meals, with almost no change occurring within the first hour after a carbohydrate meal (e.g., Lieberman *et al.*, 1986a; Rosenthal *et al.*, 1989). Furthermore, the range in macronutrient compositions of meals typical of most diets is unlikely to produce any very distinct differences in post-prandial plasma amino acid ratios, because the presence of a small amount of protein (perhaps as little as 4% energy as protein) in a high-carbohydrate meal is sufficient to block any meal-induced increases in the Trp:ΣLNAA concentration (Teff *et al.*, 1989a, see also Wurtman *et al.*, 1981).

Even more striking are the results of a study by Teff *et al.* (1989b) in which samples of cerebrospinal fluid were collected from human subjects 2.5 hours after they had consumed either 100 g of carbohydrate, a high protein load, or water. Compared with the effects of water, the nutrient loads did not alter the cerebrospinal fluid concentrations of either tryptophan or the serotonin metabolite 5-hydroxyindoleacetic acid. On the other hand, plasma Trp:ΣLNAA concentrations were affected in a similar manner to previous studies. This result would therefore support the view that in human beings differences in meal macronutrient composition do not alter plasma amino acid ratios sufficiently to cause appreciable changes in brain tryptophan levels or serotonin synthesis (but see Fernstrom, 1994).

A further issue concerns the use of the term 'craving'. Food craving is usually described as a strong desire to eat a particular food or particular types of food (crave: 'to long for, to desire intensely, to need greatly or urgently', *Collins English Dictionary*, 1986; see also Weingarten & Elston, 1991; Rogers, 1994). The best evidence demonstrating physiologically related food cravings is reported craving for salt in untreated patients with Addison's disease. In this disease the adrenal cortex is damaged and the ability to retain sodium is impaired. Less dramatically, while experimental sodium depletion in healthy subjects by a very low sodium diet and diuretics did not cause strong cravings for salt, it did result in moderate increases in the desirability of salty foods (Beauchamp *et al.*, 1991a). In studies of CCO, however, carbohydrate craving has been defined primarily on the basis of the frequent consumption of 'snacks' high in carbohydrate and fat, but low in protein. For example, in the study by Wurtman *et al.* (1987) the carbohydrate cravers ate on average 7 such snacks per day. In the same study there was also a smaller number of obese 'noncarbohydrate cravers' who acted as a control group. They had a similar frequency of snacking, divided about equally between high protein and high carbohydrate snacks. The question is whether craving is the appropriate term to describe the CCO subjects' behaviour, since there is no information on their subjective experience of appetite for carbohydrates, or how this experience contrasts with that of the obese noncarbohydrate cravers, whose actual eating behaviour did not differ very much from that of the carbohydrate cravers. In other words, there is little direct evidence to support the claim that increased carbohydrate and fat intake in CCO (Wurtman & Wurtman, 1992) is due specifically to an increased desire to eat carbohydrates. Furthermore, dietary intake data reveal fairly consistent negative associations between carbohydrate intakes and fatness (Section 6.3), and feeding trials and metabolic studies generally support a beneficial rather than damaging influence of carbohydrate consumption on weight control (Chapter 5). Thus the notion of CCO seems to contradict other results on food composition, eating behaviour and weight control.

The existence of carbohydrate craving has also been challenged on the grounds that high fat content is itself an essential feature of frequently craved foods (Drewnowski *et al.*, 1992a; see also Drewnowski, 1992; Hetherington *et al.*, 1994; van der Ster Wallin *et al.*, 1994; Hill & Heaton-Brown, 1995). Craving for foods high in fat and/or (sweet) carbohydrate has, moreover, been linked with activity of the endogenous opioid system rather than serotonergic mediation (Drewnowski, 1992). Thus Drewnowski (1992) has argued that overeating and reported cravings for foods high in sugar and fat may share a common mechanism with opiate drug addiction. Similarly, Blass (1987) earlier suggested that consumption of sweet and other palatable foods may be motivated in part by their capacity to relieve stress. These ideas are supported by results indicating that opioids are released in response to the ingestion of sweet and other palatable foods (Fullerton *et al.*, 1985; Blass 1991; Section 2.3.2), and the finding that the opioid antagonist drug naloxone is highly effective in reducing food intake in binge eaters, due largely to an effect on the consumption of sweet, high-fat foods such as chocolate and biscuits (Drewnowski *et al.*, 1992a). It is also claimed that opioid antagonists suppress stress-induced overeating (Fullerton *et al.*, 1985). There is good evidence that endogenous opioids are involved in mediating hedonic responses during eating (Kirkham & Cooper, 1991); however, whether or not the same systems are implicated in the development of food craving, compulsive eating, or obesity is less certain. An alternative view of what makes sweet, high-fat foods such as chocolate, cakes, ice-cream and biscuits special is the role these foods are perceived to have in the diet (Rogers, 1994). This is discussed in Section 9.4.2, while the next section first examines evidence for and against a biological basis for chocolate craving.

9.4   BIOLOGICAL, COGNITIVE AND SOCIO-CULTURAL DIMENSIONS OF FOOD 'ADDICTION'

9.4.1   Chocolate and 'chocoholism'

In the popular media chocolate is possibly the most discussed and written about of all foods. The question of why people like, consume and crave chocolate has also been addressed in the scientific literature; however, much of this discussion has been largely speculative and it has contained relatively little scientifically valid research. Closely connected with chocolate craving are notions concerning the effects of potentially psychoactive constituents of chocolate and chocolate 'addiction'. Chocolate is a frequent focus of reported food cravings, especially among women

(Weingarten & Elston, 1991; Rodin *et al.*, 1991). However, in itself this and other circumstantial evidence, for example the existence of groups such as Chocoholics Anonymous, is not sufficient to demonstrate addiction to chocolate (Rogers, 1994). Indeed, it is obvious that very many people eat chocolate without becoming 'addicted' (see below). Nevertheless, eating chocolate can have significant influences on mood, generally leading to an increase in pleasant feelings and a reduction in tension, although increased 'guilt' may be a penalty for some individuals (e.g., Hill *et al.*, 1991a; Hill & Heaton-Brown, 1995; Macdiarmid & Hetherington, 1995). Also, craving for various foods, including chocolate, is associated with negative moods, including boredom, tension, anger, depression and tiredness (Schlundt *et al.*, 1993b; Rogers *et al.*, 1994).

Serious reviews have generally concluded that there is no support for the suggestion that liking and craving for chocolate are related to the presence of psychoactive constituents (Tarka, 1982; Max, 1989; Rozin *et al.*, 1991). For example, although chocolate can contain relatively high concentrations of theobromine, this is a relatively weak central nervous system stimulant and does not have strong subjective effects (Mumford *et al.*, 1994). The related methylxanthine, caffeine, is also found in chocolate but in much lower concentrations. Compared with coffee and tea, chocolate is an insignificant source of dietary caffeine (Gilbert, 1984). There also appears to be a lack of any generally significant relationship between reported chocolate craving and the liking and consumption of other xanthine-containing substances (Rozin *et al.*, 1991). Other substances present in chocolate which have been discussed as potentially pharmacologically significant include histamine, serotonin, tryptophan, phenylethylamine, tyramine, magnesium and cannabinoids (e.g., Cockcroft, 1993; Michener & Rozin, 1994; di Tomaso *et al.*, 1996), though many of these compounds exist in higher concentrations in other foods with less appeal than chocolate (Robinson & Ferguson, 1992). The same is true for certain bioactive peptides, such as casomorphins which can act as opioid agonists and occur in a variety of food sources, for example, milk and gluten (Morley *et al.*, 1983; Gardner, 1984).

In any case, identifying a compound in a food is only a first step towards demonstrating that this can have psychoactive effects as consumed in everyday life, and that in turn these effects play a role in influencing liking for that food. Recent research on caffeine has demonstrated significant preference-reinforcing effects, at least at the levels of caffeine found in coffee and tea (Rogers *et al.*, 1995b; Richardson, 1996; Section 2.3.3), but this method has not yet been applied in the investigation of other such constituents of foods and drinks (except alcohol; P. J. Rogers & P. Polet, unpublished results). The most relevant published study on chocolate took a less direct approach. Michener and Rozin (1994) provided chocolate 'cravers' (individuals who reported having a craving for chocolate at least once per week) with sealed boxes containing either a milk chocolate bar, a bar of white chocolate, capsules containing cocoa (and therefore many of the presumed psychoactive ingredients of chocolate), placebo capsules, white chocolate plus cocoa capsules, or nothing. The subjects consumed, in random order, the contents of one of these boxes when they experienced a craving for chocolate, and just before, just after and 90 minutes after doing this they rated the intensity of that craving. The results showed that only consumption of chocolate itself, either white or milk chocolate, substantially reduced the craving, suggesting that there is 'no role for pharmacological effects in the satisfaction of chocolate craving' (Michener & Rozin, 1994, page 419).

A further observation is that the most widely preferred chocolate is milk chocolate and chocolate-covered confectionery. These contain a lower amount of cocoa solids, and therefore a lower concentration of potentially psychoactive compounds, than 'dark' chocolate. It is far more plausible to suggest, therefore, that liking for chocolate, and its effects on mood, are due mainly to its principal constituents sugar and fat and their related orosensory and physiological effects (Max, 1989; Rogers, 1994; Section 2.3.2 and Chapter 6).

Generally, where the terms 'craving' and 'addiction' are used the existence of certain underlying biological mechanisms which support addictions is also implied. Addiction, however, is a difficult concept. The pleasurable effects produced by the substance and withdrawal relief play important roles in reinforcing substance use and abuse; but, addiction is not defined by these effects alone (Warburton, 1990). Thus, for example, problem drug use cannot be explained without reference to individual and social perceptions of the behaviour (e.g., Heather, 1997). In the case of reported craving and addiction for chocolate and other similar foods, these perceptions may be particularly critical.

9.4.2   The role of ambivalence and attributions

Previously we discussed the effects of external cues on eating and argued that specific appetites may come to be associated with specific cues (Section 2.2.3). In other words, the experience of the desire to eat specific foods in particular contexts or in relation to particular feelings can be regarded as a feature of normal appetite (rather than being indicative of eating pathology). One of the questions that this raises is exactly what experiences are regarded as food cravings. The desire to eat cereal at breakfast and the desire to eat chocolate when relaxing and watching television in the evening may both be examples of learned specific appetites. However, very few people are likely to label the desire to eat cereal as a food craving – unless perhaps this occurred in the evening, which culturally is a less appropriate time for eating breakfast cereal.

This suggests that attitudes to food and eating will play a fundamental role in the experience of food craving. Chocolate is highly palatable food typically consumed in addition to main meals and used variously as a gift, treat, and reward. Thus chocolate is not regarded as a staple food, and indeed its nutritional value (high sugar, fat and energy content) is often viewed negatively – as the penalty for indulging in the enjoyment of the sensory pleasure it evokes (i.e., 'nice but naughty'). In other words, chocolate is a highly desirable food, but which according to social norms should be eaten with restraint (James, 1990; Rogers, 1994). Note that feelings of fullness associated with eating chocolate are quite likely to be reported with disgust rather than satisfaction. However, attempting to resist the desire to eat chocolate only causes this desire to become more prominent, and in turn the experience is labelled as craving, rather than say hunger, because of the attitude that chocolate is an indulgence. Another, less common, description is that the food is 'moreish' (Rogers, 1994). This view of food craving has similarities with Tiffany's (1990; 1995) account of drug craving. His theory proposes that drug use is largely controlled by automatic processes and involves no noticeable urges or cravings, except when drug use is prevented or **resisted**.

The conflict or ambivalence experienced when eating chocolate and other 'treat' foods, such as cakes, biscuits and also savoury 'snack' foods, is confirmed by a number results. For instance, in an investigation of the relationship between dieting and food craving subjects kept detailed diaries of their food intake, hunger, mood and food cravings (Hill *et al.*, 1991a). Chocolate was specified as the craved food on nearly 60% of all occasions on which a craving was noted. Furthermore, dysphoric mood often preceded occurrences of craving, and for the subjects who invariably acted on their craving (i.e., ate the craved food) there was a positive shift in mood after eating, for example, toward feeling calm and relaxed. Significantly, however, subjects who attempted to resist their cravings tended to report a negative shift in mood after eating the craved food. Earlier we discussed the complex relationship between dieting and food-induced salivation (Section 8.6). Another factor that may account for part of these findings is differences in restrained and unrestrained eaters' emotional responses to food and eating (Hill *et al.*, 1995). Specifically, confronting restrained eaters and dieters with palatable, 'diet-prohibited' foods when they have recently eaten can be expected to provoke anxiety which in turn will inhibit their salivary responses (Rosen, 1981; Rogers & Hill, 1989). A similar conclusion was drawn from results showing that individuals who reported themselves to be 'chocoholics' displayed, compared with a group of age and sex matched controls, the greatest liking for chocolate, the largest increase in hunger, but the smallest increase in salivation when exposed to chocolate (Figure 9.1; Rogers *et al.*, 1994). Although the results for the salivation measure appear to contradict the other measures, and also the finding that the chocoholics had a much higher frequency of consumption of chocolate, they are consistent with the suggestion that a characteristic of these individuals is an anxiety about eating chocolate (Rogers, 1994).

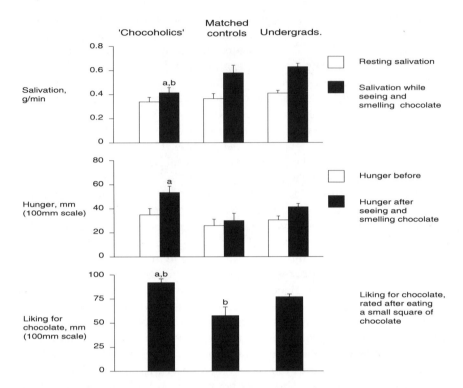

Figure 9.1 Effects of exposure to chocolate in three groups of subjects. The figures are means ± standard errors. 'a', $p < 0.05$ versus matched controls; 'b', $p < 0.05$ versus undergraduates. The chocoholics (23 women and 10 men) were 'self-diagnosed', and had responded to an advertisement in a local newspaper which began simply, 'Are you a chocoholic?' The matched control group consisted of 18 women and 6 men within the same age range (18–45 years). There were 91 women and 30 men in the undergraduate group. Subjects were tested individually using standard methods for assessing salivation, hunger, etc. (e.g., Rogers & Hill, 1989). These findings were reported in Rogers *et al.* (1994), but the data are previously unpublished.

In another study, men and women rated the 'appropriateness' of 50 foods and beverages on 50 attributes or uses (P. J. Rogers & H. G. Schutz, unpublished). Among these attributes/uses were, 'when I am unhappy', 'when I want something I really like', 'when I want something nutritious', and 'a food difficult to resist'. Chocolate ranked highest on the attribute 'difficult to resist', although it ranked only 17th in terms of frequency of consumption. Foods which were scored high on 'difficult to resist' were also highly liked (Table 9.1). Furthermore, these foods were rated as appropriate for the mood 'when I am unhappy', indicating presumably that eating these foods can improve mood. On the other hand, there was a low correlation between 'difficult to resist' and perceived nutritional value, with chocolate ranked 39th out of 50 on the use 'when I want something nutritious'. This again demonstrates the existence of ambivalent attitudes toward such foods. Additionally, eating a food to alter mood rather than to remove hunger may itself be a source of conflict – this is perceived as an inappropriate use of a food, leading to concerns about lack of self-control and self-efficacy. It is noteworthy that in this study on food appropriateness, tea and coffee were not rated highly on the attribute 'difficult to resist' (rank orders 18th and 25th, respectively), but these were the most frequently consumed items. Therefore, there would appear to relatively little ambivalence associated with tea and coffee drinking. Indeed, their use as a source of pharmacological stimulation is openly acknowledged and regarded as acceptable. In contrast to drinking tea and coffee, eating chocolate has many negative connotations. In particular, chocolate may be **perceived** as an unhealthy food, lacking in nutritional value, and is stigmatized by associations with overeating, overindulgence and obesity.

Finally, another aspect of food craving and addiction concerns the use of these terms, or the ideas that they convey, to give a particular explanation of behaviour. By saying that 'I crave chocolate' or confessing that 'I am a chocoholic' the individual is able to explain why he or she eats chocolate frequently and why he or she finds it difficult to resist. Attributing what is perceived as excessive consumption of chocolate to an addiction provides a socially (and personally) acceptable explanation for this behaviour, and thereby helps to remove individual responsibility for the difficulty. On the basis of the publicly accepted model of addictions, it implies that eating chocolate is outside the person's control, and alternatively attributes problems of control to biological effects of the food (e.g., it contains a dependence-forming substance), or possibly to an

Table 9.1 Correlations between 'a food difficult to resist' and other attributes. r = Pearson correlation coefficient (df = 48), ns = not significant ($p > 0.10$). Unpublished data from P.J. Rogers and H.G. Schutz

Attribute or use	r	p (2-tail)
When I want something I really like	0.84	< 0.001
A food I spend a lot of time thinking about	0.77	< 0.001
When I am unhappy	0.75	< 0.001
A food I feel strongly about	0.65	< 0.001
A food with which I am very involved	0.57	< 0.001
For when I eat alone	0.16	ns
For a between meal snack	0.24	< 0.1
When I am hungry	0.30	< 0.05
When I want something nutritious	−0.10	ns

individual pathology, thus invoking a medical model (Peele, 1990; Eiser, 1990). Attributions are commonsense explanations made in an attempt to understand and sometimes to excuse personal behaviour. Notions such as compulsive eating and food craving indicate an addiction model. Given the widespread salience of the concept of addiction (Peele, 1990), it is not surprising that this concept is applied to food-related behaviour. Moreover, this attribution may provide a basis for individual action which in turn will help to confirm the model. For instance, the belief that abstinence is required for recovery from addiction will lead to exactly the sort of conflict described above – between the desire to eat a food and the desire to maintain restraint. Similarly, it has been argued that attributions are significant determinants of menstrual cycle-related changes in mood and behaviour, including reports of food craving and premenstrual increases in food intake (Ussher, 1989; Rogers & Jas, 1994).

Although the lack of relevant empirical studies has meant that much of the above discussion is still speculative, it does indicate the inadequacy of exclusively biological explanations of food craving. Foods which are craved or claimed to be 'addictive' appear not to possess any unique psychopharmacological activity. Instead, the experience of food craving is probably best understood in terms of the interaction of the normal mechanisms of appetite control, the hedonic effects of certain foods, and socially and culturally determined perceptions of the role and use of those foods.

9.5 SUMMARY

The psychosomatic theory of obesity and the related idea that binge eating is reinforced by the avoidance of, or escape from, negative mood states, has received some support. Nevertheless, emotional stress also appears to affect eating through non-specific arousing effects and by disrupting dietary restraint. Another extensively investigated theory concerning dietary influences on mood was developed in the late 1970s and proposed that the balance of protein and carbohydrate consumed in a meal can affect the synthesis and activity of the brain neurotransmitter serotonin. One prediction from this theory is that meals high in protein will increase alertness. A second is that carbohydrate-rich 'snacks' or meals will relieve depressed mood. Consequently, the increased carbohydrate (and fat) intake associated with some forms of depression has been viewed as a form of nutritional self-medication and, in the case of 'carbohydrate-craving obesity' (CCO), this is proposed to be a cause of sustained weight gain. Other results, however, show that everyday variations in protein and carbohydrate intake will typically have little impact on brain serotonergic function. Additionally, the significance of carbohydrate craving is questioned by the suggestion that sweetness and/or high fat content are the essential features of frequently craved foods. Chocolate possesses these features, and there are also various claims that psychoactive compounds present in chocolate contribute to preferences and reported craving for this food, but such effects have not been demonstrated. Rather than their biological effects, what craved and 'addictive' foods appear to have most closely in common is a special role as treats ('nice but naughty'), and it is the ambivalence associated with this role which probably underlies the perception of lack of control.

Taken together, this research confirms significant influences of mood on eating and of eating on mood; however, these relationships explain less about overeating and obesity than is popularly supposed.

CHAPTER TEN

Conclusions

It has generally been assumed that appetite is regulated by a homeostatic system that serves to maintain energy balance. Accordingly, attempts to identify the physiological mechanisms underlying this homeostasis have dominated research in the area, and experimental models of obesity have been studied mainly for their potential to provide insight into these mechanisms. Contemporary reviews of the control of food intake may therefore present extensive and sophisticated models which imply multiple and sensitive mechanisms for homeostatic regulation (e.g., Bray, 1989; Weigle, 1994), akin to those established for ensuring sodium balance. Arguably, though, much of this has been of little direct relevance to understanding variance in human obesity, which appears not to be readily explained by obvious defects in any part of the many physiological or biomolecular systems examined to date.

There is clearly a strong desire within the scientific, pharmaceutical, and, indeed, the lay communities to identify **the** defect which predisposes individuals to obesity and resistance to slimming. Herman (1996) has commented on the parallels between the attributions of individuals and the interests of researchers:

> … people fall back on their own implicit theories of behavior; in the case of eating, if I ate a lot, either I must have been very hungry or the food must have tasted very good. I submit that eating researchers are not so different from the general public.
>
> Herman (1996, page 109)

Much as we suggested (Section 9.4.2) that attributions of food cravings and 'addictions' offer the eater an opportunity to lay blame outside their own control, so it is that errors of metabolism offer a more tolerable and apparently 'objective' and quantifiable organic basis for eating behaviour, rather than a complex and potentially messy interaction between the underlying physiology, individual and social psychology, and the eating environment. Hence the long and ultimately unsatisfying search for defects of energy expenditure, and (at some risk of drawing parallels) the phenomenal attention and resources drawn to the leptin system and other putative molecular genetic explanations for obesity.

In fact, we have presented extensive evidence which supports the view that the systems controlling human appetite are fairly permissive in their response to undereating and overeating, but possess a variety of features which, together with learned habits and the tendency for the individual's external environment to remain constant, typically ensure relative stability in energy balance. This is further shored by 'passive' physiological responses, such as the relationship between body mass and obligatory energy expenditure. Popular views of the causes of obesity, including 'slow metabolism' or the specific craving for and overeating of 'indulgent' and palatable foods such as sugars, chips, cakes, and confectionery, are largely not borne out by objective research.

What does the research show?

Decades of work on the effects of food composition on energy balance now seem to converge on the view that the primary route through which this major variable relates to energy balance is not directly through the (physiological) effects upon post-prandial metabolism, but via influences upon the (behavioural) act of food consumption. This places the psychobiology of appetite central to understanding the nutritional aspects of obesity. Research on appetite control, in turn, is increasingly focusing on energy-dense (and for the most part this means high-fat) diets as an important, perhaps essential factor in long-term overeating.

It is, however, facile to consider eating or physical activity as purely voluntary behaviours, given that life is dependent upon their balance. The 'voluntary' nature of eating may at times be similar to the 'voluntary' nature of scratching an itch: it can be avoided, but not ignored, and carrying out the act provides immense relief and satisfaction. That relief and satisfaction, and the anticipation of them, would seem to merit further study. There are certainly many, many physiological mediators which can consistently be shown to promote or suppress eating (but which do not necessarily explain variance in obesity). However, it is not common for individuals to reach true deprivation states in the cultures where obesity prevails, and arguably very little of normal eating occurs as a fixed response to specific hunger and feeding signals. Eating on a day-to-day basis is instead motivated and controlled more often by external factors of habit, social convention, and availability. Several pieces of research point to the possibility that irregular eating patterns may contribute to poor weight control, and this seems a natural corollary of a system which is relatively passive. Paradoxically, some of this irregularity may be a result of weight control efforts.

There is no doubt that susceptibility to obesity has strong genetic components; this may reflect relative deficits in fat oxidation, with or without a heightened preference for the sensory qualities associated with fats (or energy-dense foods), or any of a number of factors. In fact, there appears to be evidence of genetic influences for virtually every neurohumoural and behavioural factor ever linked to obesity. There is now no doubt that a very large proportion of the population is susceptible to obesity and, unfortunately, genetic research has not offered explanations for current secular trends in the disease.

Underlying the increasing prevalence of obesity in so many nations, however, is a biological system that evolved under conditions where food was less energy dense, less varied, less abundant/available, and energy expenditure much higher. Accordingly, obesity has been viewed as a product of the newly encountered aggressive or 'toxic' environment (Blundell, 1996). At the same time, the cultural preference is for a slim body shape. Considerable personal psychological and economic costs are associated with attempts to achieve an, often unrealistically, low body weight. Eating and physical activity can be deliberately modified, and the cognitive control of food intake plays a critical role in the avoidance of obesity. Nevertheless, this control can be relatively easily disrupted, predisposing the individual to ambivalent relationships with food, disordered eating patterns, and even weight gain.

Understanding of the biological systems involved in feeding and energy metabolism must therefore consider other features of the conditions in which eating behaviour develops and takes place. These conditions include powerful learned and cognitive influences which guide behaviour, and ecological constraints and opportunities afforded by social setting, lifestyle, economics, and the culture of the society in which eating occurs. The resulting psychobiological approach can then begin to effectively integrate the events occurring beneath and outside the skin. A critical feature of such an approach is that it is clearly a two-way street: shifts in one domain will influence, or be influenced by, the state of elements in another.

References

Aaron JI, Evans RE, Mela DJ. 1995. Paradoxical effect of a nutrition labelling scheme in a student cafeteria. Nutrition Research 15: 1251–1261.

Abbott WGH, Howard BV, Christin L, Freymond D, Lillioja S, Botce VL, Anderson TE, Bogardus C, Ravussin E. 1988. Short-term energy balance: Relationship with protein, carbohydrate, and fat balances. American Journal of Physiology 255: E332–E337.

Acheson KJ, Flatt J-P, Jéquier E. 1982. Glycogen synthesis versus lipogenesis after a 500 gram carbohydrate meal in man. Metabolism 31: 1234–1240.

Acheson KJ, Schutz Y, Bessard T, Anantharaman K, Flatt J-P, Jéquier E. 1988. Glycogen storage capacity and de novo lipogenesis during massive carbohydrate overfeeding in man. American Journal of Clinical Nutrition 48: 240–247.

Acheson KJ, Schutz Y, Bessard T, Ravussin E, Jéquier E. 1984. Nutritional influences on lipogenesis and thermogenesis after a carbohydrate meal. American Journal of Physiology 246: E62–E70.

Achour I, Flourié B, Briet F, Pellier P, Marteau P, Rambaud J-C. 1994. Gastrointestinal effects and energy value of polydextrose in healthy nonobese men. American Journal of Clinical Nutrition 59: 1362–1368

Ackerman SH, Albert M, Shindledecker RD, Gayle C, Smith GP. 1992. Intake of different concentrations of sucrose and corn oil in preweanling rats. American Journal of Physiology 262: R624–R627.

Ackroff K, Vigorito M, Sclafani A. 1990. Fat appetite in rats: The response of infant and adult rats to nutritive and non-nutritive oil emulsions. Appetite 15:171–188.

Adams CE, Morgan KJ. 1981. Periodicity of eating: Implications for human food consumption. Nutrition Research 1: 525–550.

Ali R, Staub H, Leveille GA, Boyle PC. 1982. Dietary fiber and obesity: A review. In: Vahouny GV, Kritchevsky D, eds. Dietary fiber in health and disease. New York: Plenum. pp. 139–149.

Allison DB, Kaprio J, Koskenvuo M, Neale MC, Hayakawa K. 1996. The heritability of body mass index among an international sample of monozygotic twins reared apart. International Journal of Obesity 20: 501–506.

Amatruda JM, Statt MC, Welle SL. 1993. Total and resting energy expenditure in obese women reduced to ideal body weight. Journal of Clinical Investigation 92: 1236–1242.

American Psychiatric Association. 1994. Diagnostic and Statistical Manual of Mental Disorders (DSM–IV). Washington, DC: APA Press.

Anand BK, Brobeck JR. 1951. Hypothalamic control of food intake in rats and cats. Yale Journal of Biology and Medicine 24: 123–140.

Anderson GH. 1995. Sugars, sweetness, and food intake. American Journal of Clinical Nutrition 62(suppl): 195S–202S.

Anderson GH, Leiter LA. 1996. Sweeteners and food intake: relevance to obesity. In: Angel A, Anderson GH, Bouchard C, Lau D, Leiter L, Mendelson R, eds. Progress in obesity research: 7. London: John Libbey & Co. pp. 345–349.

Anil MH, Forbes JM. 1987. Neural control and neurosensory functions of the liver. Proceedings of the Nutrition Society 46: 125–133.

Armstrong S, Shahbaz C, Singer G. 1981. Inclusion of meal-reversal in a behaviour modification program for obesity. Appetite 2: 1–5.

Arnold L, Ball MJ, Duncan AW, Mann J. 1993. Effect of isoenergetic intake of three or nine meals on plasma lipoproteins and glucose metabolism. American Journal of Clinical Nutrition, 57: 446–451.

Ashley DVM, Liardon R, Leathwood PD. 1985. Breakfast meal composition influences plasma tryptophan to large neutral amino acid ratios of healthy lean young men. Journal of Neural Transmission 63: 271–283.

Astrup A. 1993. Diet composition, substrate balances and body fat in subjects with a predisposition to obesity. International Journal of Obesity 17(Suppl 3): S32–S36.

Astrup A. 1996. Obesity and metabolic efficiency. In: *The origins and consequences of obesity*. Ciba Foundation Symposium 201. Chichester UK: John Wiley & Sons. pp. 159–173.

Astrup A, Buemann B, Christensen NJ, Toubro S. 1994a. Failure to increase lipid oxidation in response to increasing dietary fat content in formerly obese women. American Journal of Physiology 266: E592–E599.

Astrup A, Buemann B, Toubro S, Raben A. 1996. Defects in substrate oxidation involved in the predisposition to obesity. Proceedings of the Nutrition Society 55: 817–828.

Astrup A, Buemann B, Western P, Toubro S, Raben A, Christensen NJ. 1994b. Obesity as an adaptation to a high fat diet: Evidence from a cross-sectional study. American Journal of Clinical Nutrition 59: 350–355.

Baeke JAH, van Staveren WA, Burema J. 1983. Food consumption, habitual physical activity, and body fatness in young Dutch adults. American Journal of Clinical Nutrition 37: 278–286.

Baeyens F, Eelen P, Van den Bergy O, Crombez G. 1990. Flavour-flavour and colour-flavour conditioning in humans. Learning and Motivation 21: 434–455.

Baghurst KI, Baghurst PA, Record SJ. 1994. Demographic and dietary profiles of high and low fat consumers in Australia. Journal of Epidemiology & Community Health 48: 26–32.

Ballard-Barbash R, Thompson FE, Graubard BI, Krebs-Smith SM. 1994. Variability in percent energy from fat throughout the day: Implications for application of total diet goals. Journal of Nutrition Education 26: 278–283.

Bandini LG, Schoeller DA, Cyr HN, Dietz WH. 1990; Validity of reported energy intake in obese and nonobese adolescents. American Journal of Clinical Nutrition 52: 421–425.

Barkeling B, Rössner S, Björvell H. 1990. Efficiency of a high-protein meal (meat) and a high carbohydrate meal (vegetarian) on satiety measured by automated computerized monitering of subsequent food intake, motivation to eat and food preferences. International Journal of Obesity 14: 743–751.

Barkeling B, Rössner S, Sjöberg A. 1995. Methodological studies on single meal food intake characteristics in normal weight and obese men and women. International Journal of Obesity 19: 284–290.

Barr RG, Quek VSH, Cousineau D, Oberlander TF, Brian JA, Young SN. 1994. Effects of intra-oral sucrose on crying, mouthing and hand-mouth contact in newborn and six-week-old infants. Developmental Medicine and Child Neurology 36: 608–618.

Bartoshuk LM. 1979. Bitter taste of saccharin related to the genetic ability to taste the bitter substance 6-n-propylthiouracil. Science 205: 934–935.

Bartoshuk L, Duffy VB, Reed D, Williams A. 1996. Supertasting, earaches, and head injury: Genetics and pathology alter our taste worlds. Neuroscience and Biobehavioral Reviews 20: 79–87.

Basdevant A, Craplet C, Guy-Grand B. 1993. Snacking patterns in obese French women. Appetite 21: 17–23.

Baucom DH, Aiken PA. 1981. Effect of depressed mood on eating among obese and nonobese dieting and nondieting persons. Journal of Personality and Social Psychology 41: 577–585.

Beaton GH, Tarusak V, Anderson GH. 1992. Estimation of possible impact of non-caloric fat and carbohydrate substitutes on macronutrient intake in the human. Appetite 19: 87–103.

Beauchamp GK. 1994. The chemical senses and pleasure. In: Warburton DM, ed. *Pleasure: The Politics and the Reality.* Chichester: Wiley. pp. 29–37.

Beauchamp GK, Bertino M, Engelman K. 1991a. Human salt appetite. In: Friedman MI, Tordoff MG, and Kare MR, eds. *Chemical senses: Volume 4, appetite and nutrition.* New York: Marcel Dekker. pp. 85–107.

Beauchamp GK, Cowart BJ, Moran M. 1986. Developmental changes in salt acceptability in human infants. Developmental Psychobiology 19: 17–25.

Beauchamp GK, Cowart BJ, Schmidt HJ. 1991b. Development of chemosensory sensitivity and preference. In: Getchell TV, Doty RL, Bartoshuk LM, Snow JB Jr., eds. Smell and taste in health and disease. New York: Raven Press. pp. 405–416.

Beauchamp GK, Wysocki CJ. 1990. Perception of the odor of androstenone: Influence of genes, development, and exposure. In: Capaldi ED, Powley TL, eds. Taste, experience, and feeding. Washington, DC: American Psychological Association. pp. 105–115.

Beaudoin R, Mayer J. 1953. Food intake of obese and non-obese women. Journal of the American Dietetic Association 29: 29–33.

Belko AZ, Barbieri TF. 1987. Effect of meal size and frequency on the thermic effect of food. Nutrition Research 7: 237–242.

Bellisle F, Le Magnen J. 1981. The structure of meals in humans: eating and drinking patterns in lean and obese subjects. Physiology & Behavior 27: 649–658.

Bellisle F, Lucas F, Le Magnen J. 1984. Deprivation, palatability and the microstructure of meals in human subjects. Appetite 5: 85–94.

Bellisle F, Monneuse M-O, Steptoe A, Wardle J. 1995. Weight concerns and eating patterns: A survey of university students in Europe. International Journal of Obesity 19: 723–730.

Bellisle F, Perez C. 1994. Low-energy substitutes for sugars and fats in the human diet: Impact on nutritional regulation. Neuroscience and Biobehavioral Reviews 18: 197–205.

Bellisle F, Rolland-Cachera MF, Deheeger M, Guilloud-Battaille M. 1988. Obesity and food intake in children: Evidence for a role of metabolic and/or behavioral daily rhythms. Appetite 11: 111–118.

Benkelfat C, Ellenbogen MA, Dean P, Palmour RM, Young SN. 1994. Mood–lowering effect of tryptophan depletion. Archives of General Psychiatry 51: 687–697.

Bennett C, Reed GW, Peters NN, Sun M, Hill JO. 1992. Short-term effects of dietary-fat ingestion on energy expenditure and nutrient balance. American Journal of Clinical Nutrition 55: 1071–1077.

Bernard C. 1878. *Leçons sur les phenomenes de la vie, communs aux animaux et aux vegetaux,* translated to *Lectures on the phenomena of life common to animals and plants.* Spingfield IL: Charles C. Thomas (1974).

Bernstein IL. 1994. Development of food aversions during illness. Proceedings of the Nutrition Society 53: 131–137.

Berridge KC. 1996. Food reward: Brain substrates of wanting and liking. Neuroscience and Biobehavioral Reviews 20: 1–25.

Birch LL, Deysher M. 1985. Conditioned and unconditioned caloric compensation: Evidence for self-regulation of food intake by young children. Learning and Motivation 16: 341–355.

Birch LL, McPhee L, Steinberg L, Sullivan S. 1990. Conditioned flavour preferences in young children. Physiology and Behavior 47: 501–505.

Birch LL, McPhee L, Sullivan S, Johnson S. 1989. Conditioned meal initiation in young children. Appetite 13: 105–113.

Björntorp P, Sjöström L. 1978. Carbohydrate storage in man: Speculations and some quantitative considerations. Metabolism 27: 1853–1865.

Black AE, Goldberg GR, Jebb SA, Livingstone MB, Cole TJ, Prentice AM. 1991. Critical evaluation of energy intake data using fundamental principles of energy physiology: 2. Evaluating the results of published surveys. European Journal of Clinical Nutrition 45: 583–599.

Blair AJ, Booth DA, Lewis VJ, Wainwright CJ. 1989. The relative success of official and informal weight reduction techniques: Retrospective correlational evidence. Psychology and Health 3: 195–206.

Blair D, Buskirk ER. 1987. Habitual daily energy expenditure and activity levels of lean and adult-onset and child-onset obese women. American Journal of Clinical Nutrition 45: 540–550.

Blass EM. 1987. Opioids, sweets and a mechanism for positive affect: Broad motivational implications. In: Dobbing J, ed. *Sweetness*. Berlin, Springer–Verlag. pp. 115–126.

Blass EM. 1991. Suckling: Opioid and nonopioid processes in mother-infant bonding. In: Friedman MI, Tordoff MG, and Kare MR, eds. Chemical senses: Volume 4, appetite and nutrition. New York: Marcel Dekker. pp. 283–302.

Blass EM, Fitzgerald E, Kehoe P. 1987. Interactions between sucrose, pain and isolation distress. Pharmacology, Biochemistry and Behavior 26: 483–489.

Blass EM, Hoffmeyer LB. 1991. Sucrose as an analgesic for newborn infants. Pediatrics 87: 215–218.

Blaxter KL. 1971. Methods of measuring the energy metabolism of animals and interpretation of the results obtained. Federation Proceedings 30: 1436–1443.

Blundell JE. 1979. Hunger, appetite and satiety – constructs in search of identities. In: Turner MR, ed. Lifestyle and Nutrition. London: Applied Sceience Publishing. pp. 21–42.

Blundell JE. 1991. Pharmacological approaches to appetite suppression. Trends in Pharmacological Sciences 12: 147–157.

Blundell JE. 1996. Food intake and body weight regulation. In: Bouchard C, Bray GA, eds. *Regulation of body weight: Biological and behavioural mechanisms.* London Willey. pp. 111–133.

Blundell JE, Cotton H, Delargy H, Green S, Greenough A, King NA, Lawton CL. 1995. The fat paradox: fat-induced satiety signals versus high fat oversonsumption. International Journal of Obesity. 19: 832–835.

Blundell JE, de Graaf C. 1993. Low-calorie foods: Relevance for body weight control. In: Khan R, ed. *Low-calorie foods and food ingredients*. London: Blackie. pp. 1–21.

Blundell JE, Green S, Burley V. 1994. Carbohydrates and human appetite. American Journal of Clinical Nutrition 62(suppl): 728S–734S.

Blundell JE, Hill AJ. 1988. On the mechanism of action of dexfenfluramine: Effect on alliesthesia and appetite motivation in lean and obese subjects. Clinical Neuropharmacology 11(Suppl. 1): S121–S134.

Blundell JE, King NA. 1996. Overconsumption as a cause of weight gain: Behavioural-physiological interactions in the control of food intake (appetite). In: *The origins and consequences of obesity*. Ciba Foundation Symposium 201. Chichester UK: John Wiley & Sons. pp. 138–158.

Blundell JE, Lawton CL, Cotton JR, Macdiarmid JI. 1996. Control of human appetite: Implications for the intake of dietary fat. Annual Review of Nutrition 16: 285–319.

Blundell JE, Rogers PJ. 1991. Hunger, hedonics, and the control of satiation and satiety. In: Friedman MI, Tordoff MG, and Kare MR, eds. *Chemical senses: Volume 4, appetite and nutrition*. New York: Marcel Dekker. pp. 127–148.

Blundell JE, Rogers PJ. 1994. Sweet carbohydrate substitutes (intense sweeteners) and the control of appetite: Scientific issues. In: Fernstrom JD, Miller GD, eds. *Appetite and Body Weight Regulation*. Boca Raton: CRC Press. pp. 113–124.

Bogardus C, Lillioja S, Ravussin E, Abbott W, Zawadski JK, Young A, Knowler WC, Jacobowitz R, Moll PP. 1986. Familial dependance of the resting metabolic rate. New England Journal of Medicine 315: 96–100.

Bolton-Smith C, Woodward M. 1994. Dietary composition and fat to sugar ratios in relation to obesity. International Journal of Obesity 18: 820–828.

Bolton-Smith C, Woodward M. 1995. Intrinsic, non-milk extrinsic and milk sugar consumption by Scottish adults. Journal of Human Nutrition and Dietetics 8: 35–49.

Booth DA. 1977. Satiety and appetite are conditioned reactions. Psychosomatic Medicine 39: 76–81.

Booth DA. 1978. Acquired behaviour controlling energy intake and output. Psychiatric Clinics of North America 1: 545–579.

Booth DA. 1988. Mechanisms from models – actual effects from real life: the zero–calorie drink-break option. Appetite 11(suppl): 94–102.

Booth DA. 1991. Protein- and carbohydrate-specific cravings: neuroscience and sociology. In: Friedman MI, Tordoff MG, and Kare MR, eds. *Chemical senses: Volume 4, appetite and nutrition*. New York: Marcel Dekker. pp. 262–276.

Booth DA. 1994. *Psychology of Nutrition*. London: Taylor and Francis.

Booth DA, Chase A, Campbell AT. 1970. Relative effectiveness of protein in the later stages of appetite suppression in man. Physiology and Behavior 5: 1299–1302.

Booth DA, Mather, P. 1978. Prototype model of human feeding, growth and obesity. In: Booth DA, ed. *Hunger Models: Computable Theory of Feeding Control*. Academic Press, London. pp. 279–322.

Booth DA, Mather P, Fuller J. 1982. Starch content of ordinary foods associatively conditions human appetite and satiation, indexed by intake and eating pleasantness of starch-paired flavours. Appetite 3: 163–184.

Bornet FRJ. 1994. Undigestible sugars in food products. American Journal of Clinical Nutrition 59(suppl): 763S–769S.

Bortz WM, Wroldsen A, Issekutz B, Rodahl K. 1966. Weight loss and frequency of feeding. New England Journal of Medicine 274: 376–379.

Bouchard C. 1989. Genetic factors in obesity. Medical Clinics of North America 73: 67–81.

Bouchard C. 1991a. Current of the etiology of obesity: Genetic and nongenetic factors. American Journal of Clinical Nutrition 53: 1561S–1565S.

Bouchard C. 1991b. Heredity and the path to overweight and obesity. Medicine and Science in Sports and Exercise 23: 285–291.

Bouchard C. 1993. Genes and body fat. American Journal of Human Biology 5: 425–432.

Bouchard C, Pérusse L. 1993. Genetics of obesity. Annual Review of Nutrition. 13: 337–354.

Bouchard C, Pérusse L, Dériaz O, Després J-P, Tremblay A. 1993. Genetic influences on energy expenditure in humans. Critical Reviews in Food Science and Nutrition 33: 345–350.

Bouchard C, Tremblay A, Després J-P, Nadeau A, Lupien PJ, Thériault G,

Dussault J, Moorjani S, Pinault S, Fornier G. 1990. The response to long-term overfeeding in identical twins. New England Journal of Medicine 322: 1477–1482.

Bouchard C, Tremblay A, Després J-P, Poehlman ET, Thériault G, Nadeau A, Lupien P, Moorjani S, Dussault J. 1988. Sensitivity to overfeeding: The Quebec experiment with identical twins. Progress in Food and Nutrition Science 12: 45–72.

Bouchard C, Tremblay A, Nadeau A, Després J-P, Thériault G, Boulay MR, Lortie G, Leblanc C, Fornier G. 1989. Genetic effect in resting and exercise metabolic rates. Metabolism 38: 364–370.

Boyd NF, Cousins M, Beaton M, Kriukov V, Lockwood G, Tritchler D. 1990. Quantitative changes in dietary fat intake and serum cholesterol in women: Results from a randomized, controlled trial. American Journal of Clinical Nutrition 52: 470–476.

Braitman LE, Adlin EV, Stanton JL. 1985. Obesity and caloric intake: The National Health and Nutrition Examination Survey of 1971–1975 (HANES I). Journal of Chronic Diseases 38: 727–732.

Bray GA. 1989. Nutrient balance and obesity: An approach to control of food intake in humans. Medical Clinics of North America 73: 29–45.

Bray GA. 1995. Luxuskonsumption – myth or reality? Obesity Research 3: 491–494.

Bray GA. 1997. Energy expenditure using doubly labeled water: The unveiling of objective truth. Obesity Research 5: 71–77.

Bray MS, Boerwinkle E, Hanis CL. 1996. OB gene not linked to human obesity in Mexican American affected sib pairs from Starr County, Texas. Human Genetics 98: 590–595.

British Nutrition Foundation. 1990. *Complex carbohydrates in foods*. The Report of the British Nutrition Foundation's Task Force. London: Chapman and Hall.

Brobeck JR. 1955. Neural regulation of food intake. Annals of the New York Academy of Sciences 63: 44–55.

Brody S, Wolitzky DL. 1983. Lack of mood changes following sucrose loading. Psychosomatics 24: 155–162.

Brown PJ, Konner M. 1987. An anthropological perspective on obesity. Annals of the New York Academy of Sciences 499: 29–46.

Bruch H. 1961. Eating Disorders. New York: Basic Books.

Brzezinski AA, Wurtman JJ, Wurtman RJ, Gleason R, Greenfield J, Nader T. 1990. d-Fenfluramine suppresses the increased calorie and carbohydrate intakes and improves the mood of women with premenstrual depression. Obstetrics and Gynecology 76: 296–301.

Buemann B, Toubro S, Raben A, Astrup A. 1994. Substrate oxidations in post-tobese women on 72-h high fat diet. A possible abnormal postprandial response? International Journal of Obesity 18(suppl 2): 97

Burley VJ, Gatenby SJ, Anderson AO, Mela DJ. 1994. *Relationships between eating frequency, energy intake and body weight status: A critical review*. London: The Biscuit, Cake, Chocolate & Confectionery Alliance. [Technical report].

Burley VJ, Blundell JE. 1990. Action of dietary fiber on the satiety cascade. In: Kritchevsky D, Bonfield C, Anderson JW, eds. *Dietary fiber. Chemistry, physiology, and health effects*. New York: Plenum. pp. 227–246.

Burley VJ, Blundell JE. 1995. Dietary fibre and the pattern of energy intake. In: Kritchevsky D, Bonfield C, eds. *Dietary fiber in health & disease*. St. Paul, MN: Eagan Press. pp. 244–256.

Butterworth DE, Nieman DC, Butler JV, Herring JL. 1994. Food intake patterns of marathon runners. International Journal of Sport Nutrition 4: 1–7.

Cabanac M. 1971. Physiological role of pleasure. Science 173: 1103–1107.

Cabanac M. 1992. Pleasure: The common currency. Journal of Theoretical Biology 155: 173–200.

Campbell RG, Hashim SA, Van Itallie TB. 1971. Studies of food-intake regulation in man: Response to variations in nutritive density in lean and obese people. New England Journal of Medicine 285: 1402–1407.

Campfield LA, Smith FJ, Guisez Y,Devos R, Burn P. 1995. Recombinant mouse OB protein: Evidence for a peripheral signal linking adiposity and central neural networks. Science 269: 546–549.

Campfield LA, Smith FJ, Rosenbaum M, Hirsch J. 1996. Human eating: Evidence for a physiological basis using a modified paradigm. Neuroscience and biobehavioral Reviews 20: 133–137.

Cannon WB. 1932. *The wisdom of the body*. New York: Norton.

Caputo FA, Mattes RD. 1992. Human dietary responses to covert manipulations of energy, fat, and carbohydrate in a midday meal. American Journal of Clinical·Nutrition 56: 36–43.

Caputo FA, Mattes RD. 1993. Human dietary responses to perceived manipulation of fat content in a midday meal. International Journal of Obesity 17: 241–244.

Carbonnel F, Lémann M, Rambaud JC, Mundler O, Jian R. 1994. Effect of the energy density of a solid-liquid meal on gastric emptying and satiety. American Journal of Clinical Nutrition 60: 307–311

Carey DGP, Nguyen TV, Campbell LV, Chisholm DJ, Kelly P. 1996. Genetic influences on central abdominal fat: A twin study. International Journal of Obesity 20:722–726.

Carlisle HJ, Stellar E. 1969. Caloric regulation and food preference in normal, hyperphagic, and aphagic rats. Journal of Comparative and Physiological Psychology 69: 107–114.

Carlson NR. 1994. *Physiology of Behavior*. Fifth Edition. Allyn and Bacon, Boston.

Carlsson B, Lindell K, Gabrielsson B, Karlsson C, Bjarnason R, Westphat O, Karlsson U, Sjöström L, Carlsson LMS. 1997. Obese (ob) gene defects are rare in human obesity. Obesity Research 5: 30–35.

Carney BI, Jones KL, Horowitz M, Sun WM, Penagini R, Meyer JH. 1995. Gastric emptying of oil and aqueous meal components: effects of posture and on appetite. American Journal of Physiology 268: G925–G932.

Caro JF, Kolaczynski JW, Nyce MR, Ohannesian JP, Opentanova I, Goldman WH, Lynn RB, Zhang PL, Sinha MK, Considine RV. 1996. Decreased cerebrospinal-fluid/serum leptin ratio in obesity – A possible mechanism for leptin resistance. Lancet 348: 159–161.

Catt SL, Rosenblatt DB, Mela DJ. In press. Behavioral effects of fat manipulation in infant milks. Appetite (meeting abstract).

Champ M M-J. 1996. The analysis of complex carbohydrates: Relevance of values obtained in vitro. Proceedings of the Nutrition Society 55: 863–880.

Chao ESM, Smit Vanderkooy P. 1989. An overview of breakfast nutrition. Journal of the Canadian Dietetic Association 50: 225–228.

Chen L-N A, Parham ES. 1991. College students' use of high-intensity sweeteners is not consistently associated with sugar consumption. Journal of the American Dietetic Association 91: 686–690.

Chlebowski RT, Blackburn GL, Buzzard IM, Rose DP, Martino S, Khandekar JD, York RM, Jeffery RW, Elashoff RM, Wynder EL. 1993. Adherence to a dietary fat intake reduction program in postmenopausal women receiving therapy for early breast cancer. Journal of Clinical Oncology 11: 2072–2080.

Christensen L, Redig C. 1993. Effect of meal composition on mood. Behavioral Neuroscience 107: 346–353.

Cines BM, Rozin P. 1982. Some aspects of liking for hot coffee and coffee flavour. Appetite 3: 23–34.

Clark D, Tomas F, Withers RT, Brinkman M, Berry MN, Oliver JR, Owens PC, Butler RN, Ballard FJ, Nestel P. 1995. Differences in substrate metabolism between self-perceived 'large-eating' and 'small eating' women. International Journal of Obesity 19: 245–252.

Clark D, Tomas F, Withers RT, Neville SD, Nolan SR, Brinkman M, Chandler C, Clark C, Ballard FJ, Berry M, Nestel P. 1993. No major differences in energy metabolism between matched and unmatched groups of 'large-eating' and 'small eating' men. British Journal of Nutrition 70: 393–406.

Clark D, Tomas F, Withers RT, Chandler C, Brinkman M, Phillips J, Berry M, Ballard FJ, Nestel P. 1994. Energy metabolism in free-living 'large-eating' and 'small eating' women: Studies using $^2H_2^{18}O$. British Journal of Nutrition 72: 21–31.

Clement K, Garner C, Hager J, Philippi A, Leduc C, Carey A, Harris TJR, Jury C, Cardon LR, Basdevant A, Demenais F, Guy-Grand B, North M, Froguel P. 1996. Indication for linkage of the human OB gene region with extreme obesity. Diabetes 45: 687–690.

Clendenen VI, Herman CP, Polivy J. 1994. Social facilitation of eating among friends and strangers. Appetite 23: 1–13.

Coates TJ, Jeffery RW, Wing RR. 1978. The relationship between persons' relative body weights and the quality and quantity of food stored in their homes. Addictive Behaviors 3: 179–184.

Cockcroft V. 1993. Chocolate on the brain. The Biochemist Apr/May, 14–16.

Cohn C. 1963. Feeding frequency and body composition. Annals of the New York Academy of Sciences 110: 395–409.

Colditz GA, Willett WC, Stampfer MJ, London SJ, Segal MR, Speizer FE. 1990. Patterns of weight change and their relation to diet in a cohort of healthy men. American Journal of Clinical Nutrition 51: 1100–1105.

Cole TJ. 1991. Weight-stature indices to measure underweight, overweight, and obesity. In: Himes JH, ed. *Anthropometric assessment of nutritional status*. New York: Wiley-Liss. pp. 83–111.

Cole-Hamilton I, Gunner K, Leverkus C, Starr J. 1986. A study among dietitians and adult members of their households of the practicalities and implications of following proposed dietary guidelines for the UK. Human Nutriion: Applied Nutrition 40A: 365–389.

Collier GH. 1985. Satiety: An ecological perspective. Brain Research Bulletin. 14: 693–700.

Collins JE. 1978. Effects of restraint, monitoring, and stimulus salience on eating behaviour. Addictive Behaviors 3: 197–204.

Collins English Dictionary. 1986. Second Edition. London: Collins.

Comings DE, Gade R, MacMurray JP, Muhleman D, Peters WR. 1996. Genetic variants of the human obesity (*OB*) gene: Association with body mass index in young women, psychiatric symptoms, and interaction with the dopamine D_2 receptor (*DRD2*) gene. Molecular Psychiatry 1: 325–335.

Considine RV, Considine EL, Williams CJ, Hyde TM, Caro JF. 1996a. The hypothalamic leptin receptor in humans. Identification of incidental sequence polymorphisms and absence of the *db/db* mouse and *fa/fa* rat mutations. Diabetes 45: 992–994.

Considine RV, Considine EL, Williams CJ, Nyce MR, Zhang PL, Opentanova I, Ohannesian JP, Kolaczynski JW, Bauer TL, Moore JH, Caro JF. 1996b. Mutation screening and identification of of a sequence variation in the human Ob gene coding. Biochemical and Biophysical Research Communications 220: 735–739.

Considine RV, Sinha MK, Heiman ML, Kriauciunas A, Stephens TW, Nyce MR,

Ohannesian JP, Marco CC, McKee LJ, Bauer TL, Caro JF. 1995. Serum immunoreactive-leptin concentrations in normal-weight and obese humans. New England Journal of Medicine 334: 292–295.

Cooper PJ, Bowskill R. 1986. Dysphoric mood and overeating. British Journal of Clinical Psychology 25: 155–156.

Coronas R, Duran S, Gomez P, Romero H, Sastre A. 1982. Modified fasting and obesity: Results of a multicentric study. International journal of obesity 6: 463–471.

Cowen PJ, Anderson IM, Fairburn CG. 1992. Neurochemical effects of dieting: Relevance to changes in eating and affective disorders. In: Anderson GH, Kennedy SH, eds. *The Biology of Feast and Famine: Relevance to Eating Disorders.* San Diego: Academic Press. pp 269–284

Crawley H, Summerbell C. 1995. Feeding frequency and BMI among teenagers aged 16–17 years. International Journal of Obesity 21: 159–161.

Crittenden RG, Playne MJ. 1996. Production properties and applications of food-grade oligosaccharides. Trends in Food Science and Technology 7: 353–361.

Cross AT, Babicz D, Cushman LF. 1994. Snacking patterns among 1,800 adults and children. Journal of the American Dietetic Association 94: 1398–1403.

D'Allessio DA, Kavie EC, Mozzoli MA, Smalley KJ, Polansky M, Kendrick ZV, Owen LR, Bushman MC, Boden G, Owen OE. 1988. Thermic effect of food in lean and obese men. Journal of Clinical Investigation 81: 1781–1789.

Dallosso HM, Murgatroyd PR, James WPT. 1982. Feeding frequency and energy balance in adult males. Human Nutrition: Clinical Nutrition 36C: 25–39.

Danforth E Jr. 1985. Diet and obesity. American Journal of Clinical Nutrition 41: 1132–1145.

Daniel JR, Whistler RL. 1994. Carbohydrates, role in human nutrition. In Arntzen CJ, Ritter EM. *Encyclopedia of Agricultural Sciences, Volume 1.* New York: Academic Press. pp. 337–344.

Davies PSW, Day JME, Lucas A. 1991. Energy expenditure in early infancy and later body fatness. International Journal of Obesity 15:727–731.

Davies PSW, Wells JCK, Fieldhouse CA, Day JME, Lucas A. 1995. Parental body composition and infant energy expenditure. American Journal of Clinical Nutrition 61: 1026–1029.

Davis LB, Porter RH. 1991. Persistent effects of early odor exposure on human neonates. Chemical Senses 16: 169–174.

Debry G. 1978. Newer knowledge on the treatment of obesity. Bibliotheca Nutrition e Dietetica 26: 44–59.

de Castro JM. 1981. The stomach energy content governs meal patterning in the rat. Physiology and Behavior 26: 795–798.

de Castro JM. 1987. Macronutrient relationships with meal patterns and mood in the spontaneous feeding behaviour of humans. Physiology and Behavior 39: 561–569.

de Castro JM. 1988. The meal pattern of rats shifts from postprandial regulation to preprandial regulation when only five meals per day are scheduled. Physiology and Behavior 43: 739–746.

de Castro JM. 1993a. Genetic influences on daily intake and meal pattern of humans. Physiology & Behavior 53: 777–782.

de Castro JM. 1993b. Independence of genetic influences on body size, daily intake, and meal pattern of humans. Physiology & Behavior 54: 633–639.

de Castro JM. 1995. The relationship of cognitive restraint to the spontaneous food and fluid intake of free-living humans. Physiology and Behavior 57: 287–295.

de Castro JM. 1996. How can eating behaviour be regulated in the complex environments of free-living humans? Neuroscience and Biobehavioral Reviews 20: 119–131.

de Graaf C, Drijvers JJMM, Zimmermanns NJH, van het Hof KH, Westrate JA, van den Berg H, Velthuis- te Wierik EJM, Westerterp KR, Westerterp-Plantenga MS, Verboeket-van de Venne WPHG. In press. Energy and fat compensation during long-term consumption of reduced-fat products. Appetite.

de Graaf C, Hulshof T, Westrate JA, Jas P. 1992a. Short-term effects of different amounts of protein, fats, and carbohydrates on satiety. American Journal of Clinical Nutrition 55: 33–38.

de Graaf C, Jas P, van der Kooy K, Leenen R. 1993a. Circadian rhythms of appetite at different stages of a weight loss programme. International Journal of Obesity 17: 521–526.

de Graaf D, Schreurs A, Blauw YL. 1993b. Short-term effects of different amounts of sweet and nonsweet carbohydrates on satiety and energy intake. Physiology & Behavior 54: 833–843.

de Graaf C, Stafleu A, Staal P, Wijne M. 1992b. Beliefs about the satiating effect of bread with spread varying in macronutrient content. Appetite 18: 121–128.

Deijen JM, Heemstra ML, Orlebeke JF. 1989. Dietary effects on mood and performance. Journal of Psychiatric Research 23: 275–283.

Delwiche J. 1996. Are there 'basic' tastes? Trends in Food Science & Technology 7: 411–415.

Department of Health. 1991. *Dietary reference values for food energy and nutrients for the United Kingdom*. Report of the Panel on Dietary Reference Values of the Committee on Medical Aspects of Food Policy. [Report on Health and Social Subjects 41.] London: HMSO.

de Peuter R, Withers RT, Brinkma M, Tomas FM, Clark DG. 1992. No differences in rates of energy expenditure between post-obese women and their matched, lean controls. International Journal of Obesity 16: 801–808.

Deutsch JA, Moore BO, Heinrichs SC. 1989. Unlearned specific appetite for protein. Physiology and Behavior 46: 619–624.

de Vries JHM, Zock PL, Mensink RP, Katan MB. 1994. Underestimation of energy intake by 3-d records compared with energy intake to maintain body weight in 269 nonobese adults. American Journal of Clinical Nutrition 60:855–860.

Diaz E, Prentice AM, Goldberg GR, Murgatroyd PR, Coward WA. 1992. Metabolic response to experimental overfeeding in lean and overweight healthy volunteers. American Journal of Clinical Nutrition 56: 641–655.

Dietz WH. 1995. Is reduced metabolic rate associated with obesity? Journal of Pediatrics 129: 621–623.

Dietz WH. 1996. The role of lifestyle in health: The epidemiology and consequences of inactivity. Proceedings of the Nutrition Society 55: 829–840.

di Tomaso E, Beltramo M, Piomelli D. 1996. Brain cannabinoids in chocolate. Nature 382: 677–678.

Donato KA. 1987. Efficiancy and utilization of various energy sources for growth. American Journal of Clinical Nutrition 45: 164–167.

Dowse GK, Hodge AM, Zimmet PZ. 1996. Paradise lost: Obesity and diabetes in Pacific and Indian Ocean populations. In: Angel A, Anderson H, Bouchard C, Lau D, Leiter L, Mendelson R, eds. *Progress in obesity research 7*. London: John Libbey & Co. pp. 227–238.

Dreon DM, Frey-Hewitt B, Ellsworth N, Williams PT, Terry RB, Wood PD. 1988. Dietary fat:carbohydrate ratio and obesity in middle-aged men. American Journal of Clinical Nutrition 47: 995–1000.

Drewnowski A. 1985. Food perceptions and preferences of obese adults: A multidimensional approach. International Journal of Obesity 9: 201–212.

Drewnowski A. 1992. Food preferences and the opioid peptide system. Trends in Food Science and Technology 3: 97–99.

Drewnowski A. 1995. Intense sweeteners and the control of appetite. Nutrition Reviews 53: 1–7

Drewnowski A, Brunzell JD, Sande K, Iverius PH, Greenwood MRC. 1985. Sweet tooth reconsidered: Taste responsiveness in human obesity. Physiology & Behavior 35: 617–622.

Drewnowski A, Grinker JA, Hirsch J. 1982. Obesity and flavor perception: Multidimensional scaling of soft drinks. Appetite 3: 361–368.

Drewnowski A, Krahn DD, Demitrack MA, Nairn K, Gosnell BA. 1992a. Taste responses and preferences for sweet high-fat foods: evidence for opioid involvement. Physiology and Behavior 51: 371–379.

Drewnowski A, Kurth C, Holden-Wiltse J, Saari, J. 1992b. Food preferences in human obesity: carbohydrate versus fats. Appetite 18: 207–221.

Drewnowski A, Kurth CL, Rahaim JO. 1991. Taste preferences in human obesity: Environmental and familial factors. American Journal of Clinical Nutrition 54: 635–641.

Duggan JP, Booth DA. 1986. Obesity, overeating, and rapid gastric emptying in rats with ventromedial hypothalamic lesions. Science 231: 609–611.

Duggirala R, Blangero J, Leibel R, O'Connell P, Stern M. 1995. Linkage of markers on human chromosome 7 with obesity related traits in Mexican Americans. Obesity Research 3 (Suppl 3): 360S.

Duncan KH, Bacon JA, Weinsier RL. 1983. The effects of high and low energy density diets on satiety, energy intake, and eating time of obese and nonobese subjects. American Journal of Clinical Nutrition 37:763–767.

Durrant M. 1981. Salivation: A useful research tool? Appetite 2: 362–365.

Durrant ML, Royston P, Wloch RT. 1982. Effect of exercise on energy intake and eating patterns in lean and obese humans. Physiology and Behavior 29: 449–454.

Durrant ML, Stalley SF, Warwick PM, Garrow JS. 1978. The effects of meal frequency on body composition and hunger during weight reduction. Clinical Science 54: 4P.

Dwyer JT, Feldmam JJ, Myer J. 1970. The social psychology of dieting. J Health and Social Behaviour 11: 269–287.

Eck LH, Hackett-Renner C, Klesges LM. 1992a. Impact of diabetic status, dietary intake, physical activity, and smoking status on body mass index in NHANES II. American Journal of Clinical Nutrition 56: 329–333.

Eck LH, Klesges RC, Klesges LM, Hanson CL, Slawson D. 1992b. Children at familial risk of obesity: An examination of dietary intake, physical activity and weight status. International Journal of Obesity 16: 71–78.

Eck LH, Pascale RW, Klesges RC, White Ray JA, Klesges LM. 1995. Predictors of waist circumference changein healthy young adults. International Journal of Obesity 19: 765–769.

Edelstein SL, Barrett-Connor EL, Wingard DL, Cohn BA. 1992. Increased meal frequency associated with decreased cholesterol concentrations; Rancho Bernado, CA, 1984–1987. American Journal of Clinical Nutrition 55: 664–69.

Eiser JR. 1990. Social cognition and comparative sustance use, In: Warburton DM, ed. *Addiction controversies*. Chur Switzerland: Harwood. pp.271–282.

Elizalde G, Sclafani A. 1988. Starch-based conditioned flavour preferences in rats: Influence of taste, calories, and CS-US delay. Appetite 11: 179–200.

Elizilde G, Sclafani A. 1990a. Fat appetite in rats: Flavor preferences conditioned by nutritive and non-nutritive oil emulsions. Appetite 15: 189–197.

Elizalde G, Sclafani A. 1990b. Flavour preferences conditioned by intragastric infusions: a detailed analysis using an electronic esophagus preparation. Physiology and Behavior 47: 63–77.

Fábry P, Fodor J, Hejl Z, Braun T, Zvolánková K. 1964. The frequency of meals. Its relation to overweight, hypercholesterolaemia, and decreased glucose-tolerance. Lancet II: 614–615.

Fábry P, Hejda S,Černẏ K, O šancová K, Pechar J. 1966. Effect of meal frequency in schoolchildren. Changes in weight-height proportion and skinfold thickness. American Journal of Clinical Nutrition 18: 358–361.

Fábry P, Petrasek R, Horakova E, Konopasek E, Braun T. 1963. Energy metabolism and growth in rats adapted to intermittent starvation. British Journal of Nutrition 17: 295–301.

Fábry P, Tepperman J. 1970. Meal frequency – a possible factor in human pathology. American Journal of Clinical Nutrition 23: 1059–1068.

Fabsitz RR, Carmelli D, Hewitt JK. 1992. Evidence for independent genetic influences on obesity in middle age. International Journal of Obesity 16: 657–666.

Fabsitz RR, Garrison RJ, Feinleib M, Hjortland M. 1978. A twin analysis of dietary intake: Evidence of a need to control for possible environmental differences in MZ and DZ twins. Behavioral Genetics 8: 15–25.

Fedoroff IC, Polivy J, Herman CP. 1997. The effect of pre-exposure to food cues on the eating behaviour of restrained and unrestrained eaters. Appetite 28: 33–47.

Fehily AM, Phillips KM, Yarnell JWG. 1984. Diet, smoking, social class and body mass index in the Cerphilly Heart Disease Study. American Journal of Clinical Nutrition 40: 827–883.

Feldman M, Richardson CT. 1986. Role of thought, sight, smell, and taste of food in the cephalic pohase of gastric acid secretion in humans. Gastroenterology 90: 428–433.

Fernstrom JD. 1994. Dietary amino acids and brain function. Journal of the American Dietetic Association 94: 71–77.

Fernstrom JD, Wurtman RJ. 1971a. Brain serotonin content: Increase following ingestion of carbohydrate diet. Science 174: 1023–1025.

Fernstrom JD, Wurtman RJ. 1971b. Brain serotonin content: Physiological dependence on plasma tryptophan levels. Science 173: 149–152.

Fernstrom JD, Wurtman RJ. 1972. Brain serotonin content: Physiological regulation by plasma neutral amino acids. Science 178: 414–416.

Finkelstein B, Fryer BA. 1971. Meal frequency and weight reduction of young women. American Journal of Clinical Nutrition 24: 465–468.

Finley JW, Klemann LP, Levielle GA, Otterburn MS, Walchak CG. 1994. Caloric availability of SALATRIM in rats and humans. Journal of Agricultural & Food Chemistry 42: 474–483.

Fisher JO, Birch LL. 1995. Fat preference and fat consumption of 3- to 5-year-old children are related to parental adiposity. Journal of the American Dietetic Association 95: 759–764.

Flatt JP. 1987a. Dietary fat, carbohydrate balance, and weight maintenance: effects of exercise. American Journal of Clinical Nutrition 45: 296–306.

Flatt JP. 1987b. The difference in storage capacities for carbohydrate and for fat, and its implications in the regulation of body weight. Annals of the New York Academy of Sciences 499: 104–123.

Flatt JP. 1995. Use and storage of carbohydrate and fat. American Journal of Clinical Nutrition 61(suppl): 952S–959S.

Flatt JP, Ravussin E, Acheson KJ, Jéquier E. 1985. Effects of dietary fat on postprandial substrate oxidation and on carbohydrate and fat balances. Journal of Clinical Investigation 76: 1019–1024.

Foltin RW, Fischman MW, Emurian CS, Rachlinski JJ. 1988. Compensation for caloric dilution in humans given unrestricted access to food in a residential laboratory. Appetite 10: 13–24.

Foltin RW, Fischman MW, Moran TH, Rolls BJ, Kelly TH. 1990. Caloric compensation for lunches varying in fat and carbohydrate content by humans in a residential laboratory. American Journal of Clinical Nutrition 52: 969–980.

Foltin RW, Kelly TH, Fischman MW. 1993. Ethanol as an energy source in humans: Comparison with dextrose-containing beverages. Appetite 20: 95–110.

Foltin RW, Rolls BJ, Moran TH, Kelly TH, McNelis AL, Fischman MW. 1992. Caloric, but not macronutrient compensation by humans for required eating occasions with meals and snacks varying in fat and carbohydrate. American Journal of Clinical Nutrition 55: 331–342.

Fontaine E, Savard R, Tremblay A, Després J-P, Poehlman ET, Bouchard C. 1985. Resting metabolic rate in monozygotic and dizygotic twins. Acta Geneticae Medicae et Gemellologiae 34: 41–47.

Fontvieille AM, Ravussin E. 1993. Metabolic rate and body composition of Pima Indian and caucasian children. Critical Reviews in Food Science and Nutrition 33: 363–368.

Forbes GB. 1987a. *Human body composition.* New York: Springer-Verlag.

Forbes GB. 1987b. Lean body mass-body fat interrelationships in humans. Nutrition Reviews 45:225–231.

Forbes GB. 1990. Do obese individuals gain weight more easily than nonobese individuals? American Journal of Clinical Nutrition 52: 224–227.

Forbes JM. 1988. Metabolic aspects of the regulation of voluntary food intake and appetite. Nutrition Research Reviews 1: 145–168.

Forbes JM, Rogers PJ. 1994. Food selection. Nutrition Abstracts and Reviews 64: 1065–1078.

Foster GD, Wadden TA, Vogt RA. 1997. Resting energy expenditure in obese African American and Caucasian women. Obesity Research 5: 1–8.

Frayn KN. 1996. *Metabolic regulation: A human perspective.* Portland Press, London

French SJ, Murray B, Runsey RDE, Sepple CP, Read NW. 1993. Preliminary studies on the gastrointestinal responses to fatty meals in obese people. International Journal of Obesity 17: 295–300.

French SJ, Read NW. 1994. Effect of guar gum on hunger and satiety after meals of differing fat content: Relationship with gastric emptying. American Journal of Clinical Nutrition 59: 87–91.

Fricker J, Baelde D, Igoin-Apfelbaum L, Huet J-M, Apfelbaum M. 1992. Underreporting of food intake in obese 'small eaters'. Appetite 19: 273–283.

Fricker J, Chapelot D, Pasquet P, Rozen R, Apfelbaum M. 1995. Effect of a covert fat dilution on the spontaneous food intake by lean and obese subjects. Appetite 24: 121–138.

Fricker J, Giroux S, Fumeron F, Apfelbaum M. 1990. Circadian rhythm of energy intake and corpulence status in adults. International Journal of Obesity 14: 387–393.

Friedman MI. 1991. Metabolic control of food intake. In: Friedman MI, Tordoff MG, and Kare MR, eds. *Chemical senses: Volume 4, appetite and nutrition.* New York: Marcel Dekker. pp. 19–38.

Friedman MI. 1995. Control of energy intake by energy metabolism. American Journal of Clinical Nutrition 62(suppl): 1096S–1100S.

Friedman MI, Mattes RD. 1991. Chemical senses and nutrition. In: Getchell TV, Doty RL, Bartoshuk LM, Snow JB Jr., eds. *Smell and taste in health and disease.* New York: Raven Press. pp. 391–404.

Friedman MI, Ramirez I, Tordoff MG. 1996. Gastric emptying of ingested fat emulsion in rats: Implications for studies of fat-induced satiety. American Journal of Physiology 270: R688–R692.

Friedman MI, Stricker EM. 1976. The physiological psychology of hunger: A physiological perspective. Psychological Review 83: 409–431.

Frijters JER, Rasmussen-Conrad EL. 1982. Sensory discrimination, intensity perception, and affective judgment of sucrose-sweetness in the overweight. Journal of General Psychology 107: 233–247.

Frye CA, Crystal S, Ward KD, Kanarek RB. 1994. Menstrual cycle and dietary restraint influence taste preferences in young women. Physiology & Behavior 55: 561–567.

Fullerton DT, Getto CJ, Swift WJ, Carlson IH. 1985. Sugar, opioids and binge eating. Brain Research Bulletin 14: 673–680.

Gallacher JEJ, Fehily AM, Yarnell JWG, Butland BK. 1988. Type A behaviour, eating pattern and nutrient intake: the Caerphilly study. Appetite 11: 129–136.

Garb JL, Stunkard AJ. 1974. Taste aversions in man. American Journal of Psychiatry 131: 1204–1207.

Garcia J, Hankins WG, Rusiniak KW. 1974. Behavioural regulation of the milieu interne in man and rat. Science 185: 824–831.

Gardner MLG. 1984. Intestinal assimilation of intact peptides and proteins from the diet: A neglected field? Biological Review 59: 289–331.

Garn SM, Leonard WR. 1989. What did our ancestors eat? Nutrition Reviews 47: 337–345.

Garn SM, Leonard WR, Hawthorne VM. 1986. Three limitations of the body mass index. American Journal of Clinical Nutrition 44: 996–997.

Garn SM, Solomon MA, Cole PE. 1980. Sugar-food intake of obese and lean adolescents. Ecology of Food and Nutrition 9: 219–222.

Garner DM. 1993. Pathogenesis of anorexia nervosa. Lancet 341: 1631–1635.

Garner DM, Olmstead MP, Polivy J. 1983. Development and validation of a multidimensional eating disorder inventory for assessing anorexia nervosa and bulimia. International Journal of Eating Disorders 2: 15–35.

Garrow JS. 1988. *Obesity and related diseases.* London: Churchill Livingstone.

Garrow JS, Durrant ML, Blaza S, Wilkins D, Royston P, Sunkin S. 1981. The effect of meal frequency and protein concentration on the composition of weight lost by obese subjects. British Journal of Nutrition 45: 5–15.

Garrow JS, Webster J. 1983. Quetelet's index (W/H^2) as a measure of fatness. International Journal of Obesity 9: 147–153.

Gatenby SJ, Aaron JI, Jack VM, Mela DJ. 1997. Extended use of foods modified in fat and sugar content: Nutritional implications in a free-living female population. American Journal of Clinical Nutrition 65: 1867–1873.

Gatenby SJ, Aaron JI, Morton G, Mela DJ. 1995. Nutritional implications of reduced-fat food use by free-living consumers. Appetite 25: 241–252.

Gatenby SJ, Anderson AO, Walker AD, Southon S, Mela DJ. 1994. 'Meals' and 'snacks' – Implications for eating patterns in adults. Appetite 23: 292.

Gates JC, Huenenann RL, Brand RJ. 1975. Food choices of obese and non-obese persons. Journal of the American Dietetic Association 67: 339–343.

Gazzaniga JM, Burns TL. 1993. Relationship between diet composition and body fatness, with adjustment for resting energy expenditure and physical activity, in preadolescent children. American Journal of Clinical Nutrition 58: 21–28

Geiselman PJ, Novin D. 1982. The role of carbohydrates in appetite, hunger and obesity. Appetite 3: 203–223.

Geldszus R, Mayr B, Horn R, Geisthövel F, von zur Mhlen A, Brabent G. 1996. Serum leptin and weight reduction in female obesity. European Journal of Endocrinology. 135: 659–662.

Geliebter AA. 1979. Effects of equicaloric loads of protein, fat and carbohydrate on food intake in the rat and man. Physiology & Behavior 22: 267–273.

George V, Tremblay A, Després J-P, Leblanc C, Bouchard C. 1990. Effect of dietary fat content on regional adiposity in men and women. International Journal of Obesity 14: 1085–1094.

Geracioti TD, Liddle RA, Altemus M, Demitrack MA, Gold PW. 1992. Regulation of appetite and cholecystokinin secretion in anorexia nervosa. american journal of psychiatry 149: 958–961.

Gibney MJ. 1990. Dietary guidelines: A critical appraisal. Journal of Human Nutrition & Dietetics 3: 245–254.

Gibney MJ. 1995. Consumption of sugars. American Journal of Clinical Nutrition 62(suppl): 178S–194S

Gibson SA. 1993. Consumption and sources of sugars in the diets of British schoolchildren: Are high-sugar diets nutritionally inferior? Journal of Human Nutrition & Dietetics 6: 355–371.

Gibson SA. 1996. Are diets high in non-milk extrinsic sugars conducive to obesity? An analysis from the Dietary and Nutritional Survey of British Adults. Journal of Human Nutrition & Dietetics 9: 283–292.

Gibson EL, Wainwright CJ, Booth DA. 1995. Disguised protein in lunch after low-protein breakfast conditions food-flavor preferences dependent on recent lack of protein intake. Physiology & Behavior 58: 363–371.

Gibson GR, Willems A, Reading S, Collins MD. 1996. Fermentation of non-digestible oligosaccharides by human colonic bacteria. Proceedings of the Nutrition Society 55: 899–912.

Gilbert RM. 1984. Caffeine consumption. In The Methylxanthine Beverages and Foods: Chemistry, Consumption and Health, pp 185–214 [G. A. Spiller, editor]. New York: Alan R. Liss.

Golay A, Allaz A-F, Morel Y, de Tonnac N, Tankova S, Reaven G. 1996a. Similar weight loss with low- or high-carbohydrate diets. American Journal of Clinical Nutrition 63: 174–178.

Golay A, Eigenheer C, Morel Y, Kujawski P, Lehmann T, de Tonnac N. 1996b. Weight-loss with lower high carbohydrate diet? International Journal of Obesity 20: 1067–1072.

Goldberg GR, Black AE, Jebb SA, Cole TJ, Murgatroyd PR, Coward WA, Prentice AM. 1991. Critical evaluation of energy intake data using fundamental principles of energy physiology: 1. Derivation of cut-off limits to identify under-recording. European Journal of Clinical Nutrition 45: 569–581.

Goodwin GM, Cowen PJ, Fairburn CG, Parry-Billings M, Calder PC, Newsholme EA. 1990. Plasma concentrations of tryptophan and dieting. British Medical Journal 300: 1499–1500.

Goodwin GM, Fairburn CG, Cowen PJ. 1987. Dieting changes serotonergic function in women, not men: implications for the aetiology of anorexia nervosa? Psychological Medicine 17: 839–842.

Goran MI, Carpenter WH, McGloin A, Johnson R, Hardin JM, Weinsier RL. 1995. Energy expenditure in children of lean and obese parents. American Journal of Physiology 268: E917–E924.

Green BG. 1996. Chemesthesis: Pungency as a component of flavor. Trends in Food Science & Technology 7: 415–420.

Green SM, Blundell JE. 1996. Subjective and objective indices of the satiating effect of foods. Can people tell how filling a food will be? Eur J Clin Nutr 50: 798–806.

Green MW, Rogers PJ. 1993. Selective attention to food and body shape words in dieters and restrained nondieter. International Journal of Eating Disorders 14: 515–517.

Green MW, Rogers PJ, 1995. Impaired cognitive functioning in dieters during dieting. Psychological Medicine 25: 1003–1010.

Green MW, Rogers PJ, Elliman NA, Gatenby SJ, 1994. Impairment of cognitive performance associated with dieting and high levels of dietary restraint. Physiology and Behavior 55: 447–452.

Greenberg D, Gibbs J, Smith GP. 1989. Infusions of lipid into the duodenum elicit satiety in rats while similar infusions into the vena cava do not. Appetite 12: 213.

Greenberg D, Smith GP. 1996. The controls of fat intake. Psychosomatic Medicine 58: 559–569.

Gregory J, Foster K, Tyler H, Wiseman M. 1990. *The dietary and nutritional survey of British adults*. London: HMSO.

Grill HJ, Berridge KC. 1985. Taste reactivity as a measure of the neural control of palatability. Progress in Psychobiology and Physiological Psychology 2: 1–61.

Grilo CM, Pogue-Geile MF. 1991. The nature of environmental influences on weight and obesity: A behavior genetic analysis. Psychological Bulletin 110: 520–537.

Grinker J. 1978. Obesity and sweet taste. American Journal of Clinical Nutrition 31: 1078–1087.

Grinker JA, Gropman-Rubin J, Bose K. 1986. Sweet preference and body fatness: Neonatal data. Nutrition and Behavior 3: 197–209.

Grinker J, Hirsch J, Smith D. 1972. Taste sensitivity and susceptibility to external influence in obese and normal weight subjects. Journal of Personality and Social Psychology 22: 320–325.

Grunewald KK. 1985. Weight control in young college women: Who are the dieters? Journal of the American Dietetic Association 85: 1445–450.

Guo SS, Roche AF, Chumlea WC, Gardner JD, Siervogel RM. 1994. The predictive value of childhood body mass index values for overweight at age 35 y. American Journal of Clinical Nutrition 59: 810–819.

Halaas JL, Gajiwala KS, Maffei M, Cohen SL, Chait BT, Rabinowitz D, Lallone RL, Burley SK, Friedman JM. 1995. Weight-reducing effects of the plasma protein encoded by the obese gene. Science 269: 543–546.

Halmi KA, Sunday SR. 1991. Temporal patterns of hunger and fullness ratings and related cognitions in anorexia and bulimia. Appetite 16: 219–237.

Halmi KA, Sunday SR. 1996. Micro- and macroanalyses of patterns within a meal in anorexia and bulimia. Appetite 16: 21–36.

Hamilton CL. 1964. Rat's preference for high fat diets. Journal of Comparative and Physiological Psychology 58: 459–460.

Hamilton BS, Paglia D, Kwan AYM, Deitel M. 1995. Increased obese mRNA expression in omental fat cells from massively obese subjects. Nature Medicine 1: 953–956.

Hammer RL, Barrier CA, Roundy ES, Bradford JM, Fisher AG. 1989. Calorie-restricted low-fat diet and exercise in obese women. American Journal of Clinical Nutrition 49:77–85.

Harvey J, Wing RR, Mullen M. 1993. Effects on food cravings of a very low calorie diet or a balanced, low calorie diet. Appetite 21: 105–115.

Havel PJ, Kasim-Karakas S, Mueller W, Johnson PR, Gingerich RL, Stern JL. 1996. Relationship of plasma leptin to plasma insulin and adiposity in normal weight and overweight women: Effects of dietary fat content and sustained weight loss. Journal of Clinical Endocrinology and Metabolism 81: 4406–4413.

Hawkins RC. 1979. Meal/snack frequencies of college students: a normative study. Behavioural Psychotherapy 7: 85–90.

Heather N. 1997. A conceptual framework for explaining problem drug use and addiction. Behavioural Pharmacology, in press.

Heatherton TF, Herman CP, Polivy J, King JA, McGree ST. 1988. The (mis)measurement of restraint: an analysis of conceptual and psychometric issues. Journal of Abnormal Psychology 97: 19–28.

Heitman BT, Lissner L, Sørensen TIA, Bengtsson C. 1995. Dietary fat intake and weight gain in women genetically predisposed for obesity. American Journal of Clinical Nutrition 61: 1213–1217.

Heitmann BK, Lissner L. 1995. Dietary underreporting by obese individuals – is it specific or non-specific? British Medical Journal 311: 986–989.

Hejda S, Fábry P. 1964. Frequency of food intake in relation to some parameters of the nutritional status. Nutrition et Dieta, 6: 216.

Hellerstein MK, Christiansen M, Kaempfer S, Kletke C, Wu K, Reid JS, Mulligan K, Hellerstein NS, Shackleton CHL. 1991. Measurement of de novo hepatic lipogenesis in humans using stable isotopes. Journal of Clinical Investigation 87: 1841–1852.

Hellerstein MK. 1996. Synthesis of fat in response to alterations in diet: Insights from new stable isotope methodologies. Lipids 31(suppl): S117–S125.

Herman CP. 1978. Restrained eating. Psychiatric Clinics of North America 1: 593–607.

Herman CP. 1996. Human eating: Diagnosis and prognosis. Neuroscience and Biobehavioral Reviews 20: 107–111.

Herman CP, Mack D. 1975. Restrained and unrestrained eating. Journal of Personality 43: 647–660.

Herman CP, Polivy J. 1975. Anxiety, restraint and eating behaviour. Journal of Abnormal Psychology 6: 666–672.

Herman CP, Polivy J. 1984. A boundary model for the regulation of eating. In: Stunkard AJ, Stellar E, eds. *Eating and its disorders*. New York: Raven Press. pp. 141–156

Herman CP, Polivy, J. 1988. Restraint and excess in dieters and bulimics. In: K. M. Pirke KM,, W. Vandereycken W, Ploog D, eds. *The Psychobiology of bulimia nervosa*. Berlin: Springer-Verlag. pp.18–32.

Herman CP, Polivy J. Klajner F, Esses VM. 1981. Salivation in dieters and non-dieters. Appetite 2: 356–361.

Herskind AM, McGue M, Sørensen TIA, Harvaldd B. 1996. Sex and age specific assessment of genetic and environmental influences on body mass index in twins. International Journal of Obesity 20: 106–113.

Heshka S, Yang M-U, Wang J, Burt P, Pi-Sunyer FX. 1990. Weight loss and change in resting metabolic rate. American Journal of Clinical Nutrition 52: 981–986.

Hetherington MM, Altemus M, Nelson ML, Bernay AS, Gold PW. 1994. Eating behaviour in bulimia nervosa: multiple meal analysis. American Journal of Clinical Nutrition 60: 864–873.

Hetherington AW, Ranson SW. 1942. The spontaneous activity and food intake of rats with hypothalamic lesions. American Journal of Physiology 136: 609–617.

Hetherington MM, Rolls BJ. 1991. Eating behaviour in eating disorders: response to preloads. Physiology and Behavior 50: 101–108.

Hetherington M, Rolls BJ, Burley VJ. 1989. The time course of sensory-specific satiety. Appetite 12: 57–68.

Heymsfield SB, Darby PC, Muhlheim LS, Gallagher D, Wolper C, Allison DB. 1995. The calorie: Myth, measurement, and reality. American Journal of Clinical Nutrition 62(Suppl): 1034S–1041S.

Hickford CA, Ward T, Bulik CM. Cognitions of restrained and unrestrained eaters under fasting and nonfasting conditions. Behaviour Research and Therapy 35: 71–75.

Hill AJ. 1993. Causes and consequences of dieting and anorexia. Proceedings of the Nutrition Society 52: 211–218.

Hill AJ, Blundell JE. 1986. Macronutrients and satiety: The effects of a high-protein or high–carbohydrate meal on subjective motivation to eat and food preferences. Nutrition & Behavior 3: 133–144.

Hill AJ, Blundell JE. 1988. Role of amino acids in appetite control in man. In: Heuther G, ed. *Amino acids in health and disease*. Berlin: Springer-Verlag. pp. 239–248.

Hill AJ, Blundell JE. 1989. Comparison of the action of macronutrients on the expression of appetite in lean and obese human subject. Annals of the New York Academy of Sciences 575: 529–531.

Hill AJ, Blundell JE. 1990. Sensitivity of the appetite control system in obese subjects to nutritional and serotoninergic challenge. International Journal of Obesity 14: 219–233.

Hill AJ, Heaton-Brown L. 1995. The experience of food craving: A prospective study in healthy women. Journal of Psychosomatic Research 38: 801–814.

Hill AJ, Magson LD, Blundell JE. 1984. Hunger and palatability: tracking ratings of subjective experience before, during and after the consumption of preferred and less preferred food. Appetite 5: 361–371.

Hill AJ, Oliver S, Rogers PJ. 1992. Eating in the adult world: The rise of dieting in childhood and adolescence. British Journal of Clinical Psychology 31: 95–105.

Hill AJ, Rogers PJ, Blundell JE. 1995. Techniques for the experimental measurement of human eating behaviour and food intake: a practical guide. International Journal of obesity 19: 361–375.

Hill AJ, Weaver CFL, Blundell JE. 1991a. Food craving, dietary restraint and mood. Appetite 17: 187–197.

Hill JO, Anderson JC, Lin D, Yakubu F. 1988. Effects of meal frequency on energy utilization in rats. American Journal of Physiology 255: R616–R621.

Hill JO, Peters JC, Reed GW, Schlundt DG, Sharp T, Greene HL. 1991b. Nutrient balance in humans: effects of diet composition. American Journal of Clinical Nutrition 54: 10–17.

Hill JO, Prentice AM. 1995. Sugar and body weight regulation. American Journal of Clinical Nutrition 62(suppl): 264S–274S.

Hill SW, McCutcheon NB. 1975. Eating responses of obese and nonobese humans during dinner meals. Psychosomatic Medicine 37: 395–401.

Hill SW, McCutcheon NB. 1984. Contributions of obesity, gender, hunger, food preference, and body size to bite size, bite speed, and rate of eating. Appetite 5: 73–83.

Hirsch E, Halberg F, Goetz FC, Cressey D, Wendt H, Sothern R, Haus E, Stoney P, Minors D, Rosen G, Hill B, Hilleren M, Barett K. 1975. Body weight changes during 1 week on a single 2000-calorie meal consumed as breakfast (B) or dinner (D). Chronobiologica 2(suppl 1): 31–32.

Ho EE, Liszt A, Pudel V. 1990. The effect of energy content and sweet taste on food consumption in restrained and non-restrained eaters. Journal of the American Dietetic Association 90: 1223–1228.

Hodge AM, Dowse GK, Gareeboo H, Tuomilehto J, Alberti KGMM, Zimmet PZ. 1996. Incidence, increasing prevalence, and predictors of change in obesity and fat distribution over 5 years in the rapidly developing population of Mauritius. International Journal of Obesity 20:137–146.

Hoffman GE, Andres H, Weiss L, Kreisel C, Sander R. 1980. Lipogenesis in man. Properties and organ distribution of ATP citrate (*pro*-3S)-lyase. Biochimica et Biophysica Acta 620: 151–158.

Hogan JA. 1980. Homeostasis and behaviour. In: Toates FM, Halliday TR, eds. *Analysis of motivational processes*. London: Academic Press. pp. 3–21.

Holt SHA, Brand Miller JC. 1994. Paricle size, satiety and the glycaemic response. European Journal of Clinical Nutrition 48: 496–502.

Holt SHA, Brand Miller JC. 1995. Increased insulin responses to ingested foods are associated with lessened satiety. Appetite 24: 43–54.

Holt SHA, Brand Miller JC, Petocz P, Farmakalidis E. 1995. A satiety index of common foods. European Journal of Clinical Nutrition 49: 675–690.

Horowitz M, Jones K, Edelbroek MAL, Snout AJPM, Read NW. 1993. The effect of posture on gastric emptying and intragastric distribution of oil and aqueous meal components and appetite. Gatroenterology 105: 382–390.

Horton TJ, Drougas H, Brachey A, Reed GW, Peters JC, Hill JO. 1995. Fat and carbohydrate overfeeding in humans: Different effects on energy storage. American Journal of Clinical Nutrition 62:19–29.

Hosen JC, Hunt DA, Sims EAH, Bogardus C. 1982. Comparison of carbohydrate-containing and carbohydrate-restricted hypocaloric diets in the treatment of obesity: Effects on appetite and mood. American Journal of Clinical Nutrition 36: 463–469.

Hospers JJ, van Amelsvoort JMM, Westrate JA. 1994. Amylose-to-amylopectin ratio in pastas affects postprandial glucose and insulin responses and satiety in humans. Journal of Food Science 59: 1144–1149.

Houston BO, Sumida B. 1985. A positive feedback model for switching between two activities. Animal Behaviour 33: 315–325.

Hunt JN, Stubbs DF. 1975. The volume and content of meals as determinants of gastric emptying. Journal of Physiology (London) 245: 209–225.

Hurni M, Burnand B, Pittet PH, Jéquier E. 1982. Metabolic effects of a mixed and a high-carbohydrate low-fat diet in man, measured over 24 h in a respiration chamber. British Journal of Nutrition 47: 33–43.

Ikeda K. 1909. On a new seasoner. Journal of the Tokyo Chemical Society 30: 820–836.

Iyengar R, Gross A. 1991. Fat substitutes. In: Goldberg I, Williams R, eds. *Biotechnology and food ingredients*. New York: van Nostrand Reinhold. pp. 287–313.

Jacobs H, Thompson M, Halberg E, Halberg F, Fraeber C, Levine H, Haus E. 1975. Relative body weight loss on limited free-choice meal consumed as breakfast rather than dinner. Chronobiologica 2(suppl 1): 33.

James A. 1990. The good, the bad and the delicious: the role of confectionery in British society. Sociological Review 38: 666–688.

James WPT, Ferro-Luzzi A, Waterlow JC. 1988. Definition of chronic energy deficiency in adults. Report of a working party of the International Dietary Energy Consultancy Group. European Journal of Clinical Nutrition 42: 969–981.

Jansen A, Broekmate J, Heymans M. 1992. Cue-exposure vs. self-control in the treatment of binge eating: A pilot study. Behavior Research and Therapy 30: 235–241.

Jansen A, van den Hout, M. 1991. On being led into temptation: 'Counter-regulation' of dieters after smelling a 'preload'. Addictive Behaviors 16: 247–253.

Jebb SA. 1995. Metabolic response to slimming. In: Cottrell R, ed. *Weight control: The current perspective*. London: Chapman & Hall. pp. 48–67.

Jeffery RW, Folsom AR, Luepker RV, Jacobs DR, Gillum RF, Taylor HL, Blackburn H. 1984. Prevalence of overweight and weight loss behaviour in a metropolitan adult population: The Minnesota heart survey experience. American Journal of Public Health 74: 349–352.

Jeffery RW, Hellerstedt WL, French SA, Baxter JE. 1995. A randomized trial of counseling for fat reduction versus calorie restriction in the treatment of obesity. International Journal of Obesity 19: 132–137.

Jenson CD, Zaltas ES, Whittam JH. 1992. Dietary intakes of male endurance cyclists during training and racing. Journal of the American Dietetic Association 92: 986–988.

Jéquier E. 1992. Calorie balance versus nutrient balance. In: Kinney JM, Tucker HN, eds. *Energy metabolism: Tissue determinants and cellular corollaries*. New York: Raven Press. pp. 123–134.

Jéquier E, Schutz Y. 1983. Long-term measurements of energy expenditure in humans using a respiration chamber. American Journal of Clinical Nutrition 38: 989–998.

Johnson LR. 1991. *Gastrointestinal physiology*. St. Louis: Mosby Year Book.

Johnson RK, Goran MI, Poehlmen ET. 1994. Correlates of underreporting of energy intake in healthy older men and women. American Journal of Clinical Nutrition 59:1286–1290.

Johnson SL, McPhee L, Birch LL. 1991. Conditioned preferences: Young children prefer flavours associated with high dietary fat. Physiology and Behavior 50: 1245–1251.

Johnson WG, Keant TM, Bonar JR, Downey C. 1979. Hedonic ratings of sucrose solutions: Effect of body weight, weight loss and dietary restriction. Addictive Behaviors 4: 231–236.

Jones PJH, Namchuk GL, Pederson RA. 1995. Meal frequency influences circulating hormone levels but not lipogenesis rates in humans. Metabolism 44: 218–223.

Kanarek RB, Ryu M, Przypek J. 1995. Preferences for foods with varying levels of salt and fat differ as a function of dietary restraint and exercise but not menstrual cycle. Physiology & Behavior 57: 821–826.

Kanders BS, Lavin PT, Kowalchuck MB, Greenberg I, Blackburn GL. 1988. An evaluation of the effect of aspartame on weight loss. Appetite 11(suppl): 73–84.

Kant AK, Ballard-Barbash R, Schatzkin, A. 1995a. Evening eating and its relation to self-reported body weight and nutrient intake in women, CSFII 1985–86. Journal of the American College of Nutrition 14: 358–363.

Kant AK, Schatzkin A, Graubard BI, Ballard-Barbash R. 1995b. Frequency of eating occasions and weight change in the NHANES I Epidemiologic Follow–up Study. International Journal of Obesity 19: 468–474.

Kaplan HI, Kaplan HS. 1957. The psychosomatic concept of obesity. Journal of Nervous and Mental Disorders 125: 181–201.

Kasim SE, Martino S, Kim P-N, Khilnani S, Boomer A, Depper J, Reading BA, Heilbrun LK. 1993. American Journal of Clinical Nutrition 57: 146–153.

Kaufman NA, Poznanski R, Guggenheim K. 1975. Eating habits and opinions of teen-agers on nutrition and obesity. Journal of the American Dietetic Association 66: 264–268.

Keesey RE, 1978. Set-points and body weight regulation. Psychiatric Clinics of North America 1: 523–543.

Keim NL, Van Loan MD, Horn WF, Barbieri TF, Mayclin PL. 1997. Weight loss is greater with consumption of large morning meals and fat-free mass is preserved with large evening meals in women on a controlled weight reduction regimen. Journal of Nutrition 127: 75–82.

Kendall A, Levitsky DA, Strupp BJ, Lissner L. 1991. Weight loss on a low-fat diet: Consequence of the imprecision of the control of food intake in humans. American Journal of Clinical Nutrition 53: 1124–1129.

Kennedy GC. 1953. The role of depot fat in the hypothalamic control of food intake in rats. Proceedings of the Royal Society of London, Series B 140: 578–592.

Kern DL, McPhee L, Fisher J, Johnson S, Birch LL. 1993. The postingestive consequences of fat condition preferences for flavours associated with high dietary fat. Physiology and Behavior 54: 71–76.

Keys A, Brozek J, Henschel A. Mickelson O, Taylor HL. 1950. *The biology of human starvation: Volume 2*. Minneapolis: University of Minnesota Press.

Khan MI, Read NW. 1992. The effect of duodenal lipid infusions upon gastric pressure and sensory responses to balloon distension. Gastroenterology 102: A467.

Khan R, ed. 1993. *Low-calorie foods and food ingredients*. London: Blackie.

Kinabo JLD, Durnin JVGA. 1990. Effect of meal frequency on the thermic effect of food in women. European Journal of Clinical Nutrition 44: 389–395.

Kinney NE, Antill RW. 1996. Role of olfaction in the formation of preference for high-fat foods in mice. Physiology & Behavior 59: 475–478.

Kirkham TC, Cooper SJ. 1988. Naloxone attenuation of sham feeding is modified by manipulation of sucrose concentration. Physiology and Behaviour 44: 491–494.

Kirkham TC, Cooper SJ. 1991. Opioid peptides in relation to the treatment of obesity and bulimia. In: Bloom SR, Burnstock G eds. *Peptides: A target for new drug development*. London: IBC. pp. 28–44.

Kirkham TC, Perez S, Gibbs J. 1995. Prefeeding potentiates anorectic actions of Neuromedin B and gastrin releasing peptide. Physiology and Behavior 58: 1175–1179.

Kirsch KA, von Ameln H. 1981. Feeding patterns of endurance athletes. European Journal of Applied Physiology 47: 197–208.

Kissileff HR. 1984. Satiating efficiency and a strategy for conducting food loading experiments. Neuroscience and Biobehavioral Reviews 8: 129–135.

Kissileff HR, Pi-Sunyer XF, Thornton J, Smith GP. 1981. C-terminal octapeptide of cholecystokinin decreases food intake in man. American Journal of Clinical Nutrition 34: 154–160.

Kissileff HR, Van Itallie TB. 1982. Physiology of the control of food intake. Annual Review of Nutrition 2: 371–418.

Klajner F, Herman CP, Polivy J, Chhabra R. 1981. Human obesity, dieting, and anticipatory salivation to food. Physiology and Behavior 27: 195–198.

Kleifield EI, Lowe MR. 1990. Weight loss and sweetness preferences: The effects of recent versus past weight loss. Physiology & Behavior 49: 1037–1042.

Klein S, Goran M. 1993. Energy metabolism in repsonse to overfeeding in young adult men. Metabolism 42: 1201–1205.

Klesges RC, Klesges LM, Haddock HK, Eck LH. 1992. A longitudinal analysis of the impact of dietary intake and physical activity on weight change in adults. American Journal of Clinical Nutrition 55: 818–822.

Knittle JL. 1966. Meal eating vs. nibbling: effect on human adipose tissue metabolism. American Journal of Clinical Nutrition, 18: 310.

Kristal AR, White E, Shattuck AL, Curry S, Anderson GL, Fowler A, Urban N. 1992. Long-term maintenance of a low-fat diet: Durability of fat-related dietary habits in the Women's Health Trial. Journal of the American Dietetic Association 92: 553–559.

Kromhout D. 1983. Energy and macronutrient intake in lean and obese middle-aged men (the Zutphen Study). American Journal of Clinical Nutrition 37:295–299.

Kulesza W. 1982. Dietary intake in obese women. Appetite 3: 61–68.

Kutlu HR, Forbes JM. 1993. Self-selection of ascorbic acid in coloured foods by heat-stressed broiler chicks. Physiology and Behavior 53: 103–110.

Laessle RG, Tuschl RJ, Kotthaus BC, Pirke KM. 1989a. A comparison of the validity of three scales for the asssessment of dietary restraint. Journal of Abnormal Psychology 98: 504–507.

Laessle RG, Tuschl RJ, Kotthaus BK, Pirke KM. 1989b. Behavioural and biological correlates of dietary restraint in normal life. Appetite: 12: 83–94.

Lands WEM, Zakhari S. 1991. The case of the missing calories. American Journal of Clinical Nutrition 54: 47–48.

Lappalainen R, Sjödén P-o, Hursti T, Esa V. 1990. Hunger/craving responses and reactivity to food stimuli during fasting and dieting. International Journal of Obesity 14: 679–688.

Larson DE, Ferraro RT, Robertson DS, Ravussin E. 1995. Energy metabolism in weight-stable postobese individuals. American Journal of Clinical Nutrition 62: 735–739.

Lawson OJ, Williamson DA, Champagne CM, DeLany JP, Brooks ER, Howat PM, Wozniak PJ, Bray GA, Ryan DH. 1995. The association of body weight, dietary intake, and energy expenditure with dietary restraint and disinhibition. Obesity Research 3: 153–161.

Lean MEJ, James WPT. 1988. Metabolic effects of isoenergetic nutrient exchange over 24 hours on relation to obesity in women. International Journal of Obesity 12: 15–27.

Leathwood PD. 1987. Tryptophan availability and serotonin synthesis. Proceedings of the Nutrition Society 46: 143–156.

LeBlanc J, Mercier I, Nadeau A. 1993. Components of postprandial thermogenesis in relation to meal frequency in humans. Canadian Journal of Physiology and Pharmacology 71: 879–883.

Lee CJ, Lawler GS. 1983. Nutrient intakes in relation to body weight of nonobese and obese elderly females. Nutrition Research 3: 149–155.

Lee-Han H, Cousins M, Beaton M, McGuire V, Kriukov V, Chipman M, Boyd N. 1988. Compliance in a randomized clinical trial of dietary fat reduction in patients with breast dysplasia. American Journal of Clinical Nutrition 48: 575–586.

LeGoff DB, Leichner P, Spigelman MN. 1988. Salivary reponse to olfactory food stimuli in anorexics and bulimics. Appetite 11: 15–25.

LeGoff DB, Spigelman MN. 1987. Salivary response to olfactory food stimuli as a function of dietary restraint and body weight. Appetite 8: 29–35.

Leibel L, Hirsch J, Appel BE, Checani GC. 1992. Energy intake required to maintain body weight is not affected by wide variation in diet composition. American Journal of Clinical Nutrition 55: 350–355.

Leibel L, Rosenbaum M, Hirsch J. 1995. Changes in energy expenditure resulting from altered body weight. New England Journal of Medicine 332: 621–628.

Le Magnen J, Devos M. 1984. Meal to meal energy balance in rats. Physiology and Behavior 32: 39–44.

Le Magnen J, Tallon S. 1966. La périodicité spontanné de la prise d'aliments ad libitum du rat blanc. Journal of Physiology (Paris) 58: 323–349.

Le Magnen J. 1971. Advances in studies on the physiological control and regulation of food intake. In: Stellar E, Sprague JM, eds. *Progress in physiological psychology*, Volume 4. New York: Academic Press. pp. 203–261.

Le Magnen J. 1983. Body energy balance and food intake: a neuroendocrine regulatory mechanism. Physiological Reviews 63: 314–386.

Leveille GA. 1970. Adipose tissue metabolism: Influence of periodicity of eating and diet composition. Federation Proceedings 29: 1294–1301.

Leveille G, O'Hea EK. 1967. Influence of the periodicity of eating on energy metabolism in the rat. Journal of Nutrition, 93: 541–545.

Leveille G, Romsos, DR. 1974. Meal eating and obesity. Nutrition Today 9: 4–10.

Levi P. 1986. *The periodic table*. London: Abacus, Sphere Books Ltd.

Levine AS, Billington CJ. 1994. Dietary fiber: Does it affect food intake and body weight. In: Fernstrom JD, Miller GD, eds. *Appetite and Body Weight Regulation*. Boca Raton: CRC Press. pp. 191–200.

Levitsky DA. 1974. Feeding conditions and intermeal relationships. Physiology and Behavior 12: 779–787.

Lewis CJ, Park YK, Dexter PB, Yetley EA. 1992. Nutrient intakes and body weights of persons consuming high and moderate levels of sugars. Journal of the American Dietetic Association 92: 708–713.

Lichtman SW, Pisarka K, Berman ER, Pestone M, Dowling H, Offenbacher E, Weisel H, Heshka S, Matthews DE, Heymsfield SB. 1992. Discrepancy between self-reported and actual caloric intake and exercise in obese subjects. New England Journal of Medicine 327: 1893–1898.

Liddle RA, Goldfine ID, Williams JA. 1983. Bioassy of circulating CCK in rat and human plasma. Gastroenterology 84: 1231–1236.

Liebel RL, Rosenbaum M, Hirsch J. 1995. Changes in energy expenditure resulting from altered body weight. New England Journal of Medicine 332: 621–628.

Lieber CS. 1991. Perspectives: Do alcohol calories count? American Journal of Clinical Nutrition 54: 976–982.

Lieberman HR, Caballero B, Finer N. 1986a. The composition of lunch determines plasma tryptophan rations in humans. Journal of Neural Transmission 65: 211–217.

Lieberman H, Wurtman J, Chew B. 1986b. Changes in mood after carbohydrate consumption among obese individuals. American Journal of Clinical Nutrition 45: 772–778.

Lindeman AK. 1990. Eating and training habits of triathletes: A balancing act. Journal of the American Dietetic Association, 90: 993–995.

Lissner L. 1987. Dietary correlates of human obesity: The role of fat intake. PhD Thesis. Cornell University, Ithaca NY, USA.

Lissner L, Habicht J-P, Strupp BJ, Levitsky DA, Haas JD, Roe DA. 1989. Body composition and energy intake: Do overweight women overeat and underreport? American Journal of Clinical Nutrition 49: 320–325.

Lissner L, Heitmann BL, Bengtsson C., 1996. Low-fat diets may prevent weight gain in sedentary women: Prospective observations from the Population Study of Women in Gothenburg, Sweden. International Journal of Obesity 5:43–48.

Lissner L, Levitsky DA, Strupp BJ, Kalkwarf HJ, Roe DA. 1987. Dietary fat and the regulation of energy intake in human subjects. American Journal of Clinical Nutrition 46: 886–892.

Lissner L, Lindroos A-K. 1994. Is dietary underreporting macronutrient-specific? European Journal of Clinical Nutrition 48: 453–454.

Livesey G. 1991. Determinants of energy density with conventional foods and artificial feeds. Proceedings of the Nutrition Society 50: 371–382.

Livesey G, Johnson IT, Gee JM, Smith T, Lee WE, Hillan KA, Meyer J, Turner SC. 1993. 'Determination' of sugar alcohol and Polydextrose® absorption in humans by the breath hydrogen (H2) technique: the stoichiometry of hydrogen production and the interaction between carbohydrates assessed in vivo and in vitro. European Journal of Clinical Nutrition 47: 419–430.

Livingstone MBE, Prentice AM, Strain JJ, Coward WA, Black AE, Barker ME, McKenna PG, Whitehead RG. 1990. Accuracy of weighed dietary records in studies of diet and health. British Medical Journal 300:708–712.

Lloyd HM, Green MW, Rogers PJ. 1994. Mood and cognitive performance effects of isocaloric lunches differing in fat and carbohydrate content. Physiology and Behavior 56: 51–57.

Lloyd HM, Rogers PJ, Hedderley DI, Walker AF. 1996. Acute effects on mood and cognitive performance of breakfasts differing in fat and carbohydrate content. Appetite 27: 151–164.

Lonnquist F, Arner P, Nordford L, Schalling M. 1995. Overexpression of the obese (Ob) gene in adipose tissue of human obese subjects. Nature Medicine 1: 950–953.

Louge AW, Ophir I, Strauss KE. 1981. The acquisition of taste aversions in humans. Behaviour Research and Therapy 19: 319–333.

Louis-Sylvestre J, Giachetti I, Le Magnen J. 1984. Sensory versus dietary factors in cafeteria-induced overweight. Physiology & Behavior 32: 901–905.

Louis-Sylvestre J, Tournier A, Chapelot D, Chabert M. 1994. Effect of a fat-reduced dish in a meal on 24-h energy and macronutrient intake. Appetite 22: 165–172.

Louis-Sylvestre J, Tournier A, Verger P, Chabert M, Delorme B, Hossenlopp J. 1989. Learned caloric adjustment of human intake. Appetite 12: 95–103.

Lowe MR. 1993. The effects of dieting on eating behaviour: A three–factor model. Psychological Bulletin 114: 100–121.

Lowe MR, Kliefield E. 1988. Cognitive restraint, weight suppression, and the regulation of eating. Appetite 10: 159–168.

Lowe MR, Whitlow JW, Bellwoar V. 1991. Eating regulation: The role of restraint, dieting, and weight. International Journal of Eating Disorders 10: 461–471.

Lucas F, Sclafani A. 1996a. Food deprivation increases the rat's preference for a fatty flavor over a sweet taste. Chemical Senses 21: 169–179.

Lucas F, Sclafani A. 1996b. The composition of the maintenance diet alters flavor-preference conditioning by intragastric fat infusions in rats. Physiology & Behavior 60: 1151–1157.

Lucca PA, Tepper BJ. 1994. Fat replacers and the functionality of fat in foods. Trends in Food Science & Technology 5: 12–19.

Lyle BJ, McMahon KE, Kreutler PA. 1991. Assessing the potential dietary impact of replacing dietary fat with other macronutrients. Journal of Nutrition 122: 211–216.

Lyon X-H, Di Vetta V, Milon H, Jéquier E, Schutz Y. 1995. Compliance to dietary advice directed towards increasing the carbohydrate to fat ratio of the everyday diet. International Journal of Obesity 19: 260–269.

Mabayo RT, Okumura J-I, Hirao A, Sugita S, Sugahara K, Furose M. 1996. The role of olfaction in oil preferences in the chicken. Physiology & Behavior 59: 1185–1188.

Macdiarmid JI, Hetherington MM. 1995. Mood modulation by food: An exploration of affect and cravings in 'chocolate addicts'. British Journal of Clinical Psychology 34: 129–138.

Machinot S, Mimouni M, Lestradet H. 1975. L'alimentation spontanee de l'enfant obese au moment de la premiere consultation. Cahiers de Nutrition et de Dietetique 1: 45–46.

Maes M, Meltzer HY. 1995. The serotonin hypothesis of major depression. In: Bloom FE, Kupfer DJ, eds. *Psychopharmacology: The fourth generation of progress.* New York: Raven Press. pp. 933–944.

Maffei M, Stoffel M, Barone M, Moon B, Dammerman M, Ravussin E, Bogardus C, Ludwig DS, Flier JS, Talley M, Auerbach S, Friedman JM. 1996. Absence of mutations in the human OB gene in obese/diabetic subjects. Diabetes 45: 679–682.

Maffeis C, Pinelli L, Schutz Y. Fat intake and adiposity in 8 to 11-year-old obese children. International Journal of Obesity 20: 170–174.

Mahler R. 1972. The relationship between eating and obesity. Acta Diabetologia Latina 9: 449–465.

Manocha S, Gupta MC. 1985. Dietary intake in obese and nonobese adults. Indian Journal of Medical Research 82: 47–50.

Martin GM, Bellingham WP, Storlien LH. 1977. Effects of varied colour experience on chickens' formation of colour and texture aversions. Physiology and Behavior 8: 415–420.

Martin I, Levey A. 1994. The evaluative response: Primitive but necessary. Behaviour Research and Therapy 32: 301–305.

Martin LJ, Su W, Jones PJ, Lockwood GA, Tritchler DL, Boyd NF. 1996. Comparison of energy intakes determined by food records and doubly labelled water in women participating in a dietary-intervention trial. American Journal of Clinical Nutrition 63: 483–490.

Mattes RD. 1990. Effects of aspartame and sucrose on hunger and energy intake in humans. Physiology & Behavior 47: 1037–1044.

Mattes RD. 1991. Learned food aversions: a family study. Physiology & Behavior 50: 499–504.

Mattes RD. 1996. Dietary compensation by humans for supplemental energy provided as ethanol or carbohydrate in fluids. Physiology & Behavior 59: 179–187.

Mattes RD, Pierce CB, Friedman MI. 1988. Daily caloric intake of normal-weight adults: response to changes in dietary energy density of a luncheon meal. American Journal of Clinical Nutrition 48: 214–9.

Max B. 1989. This and that: chocolate addiction, the dual pharmacogenetics of asparagus eaters and the arithmetic of freedom. Trends in Pharmacological Science 10: 390–393.

Maxfield E, Konishi F. 1966. Patterns of food intake and physical activity in obesity. Journal of the American Dietetic Association 9: 406–408.

Mayer J. 1955. Regulation of energy intake and the body weight. The glucostatic theory and the lipostatic hypothesis. Annals of the New York Academy of Sciences 63: 15–43.

McBride A, Wise A, McNeill G, James WPT. 1990. The pattern of food consumption related to energy intake. Journal of Human Nutrition and Dietetics 3: 27–32.

McColl KA. 1988. The sugar-fat seesaw. British Nutrition Foundation Nutrition Bulletin 53: 114–118.

McCann KL, Perri MG, Nezu AM, Lowe MR. 1992. An investigation of counter-regulatory eating in obese clinic attenders. International Journal of Eating Disorders 12: 161–169.

McGrath RE, Buckwald B, Resnick EV. 1990. The effect of L-tryptophan on seasonal affective disorder. Journal of Clinical Psychiatry 51: 162–163.

McHugh PR, Moran TH. 1991. The stomach: A conception of its dynamic role in satiety. Progress in Psychobiology and Physiological Psychology 11: 197–232.

McNeill G, McBride A, Smith JS, James WPT. 1989. Energy expenditure in large and small eaters. Nutrition Research 9: 363–372.

Mehiel R, Bolles RC. 1988. Learned flavor preferences are independent of initial hedonic value. Animal Learning and Behavior 16: 383–387.

Mei. 1985. Intestinal chemosensitivity. Physiological reviews 65: 211–237.

Meiselman HL. 1977. The role of sweetness in the food preference of young adults. In: Weiffenbach JM, ed. *Taste and development. The genesis of sweet taste preference.* DHEW Publication (NIH) 77–1068. Washington DC: US Government Printing Office. pp. 269–279.

Meiselman HL, Waterman D, Symington LE. 1974. *Armed forces food preferences.* Technical Report TR-75-63-FSL. Natick, MA: U.S. Army Natick Development Center.

Meiselman HL, Wyant KW. 1981. Food preferences and flavor experiences. In: Solms J, Hall RL, eds. *Criteria of food acceptance.* Zurich: Forster Verlag AG. pp. 144–152.

Mela DJ. 1989. Gustatory function and dietary habits in users and non-users of smokeless tobacco. American Journal of Clinical Nutrition 49:482–489.

Mela DJ. 1995. Understanding fat preference and consumption: Applications of behavioural sciences to a nutritional problem. Proceedings of the Nutrition Society 54: 453–464.

Mela DJ. 1996a. Assessing the potential dietary implications of macronutrient substitutes. In: Angel A, Anderson H, Bouchard C, Lau D, Leiter L, Mendelson R, eds. *Progress in Obesity Research 7.* London: John Libbey & Co. pp. 423–430.

Mela DJ. 1996b. Eating behaviour, food preferences and dietary intake in relation to obesity and body weight status. Proceedings of the Nutrition Society 55: 803–816.

Mela DJ. 1996c. Implications of fat replacement for nutrition and food intake. Fett/Lipid 98: 50–55.

Mela DJ, Aaron JI. In press. 'Honest but invalid': What the subjects say about recording their food intake. Journal of the American Dietetic Association.

Mela DJ, Catt SL. 1996. Ontogeny of human taste and smell preferences and their implications for food selection. In: Henry CJK, Ulijaszek SJ, eds. *Long Term Consequences of Early Environment: Growth, development and the lifespan developmental perspective*. Society for the Study of Human Biology Symposium Series 37. Cambridge UK: Cambridge University Press. pp. 139–154.

Mela DJ. In press. Fat and sugar substitutes: Implications for dietary intakes and energy balance. Proceedings of the Nutrition Society.

Mela DJ. 1997. Impact of macronutrient-substituted foods on food choice and dietary intake. Annals of the New York Academy of Sciences 819: 96–107.

Mela DJ, Langley K, Martin A. 1994. Sensory assessment of fat content: Effect of emulsion and subject characteristics. Appetite 22: 67–81.

Mela DJ, Sacchetti DS. 1991. Sensory preferences for fats in foods: relationships to diet and body composition. American Journal of Clinical Nutrition 53: 908–15.

Menella J. Mother's milk: A medium for early flavor experiences. Journal of Human Lactation 11: 39–45.

Metzner HL, Lamphiear DE, Wheeler NC, Larkin FA. 1977. The relationship between frequency of eating and adiposity in adult men and women in the Tecumseh Community Health Study. American Journal of Clinical Nutrition 30: 712–715.

Michener W, Rozin P. 1994. Pharmacological versus sensory factors in the satiation of chocolate craving. Physiology and Behavior 56: 419–422.

Miller WC. 1991. Diet composition, energy intake, and nutritional status in relation to obesity in men and women. Medicine and Science in Sports and Exercise 23: 280–284.

Miller A, Barr RG, Young SN. 1994a. The cold pressor test in children: Methodological aspects and the analgesic effect of intraoral sucrose. Pain 56: 175–183.

Miller WC, Linderman AK, Wallace J, Niederpruem M. 1990. Diet composition, energy intake, and exercise in relation to body fat in men and women. American Journal of Clinical Nutrition 52: 426–430.

Miller DS, Mumford P. 1973. Luxuskonsumption. In: Apfelbaum M, ed. Regulation of energy balance in man. Paris: Masson. pp. 195–207.

Miller WC, Niederpruem M, Wallace J, Linderman AK. 1994b. Dietary fat, sugar and fiber predict body fat content. Journal of the American Dietetic Association 94: 612–615.

Millward DJ. 1995. A protein-stat mechanism for regulation of growth and maintenance of the lean body mass. Nutrition Research Reviews 8: 93–120.

Ministry of Agriculture, Fisheries and Food. 1995. *Manual of nutrition*. 10th Edition. Reference Book 342. London: HMSO.

Mizes JS. 1985. Bulimia: A review of its symptomatology and treatment. Advances in Behavior Research and Therapy 7: 91–142.

Møller SE. 1992. Serotonin, carbohydrates, and atypical depression. Pharmacology and Toxicology 71(Suppl.1): 61–71.

Molnar D. 1990. The effect of meal frequency on postprandial thermogenesis in obese children. International Journal of Obesity 14: 95.

Mook DG. 1987. *Motivation: The organization of action*. New York: Norton.

Mook DG, Votaw MC. 1992. How important is hedonism? Reasons given by college students for ending a meal. Appetite 18: 69–75.

Moore LL, Lombardi DA, White MJ, Campbell JL, Oliveria SA, Ellison SA. 1991.

Influence of parents' physical activity on the activity levels of young children. Journal of Pediatrics 118:215–219.

Moran TH, McHugh PR. 1992. Gastric mechanisms in CCK satiety. In: Dourish CT, Cooper SJ, Iversen SD, Iversen LL, eds. *Multiple Cholecystokinin Receptors in the CNS*. Oxford: Oxford University Press. pp. 183–205.

Morgan KJ, Johnson SR, Stampley GL. 1983. Children's frequency of eating, total sugar intake and weight/height stature. Nutrition Research 3: 635–652.

Morley JE, Levine AS, Yamada T, Gebhard RL, Prigge WF, Shafer RB, Goetz FC, Silvis SE. 1983. Effect of exorphins on gastrointestinal function, hormonal release and appetite. Gastroenterology 84: 1517–1523.

Mumford GK, Evans SM, Kaminski BJ, Preston KL, Sannerud CA, Silverman K, Griffiths RR. 1994. Dicriminative stimulus and subjective effects of theobromine and caffeine in humans. Psychopharmacology 115, 1–8.

Naim M, Kare MR. 1991. Sensory and postingestional components of palatability in dietary obesity: An overview. In: Friedman MI, Tordoff MG, Kare MR, eds. *Chemical senses. Volume 4: Appetite and nutrition*. New York: Marcel Dekker. pp. 109–126.

Naismith DJ, Rhodes C. 1995. Adjustment in energy intake following the covert removal of sugar from the diet. Journal of Human Nutrition & Dietetics 8: 167–175.

National Diet-Heart Study Research Group. 1968. The National Diet-Heart Study final report. Circulation 37(Suppl I): I1–I428.

Nelson LH, Tucker LA. 1996. Diet composition related to body fat in a multivariate study of 203 men. Journal of the American Dietetic Association 96: 771–777.

New SA, Grubb DA. 1996. Relationship of biscuit, cake and confectionery consumption to body mass index and energy intake in Scottish women. Proceedings of the Nutrition Society 55: 122A.

Nguyen VT, Larson DE, Johnson RK, Goran MI. 1996. Fat intake and adiposity in children of lean and obese parents. American Journal of Clinical Nutrition 63: 507–513.

Niki T, Mori H, Tamori Y, Kishimoto-Hashiramoto M, Ueno H, Araki S, Masugi J, Sawant N, Majithia HR, Rais N, Hashiramoto M, Taniguchi H, Kasuga M. 1996. Human obese gene. Molecular screening in Japanese and Asian Indian NIDDM patients associated with obesity. Diabetes 45: 675–678.

Nisbett RE. 1972. Hunger, obesity, and the ventromedial hypothalamus. Psychological Review 79: 433–453.

Norman RA, Chung WK, Power-Kehoe L, Chua SC, Leigel RL, Devoto M, Fann C, Ott J, Bogardus C, Ravussin E. 1995. Genetic linkage of homologues to rodent obesity genes in Pima Indians. Diabetes 57: A199.

Nunes WT, Canham, JE. 1963. The effect of varied periodicity of eating on serum lipids and carbohydrate tolerance in man. American Journal of Clinical Nutrition 12: 334.

Nylander I. 1971. The feeling of being fat and dieting in a school population. Acta Socia-Medica Scandinavia 1: 17–26.

Nysenbaum AN, Smart JL. 1982. Sucking behaviour and milk intake of neonates in relation to milk fat content. Early Human Development 6: 205–213.

Obarzanek E, Schreiber GB, Crawford PB, Goldman SR, Barrier PM, Frederick MM, Lakatos E. 1994. Energy intake and physical activity in relation to indexes of body fat: the National Heart, Lung, and Blood Institute Growth and Health Study. American Journal of Clinical Nutrition 60: 15–22.

Oetting RL, Vanderweele DA. 1985. Insulin suppresses intake without inducing illness in sham feeding rats. Physiology and Behavior 34: 557–562.

Ogden J, Greville L. 1993. Cognitive changes to preloading in restrained and unrestrained eaters as measured by the Stroop task. International Journal of Eating Disorders 14: 185–195.

Ogden J, Wardle J. 1991. Cognitive and emotional responses to food. International Journal of Eating Disorders 10: 297–311.

Ortega RM, Requejo AM, Andrés P, López-Sobaler AM, Redondo R, González-Fernández M. 1995. Relationship between diet composition and body mass index in a group of Spanish adolescents. British Journal of Nutrition 74: 765–773.

Ortega RM, Requejo AM, Quintas E, Sánchez-Quiles B, López-Sobaler AM, Andrés P. 1996. Estimated energy balance in female university students: differences with respect to body mass index and concern about body weight. International Journal of Obesity 20:1127–1129.

Ossenkopp K-P, Eckel LA. 1995. Toxin-induced conditioned changes in taste reactivity and the role of the chemosensitive area postrema. Neuroscience and Biobehavioral Reviews 19: 99–108.

O'Dea K. 1992. Obesity and diabetes in 'the land of milk and honey'. Diabetes/Metabolism Reviews 8: 373–388.

O'Rouke D, Wurtman JJ, Wurtman RJ, Chebli R, Gleason, R. 1989. Treatment of seasonal depression with d-fenfluramine. Journal of Clinical Psychiatry 50: 343–347.

Pangborn RM, Bos KEO, Stern JS. 1985. Dietary fat intake and taste responses to fat in milk by under-, normal, and overweight women. Appetite 6: 25–40.

Pangborn RM, Simone, M. 1958. Body size and sweetness preference. Journal of the American Dietetic Association 34: 924–928.

Parker DR, Gonzalez S, Derby CA, Gans KM, Lasater TM, Carleton RA. 1997. Dietary factors in relation to weight change among men and women from two southeastern New England communities. International Journal Of Obesity 21: 103–109.

Pasquest P, Brigant L, Froment A, Koppert GA, Bard D, de Garine I, Apfelbaum M. 1992. Massive overfeeding and energy metabolism in men: the *Guru Walla* model. American Journal of Clinical Nutrition 56: 483–490.

Passmore R, Swindells YE. 1963. Observations on the respiratory quotients and weight gain of man after eating large quantitites of carbohydrate. Br Journal Nutrition 17: 331–339.

Pavlov IP. 1927. Conditioned Reflexes. Oxford: Oxford University Press.

Peele S. 1990. Addiction as a cultural concept. Annals of the New York Academy of Sciences 602: 205–220.

Pelleymounter MA, Cullen MJ, Baker MB, Hecht R, Winters D, Boone T, Collins F. 1995. Effects of the obese gene product on body weight regulation in *ob/ob* mice. Science 269: 540–543.

Pérez C, Ackroff K, Sclafani A. 1994. Carbohydrate- and protein-conditioned flavour preferences in rats: Effects of nutrient preloads. Appetite 23: 317.

Pérusse L, Bouchard C. 1996. Identification of genes contributing to excess body fat and fat distribution. In: Angel A, Anderson H, Bouchard C, Lau D, Leiter L, Mendelson R, eds. *Progress in obesity research 7*. London: John Libbey & Co. pp. 281–289.

Pérusse L, Chagnon YC, Dionne FT, Bouchard C. 1997. The human obesity gene map: The 1996 update. Obesity Research 5: 49–61.

Pérusse L, Leblanc C, Bouchard C. 1988a. Familial resemblance in lifestyle components: Results from the Canada Fitness Survey. Canadian Journal of Public Health 79: 201–205.

Pérusse L, Leblanc C, Bouchard C. 1988b. Intergeneration transmission of physical fitness in the Canadian population. Canadian Journal of Sports Science 13: 8–14.

Pérusse L, Tremblay A, Leblanc C, Bouchard C. 1989. Genetic and environmental influences on level of habitual physical activity and exercise participation. American Journal of Epidemiology 129: 1012–1022.

Pérusse L, Tremblay A, Leblanc C, Cloninger CR, Reich T, Rice J, Bouchard C. 1988c. Familial resemblance in energy intake: Contribution of genetic and environmental factors. American Journal of Clinical Nutrition 43: 629–635.

Peters JC, Holcombe BN, Hiller LK, Webb DR. 1991. Caprenin 3. Absorption and caloric value in adult humans. Journal of the American College of Toxicology 10: 357–367.

Peterson CM, Jovanovic-Peterson L. 1995. Randomized crossover study of 40% vs. 55% carbohydrate weight loss strategies in women with previous gestational diabetes mellitus and non-diabetic women of 130–200% ideal body weight. Journal of the American College of Nutrition 14: 369–375.

Pijl H, Koppeschaar HPF, Cohen AF, Lestra JA, Schoemaker HC, Frölich M, Onkenhout W, Meinders AE. 1993. Evidence for brain serotonin-mediated control of carbohydrate consumption in normal weight and obese humans. International Journal of Obesity 17: 513–520.

Pinel JPJ. 1993. Biopsychology, Second Edition. Boston: Allyn and Bacon.

Pivonka EEA, Grunewald KK. 1990. Aspartame- or sugar-sweetened beverages: Effects on mood in young women. Journal of the American Dietetic Association 90: 250–254.

Platte P, Wurmser H, Wade SE, Mecheril A, Pirke KM. 1996. Resting metabolic rate and diet-induced thermogenesis in restrained and unrestrained eaters. International Journal of Eating Disorders 20: 33–41.

Plomin R, Daniels D. 1987. Why are children in the same family so different from one another? Behavioral and Brain Sciences 10: 1–16.

Plutchik R. 1976. Emotions and attitudes related to being overweight. Journal of Clinical Psychology 32: 21–24.

Polivy J. 1976. Perception of calories and regulation of intake in restrained and unrestrained subjects. Addictive Behaviors 1: 237–243.

Polivy J, Herman CP. 1976. Clinical depression and weight change: A complex relation. Journal of Abnormal Psychology 85: 338–340.

Polivy J, Herman CP. 1985. Dieting and binging: a causal analysis. American Psychologist 40: 193–201.

Polivy J, Herman CP, Warsh S. 1978. Internal and external components of emotionality in restrained and unrestrined eaters. Journal of Abnormal Psychology 87: 497–504.

Pond CM. 1992. An evolutionary and functional view of mammalian adipose tissue. Proceedings of the Nutrition Society 51: 367–377.

Poppitt SD, Prentice AM. 1996. Energy density and its role in the control of food intake: Evidence from metabolic and community studies. Appetite 26: 153–174.

Porrini M, Crovetti R, Riso P, Santangelo A, Testolin G. 1995. Effects of physical and chemical characteristics of food on specific and general satiety. Physiology & Behavior 57: 461–468.

Porter RH, Makin JW, Davis LB, Christensen KM. 1991. An assessment of the salient olfactory environment of formula-fed infants. Physiology and Behavior 50; 907–911.

Prentice AM. 1995a. Alcohol and obesity. International Journal of Obesity 19 (Suppl 5): S44–S50.

Prentice AM. 1995b. Are all calories equal? In: Cottrell R, ed. *Weight control: The current perspective*. London: Chapman and Hall. pp. 9–33.

Prentice AM. 1996. Food and nutrient intake and obesity. In: Angel A, Anderson GH, Bouchard C, Lau D, Leiter L, Mendelson R, eds. Progress in obesity research: 7. London: John Libbey & Co. pp. 451–457.

Prentice AM, Black AE, Coward WA, Cole TJ. 1996a. Energy expenditure in overweight and obese adults in affluent societies: An analysis of 319 doubly-labelled water measurements. European Journal of Clinical Nutrition 50: 93–97.

Prentice AM, Black AE, Murgatroyd PR, Goldberg GR, Coward WA. 1989. Metabolism or appetite: Questions of energy balance with particular reference to obesity. Journal of Human Nutrition and Dietetics 2: 95–104.

Prentice AM, Goldberg GR, Murgatroyd PR, Cole TJ. 1996b. Physical activity and obesity: Problems in correcting expenditure for size. International Journal of Obesity 20: 688–691.

Prentice AM, Jebb SA. 1995. Obesity in Britain: gluttony or sloth? British Medical Journal 311: 437–439.

Prentice AM, Sonko BJ, Murgatroyd PR, Goldberg GR. 1994. Obesity as an adaptation to a high-fat diet [letter]. American Journal of Clinical Nutrition 59: 640–641.

Prewitt TE, Schmeisser D, Bowen PE, Aye P, Dolecek TA, Langenberg P, Cole T, Brace L. 1991. Changes in body weight, body composition, and energy intake in women fed high- and low-fat diets. American Journal of Clinical Nutrition 54: 304–310.

Price RA, Gottesman II. 1991. Body fat in identical twins reared apart: Roles for genes and environment. Behavioral Genetics 21: 1–7.

Pryer JA, Vrijheid M, Nichols R, Elliott P. 1994. Who are the 'low energy reporters' in the Dietary and Nutritional Survey of British Adults? Proceedings of the Nutrition Society 53: 235A.

Raben A, Andersen HB, Christensen NJ, Madsen J, Holst JJ, Astrup A. 1994a. Evidence for an abnormal postprandial response to a high-fat meal in women predisposed to obesity. American Journal of Physiology 267: E559–E559.

Raben A, Due Jensen N, Marckmann P, Sandström B, Astrup A. 1995. Spontaneous weight loss during 11 weeks' ad libitum intake of a low fat/high fiber diet in young, normal weight subjects. International Journal of Obesity 19: 916–923.

Raben A, Tagliabue A, Christensen NJ, Madsen J, Holst JJ, Astrup A. 1994b. Resistant starch: The effect of postprandial glycemia, hormonal response, and satiety. American Journal of Clinical Nutrition 60: 544–551.

Raben A, Vasilaras TH, Møller C, Astrup A. 1996. Sucrose vs artificial sweeteners: Minor differences in body weight after 10 weeks. International Journal of Obesity 20(Suppl. 4): 51.

Ramirez I. 1990. Does dietary hyperphagia contradict the lipostatic theory? Physiology and Behavior 14: 117–123.

Ramirez I. 1992. Chemoreception for fat: Do rats sense triglycerides directly? Appetite 18: 193–206.

Ramirez I, Friedman MI. 1990. Dietary hyperphagia in rats: Role of fat, carbohydrate, and energy content. Physiology and Behavior 47: 1157–1164.

Ranganath L, Beety JM, Morgan LM, Wright WJ, Howland R, Marks V. 1996. Attenuated GLP-1 secretion in obesity: Cause or consequence?. Gut 38: 916–919.

Ranhotra GS, Gelroth JA, Glaser BK. 1993. Usable energy value of selected bulking agents. Journal of Food Science 58: 1176–1178.

Ravussin E. 1995. Low resting metabolic rate as a risk factor for weight gain: Role of the sympathetic nervous system. InternationalJournal of Obesity 19 (suppl 7): S8–S9.

Ravussin E, Lillioja S, Anderson TE, Christin L, Bogardus C. 1986. Determinants of 24-hour energy-expenditure in man. Methods and results using a respiratory chamber. Journal of Clinical Investigation 78: 1568–1578.

Ravussin E, Lillioja S, Knowler SC, Christin L, Freymond D, Abbott WGH, Boyce V, Howard BV, Bogardus C. 1988. Reduced rate of energy expenditure as a risk factor for body-weight gain . New England Journal of Medicine 318: 467–472.

Ravussin E, Schutz Y, Acheson KJ, Dusmet M, Bourquin l, Jéquier E. 1985. Short-term, mixed-diet overfeeding in man – No evidence for luxuskonsumption. American Journal of Physiology 249: E470–E477.

Ravussin E, Swinburn B. 1993. Energy metabolism. In: Stunkard AJ, Wadden TA, eds. Obesity: Theory and therapy. 2nd Edition. New York: Raven Press. pp. 97–123.

Read N, French S, Cunningham K. 1994. The role of the gut in regulating food intake in man. Nutrition Reviews 52: 1–10.

Redd M, de Castro JM. 1992. Social facilitation of eating: Effects of social instruction on food intake. Physiology and Behavior 52: 749–754.

Reddingius J. 1980. Control theory and the dynamics of body weight. Physiology and Behavior 24: 27–32.

Reed DR, Ding Y, Xu W, Cather C, Price RA. 1995. Human obesity does not segregate with the chromosomal regions of Prader-Willi, Bardet-Biedl, Cohen, Borjeson, or Wilson-Turner syndromes. International Journal of Obesity 19: 599–603.

Reed DR, Ding Y, Xu WZ, Cather C, Green ED, Price RA. 1996. Extreme obesity may be linked to markers flanking the human OB gene. Diabetes 45: 691–694.

Reed DR, Friedman MI. 1990. Diet composition alters the acceptance of fat by rats. Appetite 14: 219–230.

Retzlaff BM, Dowdy AA, Walden CE, McCann BS, Gey G, Cooper M, Knopp RH. 1991. Changes in vitamin and mineral intakes and serum concentrations among free–living men on cholesterol-lowering diets: The Dietary Alternatives Study. American Journal of Clinical Nutrition 53: 890–98.

Richardson NJ, Rogers PJ, Elliman NA. 1996. Conditioned flavour preferences reinforced by caffeine consumed after lunch. Physiology and Behavior 60: 257–263.

Ries W. 1973. Feeding behaviour in obesity. Proceedings of the Nutrition Society 32: 187–193.

Robbins TW, Fray PJ. 1980. Stress-induced eating: fact, fiction or misunderstanding? Appetite 1: 103–133.

Roberts SB. 1995. Abnormalities of energy expenditure and the development of obesity. Obesity Research 3(Suppl 2): 155s–163s.

Roberts SB, Greenberg AS. 1996. The new obesity genes. Nutrition Reviews 54: 41–49.

Roberts SB, Savage J, Coward WA, Chew B, Lucas A. 1988. Energy expenditure and intake in infants born to lean and overweight mothers. New England Journal of Medicine 318: 461–466.

Roberts SB, Young VR, Fuss P, Fiatarone MA, Richard B, Rasmussen H, Wagner D, Joseph L, Holehouse E, Evans WJ. 1990. Energy expenditure and subsequent nutrient intakes in overfed young men. American Journal of Physiology 259: R461–R469.

Robinson PH. 1989. Perceptivity and paraceptivity during measurement of gastric emptying in anorexia and bulimia nervosa. British Journal of Psychiatry 154: 400–405.

Robinson J, Ferguson A. 1992. Food sensitivity and the nervous system: hyperactivity, addiction and criminal behaviour. Nutrition Research Reviews 5: 203–223.

Robinson S, Hill AJ, Rogers PJ. 1983. Breakdown of restraint following the imagination of food but not after a highly palatable preload. International Journal of Obesity 7: 89–91.

Rodin J. 1975a. Effects of obesity and set point on taste responsiveness and ingestion in humans. Journal of Comparative Physiology and Psychology 89: 1003–1009.

Rodin J. 1975b. Has the distinction between internal versus external control of feeding outlived its usefulness? In: Bray GA, ed. Recent advances in obesity research, volume 2. London: Newman. pp. 75–85.

Rodin J. 1976. The relationship between external responsiveness and the development and maintenance of obesity. In: Novin D, Wyrwicka W, Bray G, eds. *Hunger: Basic mechanisms and treatment.* New York: Raven Press. pp. 409–419.

Rodin J. 1980. Changes in perceptual responsiveness following jejunoileostomy: Their potential role in reducing food intake. American Journal of Clinical Nutrition 33: 457–464.

Rodin J. 1981. Current status of the internal-external hypothesis for obesity: What went wrong? American Psychologist 36: 361–372.

Rodin J, Mancuso J, Granger J, Nelbach E. 1991. Food cravings in relation to body mass index, restraint and estradiol levels: a repeated measures study in healthy women. Appetite 17: 177–185.

Rodin J, Moskowitz HR, Bray GA. 1976. Relationship between obesity weight loss, and taste reponsiveness. Physiological Psychology 17:591–597.

Rodin J, Schank D, Striegel-Moore R. 1989. Psychological features of obesity. Medical Clinics of North America 73: 47–66.

Rodin J, Slochower J. 1976. Externality in the non-obese: Effects of environmental responsiveness on weight gain. Journal of Personality and Social Psychology 33: 338–344.

Rogers PJ. 1983. An investigation of the effects of dietary manipulations, obesity and hunger on feeding behaviour. Ph.D. thesis, University of Leeds, UK.

Rogers PJ. 1985. Returning 'cafeteria-fed' rats to a chow diet: Negative contrast and effects of obesity on feeding behaviour. Physiology and Behavior 35: 493–499.

Rogers PJ. 1988. Interrelationships between feeding patterns and obesity in humans and animals. Proceedings of the 1st European Congress on Obesity, Stockholm.

Rogers PJ. 1990. Why a palatability construct is needed. Appetite 14: 167–170.

Rogers PJ. 1993. The experimental investigation of human eating behaviour. In: Hindmarch I, Stonier PD, eds. *Human Psychpharmacology: Measures and methods, volume 4.* Chichester: Wiley. pp.123–142.

Rogers PJ. 1994. Mechanisms of moreishness and food craving. In: Warburton DM, ed. *Pleasure: The politics and the reality.* Chichester: Wiley. pp. 38–49.

Rogers PJ. 1995. Food, mood and appetite. Nutrition Research Reviews 8: 243–269.

Rogers PJ, Anderson AO, Finch GM, Jas P, Gatenby SJ. 1994. Relationships between food craving and anticipatory salivation, eating patterns, mood and body weight in women and men. Appetite 23: 319.

Rogers PJ, Blundell JE. 1984. Meal patterns and food selection during the development of obesity in rats fed a cafeteria diet. Neuroscience and Biobehavioral Reviews 8: 441–453.

Rogers PJ, Blundell JE. 1989a. Evaluation of the influence of intense sweeteners on the short-term control of appetite and caloric intake: A psychobiological approach. In: Grenby TH, ed. *Progress in sweeteners.* London: Elsevier Applied Science. pp. 267–289.

Rogers PJ, Blundell JE. 1989b. Separating the actions of sweetness and calories: effects of saccharin and carbohydrates on hunger and food intake in human subjects. Physiology & Behavior 45: 1093–1099.

Rogers PJ, Blundell JE. 1990. Psychobiological bases of food choice. British Nutrition Foundation Nutrition Bulletin 15(Suppl. 1): 31–40.

Rogers PJ, Blundell JE. 1991. Mechanisms of diet selection: The translation of need into behaviour. Proceedings of the Nutrition Society 50: 65–70.

Rogers PJ, Blundell JE. 1993. Intense sweeteners and appetite. American Journal of Clinical Nutrition. 83:120–121.

Rogers, PJ, Burley VJ, Alikhanizadeh LA, Blundell JE. 1995a. Postingestive inhibition of food intake by aspartame: Importance of interval between aspartame administration and subsequent eating. Physiology & Behavior 57: 489–493.

Rogers PJ, Carlyle J, Hill AJ, Blundell JE. 1988. Uncoupling sweet taste and calories: Comparison of the effects of glucose and three high intensity sweeteners on hunger and food intake. Physology & Behavior 43: 457–452.

Rogers PJ, Edwards S, Green MW, Jas P. 1992. Nutritional influences on mood and cognitive performance: The menstrual cycle, caffeine and dieting. Proceedings of the Nutrition Society 51: 343–351.

Rogers PJ, Green MW. 1993. Dieting, dietary restraint and cognitive performance. British Journal of Clinical Psychology 32: 113–116.

Rogers PJ, Hill AJ. 1989. Breakdown of dietary restraint following mere exposure to food stimuli: interrelationships between restraint, hunger, salivation, and food intake. Addictive Behaviors 14: 387–397.

Rogers PJ, Jas P. 1994. Menstrual cycle effects on mood, eating and food choice. Appetite 23: 289.

Rogers PJ, Mela DJ. 1992. Biology and the senses: Do you eat what you like or like what you eat? In: National Consumer Council, ed. *Your food: Whose choice?* London: HMSO.

Rogers PJ, Pleming HC, Blundell JE. 1990. Aspartame consumed without tasting inhibits hunger and food intake. Physiology & Behavior 47: 1239–1243.

Rogers PJ, Richardson NJ. 1993. Why do we like drinks that contain caffeine? Trends in Food Science and Technology 4: 108–111.

Rogers PJ, Richardson NJ, Elliman, NA. 1995b. Overnight caffeine abstinence and negative reinforcement of preference for caffeine-containing drinks. Psychopharmacology 120: 457–462.

Rogers PJ, Schutz HG. 1992. Influence of palatability on subsequent hunger and food intake: a retrospective replication. Appetite 19: 155–156.

Rolland-Cachera M-F, Bellisle F. 1986. No correlation between adiposity and food intake: Why are working class children fatter? American Journal of Clinical Nutrition 44:779–787.

Rolland-Cachera M-F, Bellisle F, Tichet J, Chantrel A-M, Guilloud-Batielle M, Vol S, Pequignot G. 1990. Relationship between adiposity and food intake: An example of pseudo-contradictory results obtained in case-control versus between-populations studies. International Journal of Epidemiology 19: 571–577.

Rolland-Cachera M-F, Deheeger M, Akrout M, Bellisle F. 1995. Influence of macronutrients on adiposity development: A follow up study of nutrition and growth from 10 months to 8 years of age. International Journal of Obesity 19: 573–578.

Rolls BJ. 1991. Effects of intense sweeteners on hunger, food intake, and body weight: A review. American Journal of Clinical Nutrition 53: 872–878.

Rolls BJ, Duijvenvoorde PM, Rolls ET. 1984. Pleasantness changes and food intake in a varied four course meal. Appetite 5: 337–348.

Rolls BJ, Gnizak N, Summerfelt A, Laster LJ. 1988a. Food intake in dieters and non-dieters after a liquid meal containing medium-chain triglycerides. American Journal of Clinical Nutrition 48: 66–71.

Rolls BJ, Hammer VA. 1995. Fat, carbohydrate, and the regulation of energy intake. American Journal of Clinical Nutrition 62(suppl): 1086S–1095S.

Rolls BJ, Hetherington M, Burley VJ. 1988b. The specificity of satiety: The influence of different macronutrient contents on the development of satiety. Physiology & Behavior 43: 145–153.

Rolls BJ, Kim S, McNelis AL, Fischman MW, Foltin RW, Moran TH. 1991. Time course effects of preloads high in fat or carbohydrate on food intake and hunger ratings in humans. American Journal of Physiology 260: R756–R763.

Rolls BJ, Kim-Harris S, Fischman MW, Foltin RW, Moran TH, Stoner SA. 1994. Satiety after preloads with different amounts of fat and carbohydrate: Implications for obesity. American Journal of Clinical Nutrition 60: 476–487.

Rolls BJ, Laster LJ, Summerfelt A. 1989. Hunger and food intake following consumption of low-calorie foods. Appetite 13: 115–127.

Rolls BJ, Pirraglia PA, Jones MB, Peters JC. 1992. Effects of olestra, a non-caloric fat substitute, on daily energy and fat intake in lean men. American Journal of Clinical Nutrition 56: 84–92.

Rolls BJ, Rolls ET, Rowe, EA, Sweeney K. 1981. Sensory specific satiety in man. Physiology and Behavior 27: 137–142.

Rolls BJ, Rowe EA, Turner RC. 1980. Persistent obesity in rats following a period of consumption of a mixed, high energy diet. Journal of Physiology 298: 415–427.

Romieu I, Willett WC, Stampfer MJ, Colditz GA, Sampson L, Rosner B, Hennekens CH, Speizer FE. 1988. Energy intake and other determinants of relative weight. American Journal of Clinical Nutrition 47: 406–412.

Rönnemaa T, Karonen S-L, Rissanen A, Koskenvuo M, Koivisto VA. 1997. Relation between plasma leptin levels and measures of body fat in identical twins discordant for obesity. Annals of Internal Medicine 126: 26–31.

Rosen JC. 1981. Effects of low-calorie dieting and exposure to diet-prohibited food on appetite and anxiety. Appetite 2: 366–369.

Rosen JC, Gross J, Loew A, Sims EAH. 1985. Mood and appetite during minimal-carbohydrate and carbohydrate-supplemented hypocaloric diets. American Journal of Clinical Nutrition 42: 371–379.

Rosen JC, Hunt DA, Sims EAH, Bogardus C. 1982. Comparison of carbohydrate-containing and carbohydrate-restricted hypocaloric diets in the treatment of obesity: Effects on appetite and mood. American Journal of Clinical Nutrition 36: 463–469.

Rosenthal NE, Genhart MJ, Caballero B, Jacobsen FM, Skwerer RG, Coursey RD, Rogers S, Spring BJ. 1989. Psychobiological effects of carbohydrate- and protein-rich meals in patients with seasonal affective disorder and normal controls. Biological Psychiatry 25: 1029–1040.

Rosenthal NE, Genhart MJ, Jacobson FM, Skwerer RG, Weht TA. 1987. Disturbances of appetite and weight regulation in seasonal affective disorder. Annals of the New York Academy of Sciences 499: 216–223.

Rosenthal NE, Hefferman MM. 1986. Bulimia, carbohydrate craving, and depression: A central connection? In: Wurtman RJ, Wurtman JJ. eds. *Nutrition and the brain, volume 7.* New York: Raven. pp. 139–166.

Roust LR, Hammel KD, Jensen MD. 1994. Effects of isoenergetic, low–fat diets on energy metabolism in lean and obese women. American Journal of Clinical Nutrition 60: 470–475.

Rowland NE, Morien A, Bai-han L, 1996. The physiology and brain mechanisms of feeding. Nutrition 12: 626–639.

Rozin P. 1977. The significance of learning in food selection: Some biology, psychology and sociology of science. In: Barker LM, Best M, Domjan M, eds. *Learning mechanisms in food selection.* Waco, Texas: Baylor University Press. pp.557–589.

Rozin P. 1982. 'Taste smell confusions' and the duality of the olfactory sense. Perception and Psychophysics 31: 397–401.

Rozin P. 1996. Sociocultural influences on human food selection. In: Capaldi ED, ed. Why we eat what we eat. Washington DC: American Psychological Association. pp.233–263.

Rozin P, Levine E, Stoess C. 1991. Chocolate craving and liking. Appetite 17: 199–212.

Ruderman AJ. 1985. Dysphoric mood and overeating: A test of restraint theory's disinhibition hypothesis. Journal of Abnormal Psychology 94: 78–85.

Ruderman AJ. 1986. Dietary restraint: A theoretical and empirical review. Psychological Bulletin 99, 247–262.

Ruderman AJ, Wilson GT. 1979. Weight, restraint, cognitions, and counterregulation. Behaviour Research and Therapy 17: 581–590.

Rumpler WV, Rhodes DG, Baer DJ, Conway JM, Seale J. 1996. Energy value of moderate alcohol consumption by humans. American Journal of Clinical Nutrition 64: 108–114.

Rumpler WV, Seale JL, Miles CW, Bodwell CE. 1991. Energy-intake restriction and diet-composition effects on energy expenditure in men. American Journal of Clinical Nutrition 53: 430–436.

Russek M. 1981. Current status of the hepatostatic theory of food intake control. Appetite 2: 137–143.

Ruxton CHS, Kirk TR, Belton NR. 1996. The contribution of specific dietary patterns to energy and nutrient intakes in 7–8-year-old Scottish schoolchildren. III. Snacking habits. Journal of Human Nutrition and Dietetics 9: 23–31.

Ryttig KR, Leeds AR, Rössner S. 1989. Dietary fibre in the management of overweight. In: Leeds AR, Burley VJ, eds. Dietary fibre perspectives: Reviews and bibliography 2. London: John Libbey & Co. pp. 87–99.

Sahakian BJ, Lean MEJ, Robbins TW, James WPT. 1981. Salivation and insulin secretion in response to food in non-obese men and women. Appetite 2: 209–216.

Sallis JF, Broyles SL, Frank-Spohrer G, Berry CC, Davis TB, Nader PR. 1995. Child's home environment in relation to the mother's adiposity. International Journal of Obesity 19: 190–197.

Saltzman E, Roberts SB. 1995. The role of energy expenditure in energy regulation: Findings from a decade of research. Nutrition Reviews 53: 209–220.

Sandhofer F, Bolzano K, Sailer S, Braunsteiner H. 1969. Quantitative Untersuchungen über den Einbau von Plasmaglucose-Kohlenstoff in Plasmatriglyceride und die Veresterungstrate von freien Fettsäuren des Plasmas zu Plasmatriglyceriden während oraler Zufuhr von Glucose bei primärer kohlenhydratinduzierter Hypertriglyceridämie. Klin Woch 47: 1086–1094.

Sandström B, Marckmann P, Bindslev N. 1992. An eight-month controlled study of a low-fat high-fibre diet: Effects on blood lipids and blood pressure in healthy young subjects. European Journal of Clinical Nutrition 46: 95–109.

Sawaya AL, Tucker RK, Tsay R, Willett W, Saltxman E, Dallal GE, Roberts SB. 1996. Evaluation of four methods for determining energy intake in young and older women: comparison with doubly labeled water measurements of total energy expenditure. American Journal of Clinical Nutrition 63:491–499.

Scarr S, Webber PL, Weinberg RA, Wittig MA. 1981. Personality resemblance among adolescents and their parents in biologically related and adoptive families. Journal of Personality and Social Psychology 40: 885–898.

Schachter S. 1971a. Emotion, obesity and crime. New York: Academic Press.

Schachter S. 1971b. Some extraordinary facts about obese humans and rats. American Psychologist 26: 129–144.

Schachter S, Rodin J. 1974. Obese humans and rats. Washington DC: Erlbaum/Halsted.

Schaefer EJ, Lichtenstein AH, Lamon-Fava S, McNamara JR, Schaefer MM, Rasmussen H, Ordovas JM. 1995. Body weight and low-density lipoprotein cholesterol changes after consumption of a low-fat ad libitum diet. Journal of the American Medical Association 274: 1450–1455.

Schectman G, McKinney P, Pleuss J, Hoffman RG. 1990. Dietary intake of Americans reporting adherance to a low cholesterol diet (NHANES II). American Journal Publ Hlth 80: 698–703.

Schemmel R, Mickelsen O, Gill JL. 1970. Dietary obesity in rats: Body weight and body fat accretion in seven strains of rats. Journal of Nutrition 100: 1041–1048.

Schiffman SS, Gatlin CA. 1993. Sweeteners – state of knowledge review. Neuroscience and Biobehavioral Reviews 17: 313–345.

Schlundt DG, Hill JO, Pope-Cordle J, Arnold D, Virts KL, Katahn M. 1993a. Randomized evaluation of a low fat ad libitum carbohydrate diet for weight reduction. International Journal of Obesity 17: 623–629.

Schlundt DG, Hill JO, Sbrocco T, Pope-Cordle J, Kasser T. 1990. Obesity: A bio-genetic or biobehavioral problem? International Journal of Obesity 14: 815–828.

Schlundt DG, Virts KL, Sbrocco T, Pope-Cordle J, Hill JO. 1993b. A sequential behavioural analysis of craving sweets in obese women. Addictive Behaviors 18: 67–80.

Schoeller DA. 1995. Limitations in the assessment of dietary energy intake by self-report. Metabolism 44(2, Suppl. 2):18–22.

Schoeller D. 1996. No evidence for a difference in thermogenesis between obese and lean humans. In: Angel A, Anderson GH, Bouchard C, Lau D, Leiter L, Mendelson R, eds. *Progress in obesity research: 7.* London: John Libbey & Co. pp. 465–470.

Schulz LO, Schoeller DA. 1994. A compilation of total daily energy expenditure and body weights in healthy adults. American Journal of Clinical Nutrition 60: 676–681.

Schutz Y. 1995. Abnormalities of fuel utilization as predisposing to the develop-ment of obesity in humans. Obesity Research 3(suppl):173s–178s.

Schutz Y, Flatt JP, Jéquier E. 1989. Failure of dietary fat to promote fat oxidation: A factor favoring the development of obesity. American Journal of Clinical Nutrition 50: 307–314.

Schutz Y, Tremblay A, Weinsier RL, Nelson KM. 1992. Role of fat oxidation in the long-term stabilization of body weight in obese women. American Journal of Clinical Nutrition 55: 670–674.

Sclafani A. 1980. Dietary obesity. In: Bray G, ed. Hunger: *Basic mechanisms and clinical implications.* Newman: London. pp. 281–295.

Sclafani A. 1990. Nutritionally based learned flavour preferences in rats. In Capaldi ED, Powley TL, eds. *Taste, feeding and experience.* Washington, DC: American Psychological Association. pp. 139–156.

Sclafani A. 1995. How food preferences are learned: laboratory animal models. Proceedings of the Nutrition Society 54: 419–427.

Sclafani A, Lucas F, Ackroff K. 1996. The importance of taste and palatability in carbohydrate–induced overeating in rats. American Journal of Physiology 270: R1197–R1202.

Sclafani A, Nissenbaum JW. 1985. Is gastric sham feeding really sham feeding? American Journal of Physiology 248: R387–R390.

Seddon L, Berry N. 1996. Media-induced disinhibition of dietary restraint. British Journal of Health Psychology 1: 27–33.

Seidell JC, Muller DC, Sorkin JD, Andres R. 1992. Fasting respiratory exchange ratio and resting metabolic rate as predictors of weight gain: the Baltimore Longitudinal Study on Aging. International Journal of Obesity 16: 667–674.

Sensi S, Capani F. 1987. Chronobiological aspects of weight loss in obesity: effects of different meal timing regimens. Chronobiology International 4:251–261.

Serra-Majem L, Ribas L, Inglès C, Fuentes M, Lloveras G, Salleras L. 1996. Cyclamate consumption in Catelonia, Spain (1992): relationship with Body Mass Index. Food Additives and Contaminants 13: 695–703.

Setser CS, Racette WL. 1992. Macromolecule replacers in food products. Critical Reviews in Food Science and Nutrition 32: 275–297.

Shah M, McGovern P, French S, Baxter J. 1994. Comparison of a low fat, ad libitum complex-carbohydrate diet with a low–energy diet in moderately obese women. American Journal of Clinical Nutrition 59: 980–984.

Shepherd R, Farleigh CA. 1989. Sensory assessment of foods and the role of sensory attributes in determining food choice. In: Shepherd R, ed. *Handbook of the Psychophysiology of Human Eating*. Chichester, UK: Wiley. pp.25–56.

Sheppard L, Kristal AR, Kushi LH. 1991. Weight loss in women participating in a randomized trial of low-fat diets. American Journal of Clinical Nutrition 54: 821–828.

Shetty PS, Prentice AM, Goldberg GR, Murgatroyd PR, McKenna APM, Stubbs RJ, Volschenk PA. 1994. Alterations in fuel selection and voluntary food intake in response to isoenergetic manipulation of glycogen stores in humans. American Journal of Clinical Nutrition 60: 534–543.

Shide DJ, Rolls, BJ. 1995. Information about the fat content of preloads influences energy intake in healthy women. Journal of the American Dietetic Association 95: 993–998.

Shintani TT, Hughes CK, Beckham S, O'Connor HK. 1991. Obesity and cardiovascular risk intervention through the ad libitum feeding of traditional Hawiian diet. American Journal of Clinical Nutrition 53: 1647S–1651S.

Siggaard R, Raben A, Astrup A. 1996. Weight loss during 12 weeks' ad libitum carbohydrate-rich diet in overweight subjects at a Danish work site. Obesity Research 4: 347–356.

Simoes EJ, Byers T, Coates RJ, Serdula MK, Mokdad AH, Heath GW. 1995. The association between leisure-time physical activity and dietary fat in American adults. American Journal of Public Health 85: 240–244.

Simon C, Schlienger JL, Sapin R, Imler M. 1986. Cephalic phase insulin secretion in relation to food presentation in normal and overweight subjects. Physiology & Behavior 36: 465–469.

Sims EAH, Danforth E Jr, Horton ES, Bray GA, Glennon JA, Salans LB. 1973. Endocrine and metabolic effects of experimental obesity in man. Recent Progress in Hormone Research 29: 457–464.

Sipiläinen R, Uusitupa M, Heikkinen S, Rissanen A, Laakso M. 1997. Polymorphism of the 3-adrenergic receptor gene affects basal metabolic rate in obese Finns. Diabetes 46: 77–80.

Sivapalan K, Tobin G. 1987. Effects of meal frequency on energy expenditure and body weight in adult rats. Journal of Physiology 386: 62P.

Slattery ML, McDonald A, Bild DE, Caan BJ, Hilner JE, Jacobs DR, Liu K. 1992. Associations of body fat and its distribution with dietary intake, physical activity, alcohol, and smoking in black and whites. American Journal of Clinical Nutrition 55: 943–949.

Slochower JA. 1983. *Excessive eating*. New York: Human Sciences Press.

Smalley KJ, Knerr AN, Kendrick ZV, Colliver JA, Owen OE. 1990. Reassessment of body mass indices. American Journal of Clinical Nutrition 52: 405–408.

Smith BA, Fillion TJ, Blass EM. 1990. Orally mediated sources of calming in 1 to 3 day old human infants. Developmental Psychology 26: 731–737.

Smith GP, Gibbs J. 1992. The development and proof of the CCK hypothesis of satiety. In: Dourish CT, Cooper SJ, Iversen SD, Iversen LL, eds. *Multiple*

Cholecystokinin Receptors in the CNS. Oxford: Oxford University Press. pp. 166–182.

Smith GP, Gibbs J, Young RC. 1974. Cholecystokinin and intestinal satiety in the rat, Federation Proceedings 33: 1146–1149.

Smith GP, Greenberg D, Corp E, Gibbs J. 1990. Afferent information in the control of eating. In: Bray GA, ed. *Obesity: Towards a molecular approach*. New York: Alan R. Liss, Inc.

Smith–Schneider LM, Sigman-Grant MJ, Kris-Etherton P.M. 1992. Dietary fat reduction strategies. Journal of the American Dietetic Association 92: 34–38.

Snowdon CT. 1970. Gastrointestinal sensory and motor control of food intake. Journal of Comparative and Physiological Psychology 71: 59–67.

Sobal J, Stunkard AJ. 1989. Socioeconomic status and obesity: A review of the literature. Psycholical Bulletin 105: 260–275.

Sørensen TIA, Echwald SM, Holm J-C. 1996. Leptin in ,obesity. British Medical Journal 313: 953–954.

Sørensen TIA, Price RA, Stunkard AJ, Schlusinger F. 1989. Genetics of obesity in adult adoptees and their biological siblings. British Medical Journal 298: 87–90.

Specker S, Dezwaan M, Raymond N, Michell J. 1994. Psychopathology in subgroups of obese women with and without binge-eating disorder. Comprehensive Psychiatry 35: 185–190.

Spector AC, Breslin P, Grill HJ. 1988. Taste reactivity as a dependent measure of the rapid formation of a conditioned taste aversion: A tool for the neural analysis of taste-visceral associations. Behavioral Neuroscience 102: 942–952.

Spencer JA, Fremouw WJ. 1979. Binge eating as a function of restraint and weight classification. Journal of Abnormal Psychology 88: 262–267.

Spiegel TA, Jordan HA. 1978. Effects of simultaneous oral-intragastric ingestion on meal patterns and satiety in humans. Journal of Comparative and Physiological Psychology 92: 133–141.

Spitzer L, Rodin J. 1981. Human eating behaviour: A critical review of studies in normal weight and overweight individuals. Appetite 2: 293–329.

Spitzer L, Rodin J. 1987. Effects of fructose and glucose preloads on subsequent food intake. Appetite 8: 135–145.

Spring B. 1986. Effects of foods and nutrients on the behaviour of normal individuals. In: Wurtman RJ, Wurtman JJ. eds. *Nutrition and the brain, volume 7*. New York: Raven. pp. 1–47 .

Spring B, Chiodo J, Bowen DJ. 1987. Carbohydrates, tryptophan, and behavior: A methodological Review. Psychological Bulletin 102: 234–256.

Stacher G, Bauer H, Steinringer H. 1979. Cholecystokinin decreases appetite and activation evoked by stimuli arising from the preparation of a meal in man. Physiology and Behavior 23: 325–331.

Stacher G, Steinringer H, Schmierer G, Schneider C, Winkleher S. 1982. Cholecystokinin octapeptide decreases intake of solid food in man. Peptides 3: 607–612.

Steinberg S, Annable L, Young SN, Bélanger M-C. 1986. Tryptophan in the treatment of late luteal phase dyphoric disorder: A pilot study. Journal of Psychiatry and Neuroscience 19: 114–119.

Steinberg LA, O'Connell NC, Hatch TF, Picciano MF, Birch LL. 1992. Tryptophan intake influences infants' sleep latency. Journal of Nutrition 122: 1781–1791.

Steiner JE. 1987. What the neonate can tell us about umami. In: Kawamura Y, Kare MR, eds. Umami: a basic taste. Marcel Dekker: New York. pp. 97–123.

Stellar E. 1954. The physiology of motivation. Psychological Review 61: 5–22.

Stricker EM. 1982. The central control of food intake: A role for insulin. In: Hoebel BG, Novin D, eds. *The neural basis of feeding and reward*. Brunswick, ME: Haer Institute for Electrophysiological Research. pp. 227–240.

Stricker EM. 1984. Biological bases of hunger and satiety: Therapeutic implications. Nutrition Reviews 42: 333–340.

Stricker EM, Verbalis JG. 1987. Biological bases of hunger and satiety. Annals of Behavioural Medicine 9: 3–8.

Stubbs RJ, Harbron CG. 1996. Covert manipulation of the ratio of medium– to long–chain triglycerides in isoenergetically dense diets: Effect on food intake in *ad libitum* feeding men. International Journal of Obesity 20: 435–444.

Stubbs RJ, Harbron CG, Prentice AM. 1996. Covert manipulation of the dietary fat to carbohydrate ratio of isoenergetically dense diets: Effect on food intake in feeding men *ad libitum*. International Journal of Obesity 20: 651–660.

Stubbs RJ, Murgatroyd OR, Goldberg GR, Prentice AM. 1993. Carbohydrate balance and the regulation of day-to-day food intake in humans. American Journal of Clinical Nutrition 57: 897–903.

Stubbs RJ, Ritz P, Coward WA, Prentice AM. 1995. Covert manipulation of the ratio of dietary fat to carbohydrate and energy density: Effect on food intake and energy balance in free-living men eating *ad libitum*. American Journal of Clinical Nutrition 62: 330–337.

Stunkard AJ, Foch TT, Hrubec Z. 1986a. A twin study of human obesity. Journal of the American Medical Association 256: 51–54.

Stunkard AJ, Harris JR, Pedersen NL, McClearn GE. 1990. The body-mass index of twins who have been reared apart. New England Journal of Medicine 322: 1483–1487.

Stunkard AJ, Messick S. 1985. The Three-Factor Eating Questionnaire to measure dietary restraint, disinhibition and hunger. Journal of Psychosomatic Research 29: 71–78.

Stunkard AJ, Sørensen TIA, Hanis C, Teasdale TW, Chakraborty R, Schull WJ, Schulsinger F. 1986b. An adoption study of human obesity. New England Journal of Medicine 314: 193–8.

Sullivan RM, Taborsky-Barba S, Mendoza R, Itano A, Leon M, Cotman CW, Payne TF, Lott I. 1991. Olfactory classical conditioning in neonates. Pediatrics 87: 511–518.

Summerbell CD, Moody RC, Shanks J, Stock MJ, Geissler C. 1995. Sources of energy from meals versus snacks in 220 people in four age groups. European Journal of Clinical Nutrition 49: 33–41.

Surwit RS, Feinglos MN, McCaskill CC, Clay SL, Lin PH, Babyak MA, Brownlow BS, Plaisted CS. 1996. Metabolic and behavioral effects of a high sucrose diet in weight loss. Obesity Research 4(Suppl. 1): 53S.

Swindells YE, Holmes SA, Robinson MF. 1968. The metabolic response of young women to changes in the frequency of meals. British Journal of Nutrition 22: 667–679.

Tai MM, Castillo P, Pi-Sunyer FX. 1991. Meal size and frequency: effect on the thermic effect of food. American Journal of Clinical Nutrition 54: 783–787.

Taratini PA, Ravussin E. 1995. Variability in metabolic rate: biological sites of regulation. International Journal of Obesity 19(suppl 4): S102–S106.

Tarka SM. 1982. The toxicology of cocoa and methylxanthines: a review of the literature. CRC Critical Reviews of Toxicology 9: 275–312.

Tartaglia LA, Dempski M, Weng X, Deng N, Culpapper J, Devos R, Richards GJ, Campfield LA, Clark FT, Deeds J, Muir C, Sanker S, Moriarty A, Moore KJ, Smutko JS, Mays GG, Woolf EA, Monroe CA, Tepper RI. 1995. Identification and expression cloning of a leptin receptor, OB-R. Cell 83: 1263–1271.

Tatzer E, Schubert MT, Timischl W, Simburne G. 1985. Discrimination of taste preference for sweet in premature babies. Early Human Development 12: 23–30.

Taylor MA, Garrow JS. 1996. The effect of meal frequency and energy restriction on total energy expenditure and spontaneous activity in obese subjects in a chamber calorimeter. Proceedings of the Nutrition Society 55: 216A.

Teff KL, Engelman K. 1996. Palatability and dietary restraint: Effect on cephalic phase insulin release in women. Physiology & Behavior 60: 567–573.

Teff KL, Young SN, Blundell JE. 1989a. The effect of protein or carbohydrate breakfasts on subsequent plasma amino acid levels, satiety and nutrient selection in normal males. Pharmacology, Biochemistry and Behavior 34: 829–837.

Teff KL, Young SN, Marchand L, Botez MI. 1989b. Acute effect of protein or carbohydrate breakfasts on human cerebrospinal fluid monoamine precursor and metabolite levels. Journal of Neurochemistry 52: 235–241.

Teitelbaum P, Epstein AN. 1962. The lateral hypothalamic syndrome: recovery of feeding and drinking after hypothalamic lesions. Psychological Review 69: 74–90.

Tepper BJ. Dietary restraint and responsiveness to sensory-based food cues as measured by cephalic phase salivation and sensory specific satiety. Physiology and Behavior 52: 305–311.

Tepper BJ, Friedman MI. 1989. Diabetes and a high-fat/low-carbohydrate diet enhance the acceptability of oil emulsions to rats. Physiology & Behavior 45: 717–721.

Theusen L, Henriksen LB, Engby B. 1986. One-year experience with a low-fat, low-cholesterol diet in patients with coronary heart disease. American Journal of Clinical Nutrition 44: 212–219.

Thomas CD, Peters JC, Reed GW, Abumrad NN, Sun M, Hill JO. 1992. Nutrient balance and energy expenditure during ad libitum feeding of high-fat and high-carbohydrate diets in humans. American Journal of Clinical Nutrition 55: 934–42.

Thompson DA, Moskowitz HR, Campbell RG. 1976. Effects of body weight and food intake on pleasantness ratings for a sweet stimulus. Journal of Applied Physiology 41: 77–83.

Thompson DA, Moskowitz HR, Campbell RG. 1977. Taste and olfaction in human obesity. Physiology & Behavior 19: 335–337.

Tiffany ST. 1990. A cognitive model of drug urges and drug-use behaviour: The role of automatic and non-automatic processes. Psychological Review 97: 147–168.

Tiffany ST. 1995. The role of cognitive factors in reactivity to drug cues. In: Drummond DC, Tiffany ST, Glautier S, Remmington B, eds. *Addictive behaviour: Cue exposure theory and practice*. Chichester: Wiley pp. 137–165.

Toates FM. 1975. *Control theory in biology and experimental psychology*. London: Hutchinson Educational.

Toates F. 1986. *Motivational systems*. Cambridge: Cambridge University Press.

Tordoff MG. 1988. How do non-nutritive sweeteners increase food intake? Appetite 11(suppl): 5–11.

Tordoff MG, Alleva AA. 1990. Oral stimulation with aspartame increases hunger. Physiology & Behavior 47: 555–559.

Tordoff MG, Friedman MI. 1986. Hepatic-portal glucose infusions decrease food intake and increase food preference. American Journal of Physiology 251: R192–R196.

Tordoff MG, Tepper BJ, Friedman MI. 1987. Food flavour preferences produced by drinking glucose and oil in normal and diabetic rats: Evidence for conditioning based on fuel oxidation. Physiology & Behavior 41:481–487.

Tordoff MG, Ulrich PM, Sandler F. 1990. Flavour preferences and fructose: Evidence that the liver detects the unconditioned stimulus for calorie-based learning. Appetite 14: 29–44.

Treit D, Spetch ML, Deutsch JA. 1983. Variety in the flavor of food enhances eating in the rat: A controlled demonstration. Physiology & Behavior 30: 207–211.

Tremblay A, Alméras N. 1995. Exercise, macronutrient preferences and food intake. International Journal of Obesity 19(Suppl 4): S97–S101.

Tremblay A, Després J-P, Thériault G, Bouchard C. 1992a. Effect of longterm over-feeding on energy expenditure. In: Aihaud G, Guy-Grand B, Lafontan M, Ricquier D, eds. *Obesity in Europe 91*. Proceedings of the 3rd European Congress on Obesity. London: John Libbey & Co., pp. 319–321.

Tremblay A, Després J-P, Thériault G, Fournier G, Bouchard C. 1992b. Overfeeding and energy expenditure in humans. American Journal of Clinical Nutrition 56: 857–862.

Tremblay A, Levallée N, Alméras N, Allard L, Després J-P, Bouchard C. 1991a. Nutritional determinants of the increase in energy intake associated with a high-fat diet. American Journal of Clinical Nutrition 53: 1134–1137.

Tremblay A, Plourde G, Després J-P & Bouchard C. 1989. Impact of dietary fat content and fat oxidation on energy intake in humans. American Journal of Clinical Nutrition 49: 799–805.

Tremblay A, Seale J, Almeras N, Conway J, Moe P. 1991b. Energy requirements of a postobese man reporting a low energy intake at weight maintenance. American Journal of Clinical Nutrition 54: 506–508.

Tremblay A, St-Pierre S. 1996. The hyperphagic effect of a high-fat diet and alcohol intake persists after control for energy density. American Journal of Clinical Nutrition 63: 479–482.

Tucker LA, Kano MJ. 1992. Dietary fat and body fat: A multivariate study. American Journal of Clinical Nutrition 56: 616–622.

Tuobro S, Astrup A. 1996. Randomised comparison of diets for maintaining obese subjects' weight after major weight loss: Ad lib, low fat, high carbohydrate diet *v* fixed energy intake. British Medical Journal 314: 29–34.

Tuschl RJ. 1990. From dietary restraint to binge eating: Some theoretical considerations. Appetite 14: 105–109.

Tuschl RJ, Platte P, Laessle RG, Stichler W, Pirke K-M. 1990. Energy expenditure and everyday eating behavior in healthy young women. American Journal of Clinical Nutrition 52: 81–86.

Ussher J. 1989. *The psychology of the female body*. London: Routledge.

Valdez R, Greenlund KJ, Wattigney WA, Bao W, Berenson GS. 1996. Use of weight-for-height indices in children to predict adult overweight: The Bogalusa Heart Study. International Journal of Obesity 20: 715–721.

van der Ster Wallin G, Norring C, Holmgren S. 1994. Binge eating versus non-purged eating in bulimics: Is there a carbohydrate craving after all? Acta Psychiatrica Scandinavia 89: 376–381.

Van Es AJH. 1991. Dietary energy density on using sugar alcohols as replacements for sugar. Proceedings of the Nutrition Society 50: 383–390.

Van Itallie TB, Kissileff HR. 1990. Human obesity: A problem in body energy economics. In: Stricker EM. ed, *Handbook of Behavioral Neurobiology. Volume 10, Neurobiology of food and fluid intake*. New York: Plenum Press. pp. 207-240.

Van Itallie TB, Vanderweele DA. 1981. The phenomenon of satiety. In: Bjorntorp P, Cairella M, Howard AN, eds. *Recent advances in obesity research*, Volume 3. London: Libbey. pp. 278–289.

van Stratum P, Lussenburg RN, van Wezel LA, Vergroesen AJ, Cremer HD. 1978. The effect of dietary carbohydrate:fat ration on energy intake by adult women. American Journal of Clinical Nutrition 31: 206–212.

van Strien T. 1996. On the relationship between dieting and 'obese' and bulimic eating patterns. International Journal of Eating Disorders 19; 83–92.

van Strein T, Frijters JER, Bergers GPA, Defares PB. 1986. The Dutch Eating Behaviour Questionnaire (DEBQ) for assessment of restrained, emotional, and external eating behaviour. International Journal of Eating Disorders 5: 295–315.

Varendi H, Porter RH, Winberg J. 1996. Attractiveness of amniotic fluid odor: evidence of prenatal olfactory learning? Act Paediatrica 85: 1223–1227.

Verboeket-van de Venne WPHG, Westerterp KR. 1993. Frequency of feeding, weight reduction and energy metabolism. International Journal of Obesity 17: 31–36.

Verboeket-van de Venne WPHG, Westerterp KR, Hermans-Limpens TJFMB, de Graaf C, van het Hof K, Westrate JA. 1996. Long term consumption of full-fat or reduced-fat products in healthy non-obese volunteers: Assessment of energy expenditure and substrate oxidation. Metabolism 45:1004–1010.

Verboeket-van de Venne WPHG, Westerterp KR, Kester ADM. 1993. Effect of the pattern of food intake on human energy metabolism. British Journal of Nutrition 70: 103–115.

Vitiello MV, Woods SC. 1977. Evidence for withdrawal from caffeine in rats. Pharmacology Biochemistry and Behavior 6: 553–555.

Vogler GP, Sørensen TIA, Stunkard AJ, Srinivasan MR, Rao DC. 1995. Influences of genes and shared family environment on adult body mass index assessed in an adoption study by a comprehensive path model. International Journal of Obesity 19: 40–45.

Wadden TA, Stunkard AJ, Brownell KD, Day SC. 1985. A comparison of two very-low-calories diets: protein-sparing modified fast versus protein-formula-liquid diet. American Journal of Clinical Nutrition 41: 533–539.

Wadden TA, Stunkard AJ, Day SC, Gould RA, Rubin CJ. 1987. Less food, less hunger: Reports of appetite and symptoms in a controlled study of a protein-sparing modified fast. International Journal of obesity 11: 239–249.

Wade J, Milner J, Krondl M. 1981. Evidence for a physiological regulation of food selection and nutrient intake in twins. American Journal of Clinical Nutrition 34:143–147.

Warburton DM. 1990. *Addiction controversies.* Chur Switzerland: Harwood.

Wardle J. 1986. The assessment of restrained eating. Behaviour Research and Therapy 24: 213–215.

Wardle J. 1987. Eating style: A validation study of the Dutch Eating Behaviour Questionnaire in normal subjects and women with eating disorders. Journal of Psychosomatic Research 34: 161–169.

Wardle J. 1990. Conditioning processes and cue exposure in the modification of excessive eating. Addictive Behaviors 15: 387–393.

Wardle J, Beinart H. 1981. Binge eating: a theoretical review. British Journal of Clinical Psychology 20: 97–109.

Warwick ZS, Hall WG, Pappas TN, Schiffman SS. 1993. Taste and smell sensations enhance the satiating effect of both a high carbohydrate and a high-fat meal in humans. Physiology & Behavior 53: 553–556

Warwick ZS, Schiffman SS. 1990. Sensory evaluations of fat-sucrose and fat-salt mixtures: Relationship to age and weight status. Physiology & Behavior 48: 633–636.

Warwick ZS, Schiffman SS. 1991. Flavor-calorie relationships: Effect on weight gain in rats. Physiology & Behavior 50: 465–470.

Warwick ZS, Schiffman SS. 1992. Role of dietary fat in calorie intake and weight gain. Neuroscience and Biobehavioral Reviews 16: 585–596.

Warwick ZS, Schiffman SS, Anderson JB. 1990. Relationship of dietary fat content to food preferences in young rats. Physiology & Behavior 48: 581–586.

Weigle DS. 1994. Appetite and the regulation of body composition. FASEB Journal 8: 302–301.

Weingarten HP. 1983. Conditioned cues elicit eating in sated rats: A role for learning in meal initiation. Science 220: 431–433.

Weingarten HP. 1984a. Meal initiation controlled by learned cues: Basic Behavioural properties. Appetite 5: 147–158.

Weingarten HP. 1984b. Meal initiation controlled by learned cues: Effects of peripheral cholinergic blockade and cholecystokinin. Physiology and Behavior 32: 403–408.

Weingarten HP. 1985. Stimulus control of eating: implications for a two-factor theory of hunger. Appetite 6: 387–401.

Weingarten HP, Elston D. 1991. Food cravings in a college population. Appetite 17: 167–175.

Weingarten HP, Kulikovsky OT. 1989. Taste-to-postingestive consequence conditioning: is the rise in sham feeding with repeated experience a learned phenomenon. Physiology and Behavior 45: 471–476.

Weinsier RL, Nelson KM, Hensrud DD, Darnell BE, Hunter GR, Schutz Y. 1995. Metabolic predictors of obesity. Contribution of resting energy expenditure, thermic effect of food, and fuel utilization to four-year weight gain of post-obese and never-obese women. Journal of Clinical Investigation 95: 980–985.

Weiss L, Hoffman GE, Schrieber R, Andres H, Fuchs E, Koerber E, Kolb HJ. 1986. Fatty-acid biosynthesis in man, a pathway of minor importance. Purification, optimal assay conditions, and organ distribution of fatty-acid synthase. Biological Chemistry - Hoppe Seyler 367: 905–912.

Welch IMcL, Saunders K, Read NW. 1985. The effect of ileal and intravenous infusions of fat emulsions on feeding and satiety on human volunteers. Gastroenterology 89: 1293–1297.

Welle S, Forbes GB, Statt M, Barnard RR, Amatruda JM. 1992. Energy expenditure under free-living conditions in normal-weight and overweight women. American Journal of Clinical Nutrition 55: 14–21.

Wells JCK, Stanley M, Laidlaw AS, Day JME, Davies PSW. 1996. The relationship between components of infant energy expenditure and childhood body fatness. International Journal of Obesity 20: 848–853.

Weltzin TE, Fernstrom MH, Kaye WH. 1994. Serotonin and bulimia nervosa. Nutrition Reviews 52: 399–408.

West JA, de Looy AE. 1996. Responses to weight-reducing diets including and excluding sucrose as a sweetener. Proceedings of the Nutrition Society 55: 125A.

Westenhoefer J. 1991. Dietary restraint and disinhibition: Is restraint a homeogeneous construct? appetite 16; 45–55.

Westenhoefer J, Broeckmann P, Münch A-K, Pudel V. 1994. Cognitive control of eating behaviour and the disinhibition effect. Appetite 23: 27–41.

Westerterp KR, Pasman WJ, Yedema MJW, Wijckmans-Duijsens NEG. 1996a. Energy intake adaptation of food intake to extreme energy densities of food by obese and non-obese women. European Journal of Clinical Nutrition 50: 401–407.

Westerterp KR, Verboeket-van de Venne WPHG, Bouten CVC, de Graaf C, van het Hof K, Westrate JA. 1996b. Energy expenditure and physical activity in subjects consuming full- of reduced-fat products as part of their normal diet. British Journal of Nutrition 76: 785–795.

Westerterp KR, Verboeket-van de Venne WPHG, Kester ADM. 1993. Effect of the pattern of food intake on human energy metabolism. British Journal of Nutrition 70: 103–115.

Westerterp KR, Verboeket-van de Venne WPHG, Westerterp-Plantenga MS,

Velthuis- te Wierik EJM, de Graaf C, Westrate JA. 1996c. Dietary fat and body fat: An intervention study. International Journal of Obesity 20:1022–1026.

Westerterp-Plantenga MS, van den Heuvel E, Wouters L, ten Hoor, F. 1992. Diet-induced thermogenesis and cumulative food intake curves as a function of familiarity with food and dietary restraint in humans. Physiology & Behavior 51: 457–465.

Westerterp-Plantenga MS, Westerterp KR, Nicolson NA, Mordant A, Schoffelen PFN, ten Hoor F. 1990. The shape of the cumulative food intake curve in humans, during basic and manipulated meals. Physiology & Behavior 47: 569–576.

Westerterp-Plantenga MS, Wijckmans-Duysens NA, ten Hoor F. 1994. Food intake in the daily environment after energy-reduced lunch, related to habitual meal frequency. Appetite 22: 173–182.

Westerterp-Plantenga MS, Wijckmans-Duysens NA, Verboeket-van de Venne WPHG, de Graaf K, Westrate JA, van het Hof KH. 1997. Diet-induced thermogenesis and satiety in humans after full-fat and reduced-fat meals. Physiology & Behavior 61: 343–349.

Westerterp-Plantenga MS, Wouters L, ten Hoor F. 1991. Restrained eating, obesity, and cumulative food intake curves during four-course meals. Appetite 16: 149–158.

Westrate JA, Dopheide T, Robroch L, Deurenberg P, Hautvast JGAJ. 1990. Does variation in palatability affect the postprandial response in energy expenditure? Appetite 15: 209–219.

Whitehead R, Prentice A, eds. 1991. *New techniques in nutritional research.* [Bristol-Myers Squibb/ Mead Johnson Nutrition Symposia Volume 9.] London: Academic Press.

WHO. 1990. Diet, nutrition, and the prevention of chronic diseases. WHO Technical Report Series 797. Geneva: World Health Organization.

Wiepkema PR. 1968. Behaviour changes in CBA mice as a result of one goldthioglucose injection. Behaviour 32: 179–209.

Wiepkema PR. 1971a. Behavioural factors in the regulation of food intake. Proceedings of the Nutrition Society 30: 142–149.

Wiepkema PR. 1971b. Positive feedbacks at work during feeding. Behaviour 39: 266–273.

Wirtshafter D, Davis JD. 1977. Set points and settling points, and the control of body weight. Physiology and Behavior 19: 75–78.

Witherly SA, Pangborn RM, Stern JS. Gustatory responses and eating duration of obese and lean adults. Appetite 1: 53–63.

Woods SC, Porte D, Strubbe JH, Steffans AB. 1986. The relationships among body fat, feeding and insulin. In: Ritter RC, Ritter S, Barnes CD, eds. *Feeding Behavior: Neural and humoral controls.* Orlando: Academic press. pp. 315–327.

Wooley OW, Wooley SC. 1981. Relationship of salivation in humans to deprivation, inhibition and the encephalization of hunger. Appetite 2: 331–350.

Wooley OW, Wooley SC, Dunham RB. 1972. Can calories be perceived and do they affect hunger in obese and nonobese humans? Journal of Comparative and Physiological Psychology 80: 250–258.

Woolridge MW, Baum JD, Drewett RF. 1980. Does a change in the composition of human milk affect sucking patterns and milk intake? Lancet 2: 1292–1294.

World Health Organization. 1985. *Energy and Protein Requirements.* Report of a Joint FAO/WHO/UNU Expert Consultation. [WHO Technical Report Series 724]. Geneva: WHO.

Wurtman JJ. 1988. Carbohydrate craving, mood changes, and obesity. Journal of Clinical Psychiatry 49(Suppl): 37–39.

Wurtman JJ, Brzezinski A, Wurtman RJ, Laferrere B. 1989. Effect of nutrient intake on premenstrual depression. American Journal of Obstetrics and Gynecology 161: 1228–1234.

Wurtman RJ, Hefti F, Melamed E. 1981. Precursor control of neurotransmitter synthesis. Pharmacological Reviews 32: 315–335.

Wurtman RJ, Wurtman JJ. 1989. Carbohydrates and depression. Scientific American 260: 50–57.

Wurtman RJ, Wurtman JJ. 1992. The use of carbohydrate–rich snacks to modify mood state: a factor in the production of obesity. In: Anderson GH, Kennedy SH, eds. *The Biology of Feast and Famine: Relevance to Eating Disorders*. San Diego: Academic Press. pp. 151–156.

Wurtman J, Wurtman R, Reynolds S, Tsay R, Chew, B. 1987. Fenfluramine suppresses snack intake among carbohydrate cravers but not among noncarbohydrate cravers. International Journal of Eating Disorders 6: 687–699.

Yeomans MR. 1996. Palatability and the microstructure of feeding in humans: The appetizer effect. Appetite 27: 119–133.

Yeomans MR, Wright P. 1991. Lower pleasantness of palatable foods in nalmafene–treated human volunteers. Appetite 16: 249–259.

Yeomans MR, Wright P, Macleod HA, Critchley JAJH, 1990. Effects of nalmafene on feeding in humans: Dissociation of hunger and palatability. Psychopharmacology 100: 426–432.

Young PT. 1959. The role of affective processes in learning and motivation. Journal of General Psychology 22: 33–66.

Young SN. 1986. The clinical psychopharmacology of tryptophan. In: Wurtman RJ, Wurtman JJ. eds. *Nutrition and the brain, volume 7*. New York: Raven. pp. 49–88.

Young SN. 1991. Some effects of dietary components (amino acids, carbohydrate, folic acid) on brain serotonin synthesis, mood and behaviour, Canadian Journal of Physiology and Pharmacology 69: 893–903.

Young SN. 1993. The use of diet and dietary components in the study of factors controlling affect in humans: A review. Journal of Psychiatry and Neuroscience 18: 235–244.

Young CM, Scanlon SS, Topping CM, Simko V, Lutwak L. 1971. Frequency of feeding, weight reduction, and body composition. Journal of the American Dietetic Association 59: 466–472.

Young CM, Hutter LF, Scanlan SS, Rand CE, Lutwak L, Simko V. 1972. Metabolic effects of meal frequency on normal young men. Journal of the American Dietetic Association 61: 391–398.

Young SN, Smith, S. E, Pihl, R. O, Finn, P. 1985. Tryptophan depletion causes a rapid lowering of mood in normal males. Psychopharmacology 87: 173–177.

Zelewski M, Swierczynki L. 1990. Comparative studies on lipogenic enzyme activities in the liver of human and some animal species. Comparative Biochemistry and Physiology 95: 469–472.

Zellner DA. 1991. How foods get to be liked. In: Bolles RC, ed. The hedonics of taste. Hillside New Jersey: Erlbaum. pp. 199–217.

Zellner DA, Rozin P, Aron M, Kulish C. 1983. Conditioned enhancement of human's liking for flavour by pairing with sweetness. Learning and Motivation 14: 338–350.

Zhang Y, Proenca R, Maffei M, Barone M, Leopold L, Friedman JM. 1994. Positional cloning of the mouse obese gene and its human homologue. Nature 372: 425–432.

Zurlo F, Lillioja S, Esposito-del Puente A, Nyomba BL, Raz I, Saad MF, Swinburn BA, Knowler WC, Bogardus C, Ravussin E. 1990. Low ratio of fat to carbohydrate oxidation as predictor of weight gain: Study of 24-h RQ. American Journal of Physiology 259: E650–E657.

Zurlo F, Ravussin E. 1992. A low rate of fat utilization as a predictor of weight gain. In Belfiore F, Jeanrenaud B, Papalia D, eds. *Obesity: Basic concepts and clinical aspects*. Frontiers in Diabetes 11: 50–60.

Index

Note: page numbers in **bold** refer to figures; those in *italics* refer to tables.